Fundamental Critical Care Support

Fifth Edition

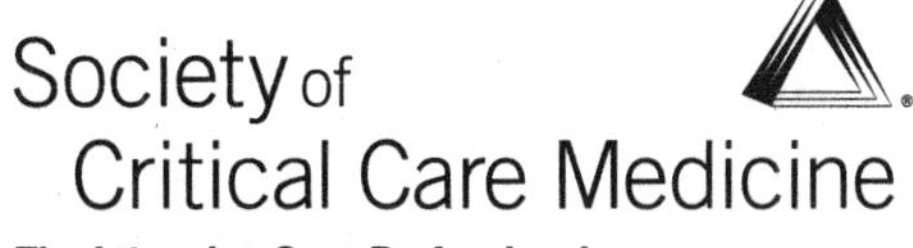

Managing Editor: Katie Brobst

Printed in the United States of America
First Printing, May 2012

Society of Critical Care Medicine
Headquarters
500 Midway Drive
Mount Prospect, IL 60056 USA
Phone +1 (847) 827-6869
Fax +1 (847) 827-6886
www.sccm.org

International Standard Book Number: 978-0-936145-78-5

Fundamental Critical Care Support
Fifth Edition

Editor

David J. Dries, MD, FCCM
Regions Hospital
Saint Paul, Minnesota, USA
No disclosures

FCCS *Fifth Edition Planning Committee*

Marie R. Baldisseri, MD, FCCM
University of Pittsburgh Medical Center
Pittsburgh, Pennsylvania, USA
No disclosures

Thomas P. Bleck, MD, FCCM
Rush Medical College
Chicago, Illinois, USA
No disclosures

Gregory H. Botz, MD, FCCM
University of Texas MD Anderson Cancer Center
Houston, Texas, USA
No disclosures

Edgar Jimenez, MD, FCCM
Orlando Regional Medical Center
Orlando, Florida, USA
No disclosures

Keith Killu, MD
Henry Ford Hospital
Detroit, Michigan, USA
No disclosures

Rodrigo Mejía, MD, FCCM
University of Texas MD Anderson Cancer Center
Children's Cancer Hospital
Houston, Texas, USA
No disclosures

Rahul Nanchal, MD
Medical College of Wisconsin
Milwaukee, Wisconsin, USA
No disclosures

Don C. Postema, PhD
Regions Hospital
Gillette Children's Specialty Healthcare
Bethel University
Saint Paul, Minnesota, USA
No disclosures

Mary J. Reed, MD, FCCM
Geisinger Medical Center
Danville, Pennsylvania, USA
No disclosures

Sophia C. Rodgers, ACNP, FCCM
University of New Mexico School of Medicine
Albuquerque, New Mexico, USA
No disclosures

John B. Sampson, MD
Harford Memorial Hospital
Havre de Grace, Maryland, USA
No disclosures

Babak Sarani, MD
George Washington University
Washington, DC, USA
No disclosures

Janice L. Zimmerman, MD, FCCM
Methodist Hospital
Houston, Texas, USA
No disclosures

Fundamental Critical Care Support
Fifth Edition

Contributors

Kent Blad, DNP, ACNP-BC, FNP-c, FAANP, FCCM
Brigham Young University
Provo, Utah
No disclosures

Steven M. Hollenberg, MD, FCCM
Cooper University Hospital
Camden, New Jersey, USA
No disclosures

Sabrina D. Jarvis, DNP, ACNP-BC, FNP-BC, FAANP
College of Nursing
Brigham Young University
Provo, Utah
No disclosures

Zahid P. Khan, MBBS, FCCM
City Hospital NHS Trust
Birmingham, UK
No disclosures

Gagan Kumar, MD
Medical College of Wisconsin
Milwaukee, Wisconsin, USA
No disclosures

Patti L. Kunkel, CNP
Henry Ford Hospital
Detroit, Michigan, USA
No disclosures

Joshua M. Levine, MD
University of Pennsylvania
Philadelphia, Pennsylvania, USA
No disclosures

Jayshil Patel, MD
Medical College of Wisconsin
Milwaukee, Wisconsin, USA
No disclosures

F. Elizabeth M. Poalillo, CCRN, MSN, RN, ARNP
Pulmonary Practice of Orlando
Orlando, Florida, USA
No disclosures

Bruce M. Potenza, MD
University of California San Diego
San Diego, California, USA
No disclosures

Nitin Puri, MD
Inova Fairfax Hospital
Falls Church, Virginia, USA
No disclosures

Amit Taneja, MD
Medical College of Wisconsin
Milwaukee, Wisconsin, USA
No disclosures

Contents

Contents

PREFACE

This is the fifth edition textbook publication of the Fundamental Critical Care Support (FCCS) program of the Society of Critical Care Medicine. Reflecting the continued growth of the FCCS program since its inception in 1994, this edition will be available in multiple languages, at hundreds of sites, in over 30 countries, and with a growing volume of online resources. As with previous editions, the success of the program is built on the efforts of individuals who have volunteered their time and talents to present the important concepts and principles of fundamental critical care.

Our volunteers' energy and compassion has been guided by key members of the SCCM staff: Gervaise Nicklas, MS, RN, Program Development Manager for FCCS; and Ms. Katie Brobst, Managing Editor, Books, both of whom diplomatically kept the contributors on task. We have expanded the disciplines represented among chapter contributors. Major input to this fifth edition came from the FCCS, Fifth Edition Planning Committee. In addition, the total list of contributors reflects input from approximately half of the international FCCS Program Committee.

As in the fourth edition, we have increased the emphasis on case-based education, with scenarios presented throughout the chapters and considerations highlighted in text boxes. Online skill station materials, which accompany the text, also feature an interactive and case-based format. Our goal is to present our students with problems that mirror clinical reality rather than emphasize the artificial confines of lecture topics.

The FCCS program continues to be a cornerstone of the Society of Critical Care Medicine's education mission. It is a concrete manifestation of our goal to provide the *Right Care, Right Now™*.

David J. Dries, MSE, MD
Editor
2010-2012 Chair, FCCS Program Committee

Chapter 1

Recognition and Assessment of the Seriously Ill Patient

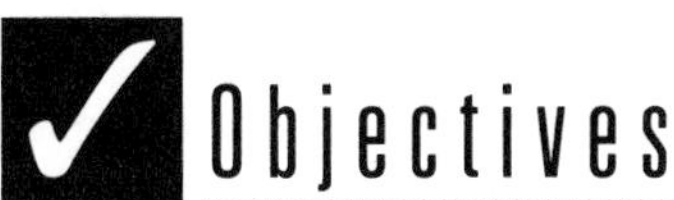

Objectives

- Explain the importance of early identification of patients at risk for life-threatening illness or injury and the importance of early intervention.
- Recognize the early signs and symptoms of critical illness.
- Discuss the initial assessment and early treatment of the critically ill or injured patient.

Case Study

A 54-year-old diabetic woman with cholelithiasis and recurrent episodes of pancreatitis undergoes a laparoscopic cholecystectomy. On the third postoperative day, she develops shortness of breath. The surgeon asks you to see the patient.

- What history is important to obtain for this patient?
- Which aspects of the physical examination would you concentrate on initially?
- Which investigations would you order for this patient?

I. INTRODUCTION

As the old adage goes, an ounce of prevention is worth a pound of cure. That principle often applies in the care of critically ill patients. Early identification of patients at risk for life-threatening illness makes it easier to manage them appropriately and prevent further deterioration. Many clinical problems, if recognized early, can be managed with simple measures such as supplemental oxygen, respiratory therapy interventions, intravenous fluids, or effective analgesia. The early identification of patients in trouble allows clinicians time to identify the main physiological problem, determine its underlying cause, and begin treatment. The longer the interval between the onset of an acute illness and the appropriate intervention, the more likely it is that the patient's condition will deteriorate, even to cardiopulmonary arrest. Several studies have demonstrated that physiological deterioration precedes many cardiopulmonary arrests by hours, suggesting that early intervention could prevent the need for resuscitation, admission to the ICU, and other sentinel events. Many hospitals are using rapid response systems to identify patients at risk and begin early treatment. (See **Appendix 1** for further information on organization and implementation of rapid response systems.) The purpose of this chapter is to describe the general principles involved in recognizing and assessing acutely ill patients.

II. RECOGNIZING THE PATIENT AT RISK

> !
>
> *Patients seldom deteriorate abruptly, even though clinicians may recognize the deterioration suddenly.*
>
> !

Recognizing that a patient is seriously ill is usually not difficult. It may be more challenging, however, if the patient is in the very early stages of the process. Young and otherwise fit patients may be much slower to exhibit the signs and symptoms of an acute illness than may elderly patients with impaired cardiopulmonary function. Individuals who are immunosuppressed or debilitated may not mount a vigorous and clinically obvious inflammatory response. Some conditions, such as cardiac arrhythmias, do not evolve with progressively worsening and easily detectable changes in physiology but present as an abrupt change of state. In most circumstances, a balance exists between the patient's physiologic reserve and the acute disease. Patients with limited reserve are more likely to be susceptible to severe illness and to experience greater degrees of organ-system impairment. Therefore, identifying patients at risk for deterioration requires assessment of their background health, their current disease process, and their current physiological condition.

A. Assessing Severity

"How sick is this patient?" is one of the most important questions a clinician must answer. Determining the response requires the measurement of vital signs and other specific physiological variables (**Appendix 1**). Acute illness typically causes predictable physiological changes that are associated with a limited range of clinical signs. For example, a patient's physiological response to a bacterial infection may result in fever, delirium, shaking chills, and tachypnea. The most important step is to recognize these signs and initiate physiologic monitoring in order to quantify the severity of disease and take appropriate action. Sick patients may present with confusion, irritability, impaired consciousness, or a sense of impending doom. They may appear short of breath and demonstrate signs of a sympathetic response, such as pallor, sweating, or cool extremities. Symptoms may be nonspecific, such as nausea and weakness, or they may identify the involvement of a particular organ system (for example, chest pain). Therefore, a high index of suspicion is required when measuring vital signs: pulse rate, blood pressure, respiratory rate, oxygenation, temperature, and urine output. Clinical monitoring helps to quantify the severity of the disease process, tracks trends and rates of deterioration, and directs attention to those aspects of physiology that most urgently need treatment. The goals at this stage of assessment are to recognize that a problem exists and to maintain physiological stability while pursuing the cause and initiating treatment.

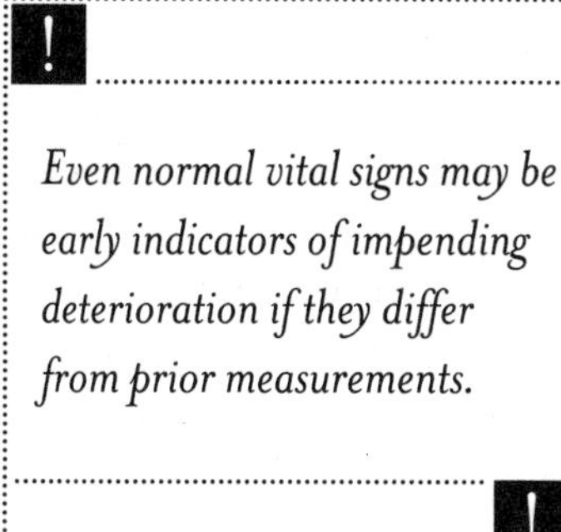

Even normal vital signs may be early indicators of impending deterioration if they differ from prior measurements.

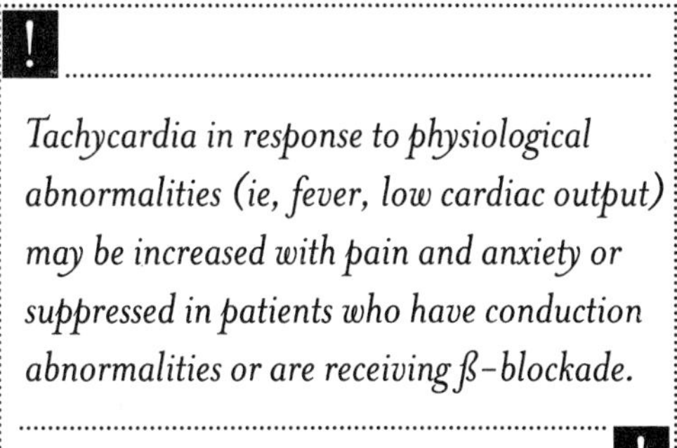

Tachycardia in response to physiological abnormalities (ie, fever, low cardiac output) may be increased with pain and anxiety or suppressed in patients who have conduction abnormalities or are receiving ß-blockade.

B. Making a Diagnosis

Making an accurate diagnosis in the acutely ill patient often must take second place to treating life-threatening physiological abnormalities. It is important to ask the question, "What physiological problem needs to be corrected now to prevent further deterioration of the patient's condition?" Correcting the problem may be as simple as providing oxygen or intravenous fluids. Time for the leisurely pursuit of a differential diagnosis is not likely to be available. However, an accurate diagnosis is essential for refining treatment options once physiological stability is achieved. The general principles of taking an accurate history, performing a brief, directed clinical examination followed by a secondary survey, and organizing laboratory investigations are fundamentally important. Good clinical skills and a disciplined approach in circumstances that may be frightening for inexperienced staff are required to accomplish these tasks.

III. INITIAL ASSESSMENT OF THE CRITICALLY ILL PATIENT

!

A primary and secondary survey approach is recommended in the assessment of a seriously ill patient.

!

A framework for assessing the acutely ill patient is provided in **Table 1-1** and discussed below. Further information on specific issues and treatments can be found in later chapters of this text.

Table 1-1 Framework for Assessing the Acutely Ill or Injured Patient

	PHASE I **Initial Contact— First Minutes** (Primary Survey) What is the main physiological problem?	**PHASE II** **Subsequent Reviews** (Secondary Survey) What is the underlying cause?
History	**Main features of circumstances and environment** • Witnesses, healthcare personnel, relatives • Main symptoms: pain, dyspnea, altered mental status, weakness • Trauma or no trauma • Operative or nonoperative • Medications and/or toxins	**More detailed information** • Present complaint • Past history, chronic diseases, surgical procedures • Hospital course (if applicable) • Psychosocial and physical independence • Medications and allergies • Family history • Ethical or legal issues, code status • Systems review
Examination	**Look, listen, feel** • Airway • Breathing and oxygenation • Circulation • Level of consciousness	**Structured examination of organ systems** • Respiratory system • Cardiovascular system • Abdomen and genitourinary tract • Central nervous and musculoskeletal systems • Endocrine and hematological systems
Chart review, documentation	**Essential physiology, vital signs** • Heart rate, rhythm • Blood pressure • Respiratory rate and pulse oximetry • Level of consciousness	**Case records and note keeping** • Examine medical records, if available • Formulate specific diagnosis or differential diagnosis • Document current events
Investigations	• Blood gas analysis (use venous if arterial access is difficult) • Blood glucose	• Laboratory blood tests • Radiology • Electrocardiography • Microbiology
Treatment	**Proceeds in parallel** • Ensure adequate airway and oxygen • Provide intravenous access ± fluids • Assess response to immediate resuscitation • CALL FOR MORE ADVICE AND ASSISTANCE FROM AN EXPERIENCED COLLEAGUE	**Refine treatment, assess responses, review trends** • Provide support for specific organ systems as required • Choose most appropriate site for care • Obtain specialist advice and assistance

A. History

The patient's history provides the greatest contribution to diagnosis. Often the current history, past medical history, and medication list must be obtained from family members, caregivers, friends, neighbors, or other healthcare providers. The risk of critical illness is increased in patients with the following characteristics:

- Emergency admission (limited information)
- Advanced age (limited reserve)
- Severe coexisting chronic illness (limited reserve, limited options for management)
- Severe physiological abnormalities (limited reserve, refractory to therapy)
- Need for, or recent history of, major surgery, especially an emergency procedure
- Severe hemorrhage or need for a massive blood transfusion
- Deterioration or lack of improvement
- Immunodeficiency
- Combination of these factors

A complete history includes the present complaint, treatment history, hospital course to the present (if applicable), past illnesses, past operative procedures, current medications, and any medication allergies. A social history, including alcohol, tobacco, or illicit drug use, and a family history, including the degree of physical and psychosocial independence, are essential and often overlooked. The history of the present complaint must include a brief review of systems that should be replicated in the examination that follows.

Critical illness is often associated with inadequate cardiac output, respiratory compromise, and a depressed level of consciousness. Specific symptoms will typically be associated with the underlying condition. Patients may complain of nonspecific symptoms such as malaise, fever, lethargy, anorexia, or thirst. Organ-specific symptoms may direct attention to the respiratory, cardiovascular, or gastrointestinal systems. Distinguishing acute from chronic disease is important at this point, as chronic conditions may be difficult to reverse and may act as rate-limiting factors during the recovery phase of critical illness.

B. Examination

Look, listen, and feel. The patient must be fully exposed for a complete examination. The initial examination must be brief, directed, and concentrated on the basic elements: airway, breathing, circulation, and level of consciousness. As the treatment proceeds, a more detailed secondary survey should be conducted to refine the preliminary diagnosis and assess the response to initial treatment. A full examination must be performed at some point and will be guided by the history and other findings. *Ongoing deterioration or development of new symptoms warrants repetition of the primary survey.*

Remember the ABCs of resuscitation: airway, breathing, circulation. The airway and respiratory system should be assessed first, as summarized in **Table 1-2**. Observe the patient's mouth and chest. There may be obvious signs suggesting airway obstruction as well as vomitus, blood, or a foreign body. The patient's respiratory rate, pattern of breathing, and use of accessory respiratory muscles will help to confirm and assess the severity of respiratory distress or airway obstruction (**Chapter 2**). Tachypnea is the single most important indicator of critical illness. Therefore, the respiratory rate must be accurately measured and documented. Although tachypnea may result from pain or anxiety, it may also indicate pulmonary disease, severe metabolic abnormalities, or infection. Look for cyanosis, paradoxical respiration, equality and depth of respiration, use of accessory muscles, and tracheal tug. An increase in the depth of respiration (Kussmaul breathing) may indicate severe metabolic acidosis. Periodic breathing (Cheyne-Stokes respiration) usually indicates severe brainstem injury or cardiac dysfunction. Agitation and confusion may result from hypoxemia, whereas hypercapnia will usually depress the level of consciousness. Low oxygen saturation can be detected with pulse oximetry, but this assessment may be unreliable if the patient is hypovolemic, hypotensive, or hypothermic. Noisy breathing (eg, grunting, stridor, wheezing, gurgling) may indicate partial airway obstruction, whereas complete airway obstruction will result in silence.

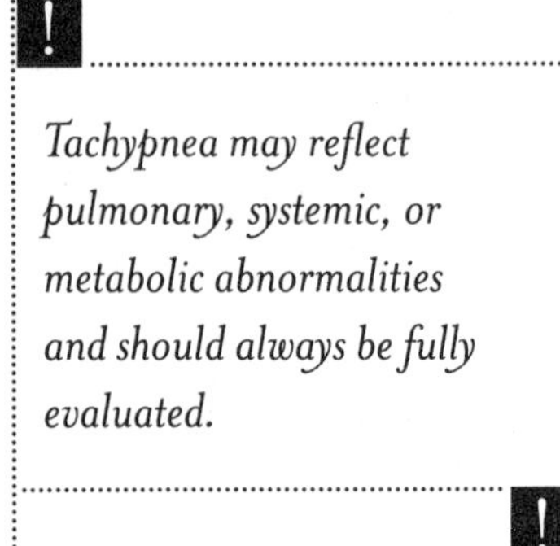
Tachypnea may reflect pulmonary, systemic, or metabolic abnormalities and should always be fully evaluated.

Table 1-2 Assessment of Airway and Breathing

	Airway
Causes of Obstruction	Direct trauma, blood, vomitus, foreign body, central nervous system depression (with soft tissue or tongue blocking airway), infection, inflammation, laryngospasm
LOOK for	Cyanosis, altered respiratory pattern and rate, use of accessory respiratory muscles, tracheal tug, altered level of consciousness
LISTEN for	Noisy breathing (grunting, stridor, wheezing, gurgling); silence indicates complete obstruction
FEEL for	Decreased or absent airflow
	Breathing
Causes of Inadequate Breathing or Oxygenation	
Depressed respiratory drive	Central nervous system depression
Decreased respiratory effort	Muscle weakness, nerve/spinal cord damage, chest wall abnormalities, pain
Pulmonary disorders	Pneumothorax, hemothorax, aspiration, chronic obstructive pulmonary disease, asthma, pulmonary embolus, lung contusion, acute lung injury, acute respiratory distress syndrome, pulmonary edema, rib fracture, flail chest
LOOK for	Cyanosis, altered level of consciousness, tracheal tug, use of accessory respiratory muscles, altered respiratory pattern, altered respiratory rate, equality and depth of breaths, oxygen saturation
LISTEN for	Dyspnea, inability to talk, noisy breathing, dullness to percussion, auscultation of breath sounds
FEEL for	Symmetry and extent of chest movements, position of trachea, crepitus, abdominal distension

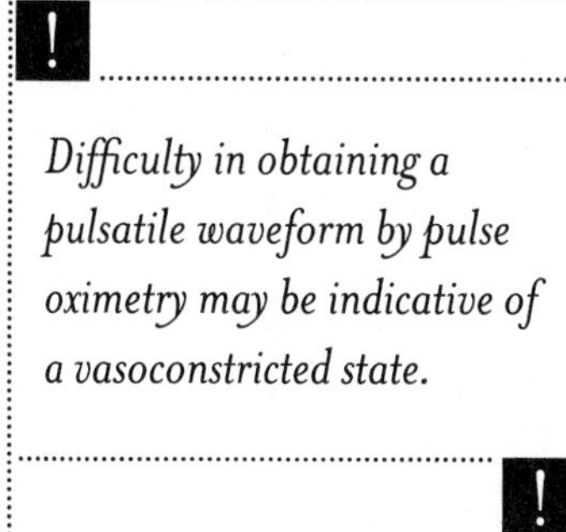

Inadequate circulation may result from primary abnormalities of the cardiovascular system or secondary abnormalities caused by metabolic disturbances, sepsis, hypoxia, or drugs (**Table 1-3**). *A drop in blood pressure may be a late sign of cardiovascular disturbance signaling failure of the compensatory mechanisms.* Central and peripheral pulses should be assessed for rate, regularity, volume, and symmetry. Patients with hypovolemia or low cardiac output will have weak and thready peripheral pulses. A bounding pulse suggests hyperdynamic circulation, and an irregular rhythm usually signifies atrial fibrillation. A ventricular premature beat is often immediately followed by a compensatory pause, and the subsequent beat often has a larger pulse volume. Pulsus paradoxus is a weakening or disappearance of the pulse with deep inspiration and can occur with profound hypovolemia, constrictive pericarditis, cardiac tamponade, asthma, and chronic obstructive pulmonary disease. The location and character of the left ventricular impulse may suggest left ventricular hypertrophy, congestive heart failure, cardiac enlargement, severe mitral regurgitation, or severe aortic regurgitation. The turbulent flow of blood through a stenotic heart valve or a septal defect may produce a palpable thrill.

Table 1-3 Assessment of Circulation

Causes of Circulatory Inadequacy	
Primary—directly involving the heart	Ischemia, arrhythmias, valvular disorders, cardiomyopathy, pericardial tamponade
Secondary—pathology originating elsewhere	Drugs, hypoxia, electrolyte disturbances, dehydration, sepsis, acute blood loss, anemia
LOOK for	Reduced peripheral perfusion (pallor), hemorrhage (obvious or concealed), altered level of consciousness, dyspnea, decreased urine output, jugular venous distension
LISTEN for	Additional or altered heart sounds, carotid bruits
FEEL for	Precordial cardiac pulsation, central and peripheral pulses (assessing rate, quality, regularity, symmetry), cool extremities

In addition to the ABCs, a quick external examination should look for pallor, cyanosis, diaphoresis, jaundice, erythema, or flushing. The skin may be moist or dry, thin, edematous, or bruised, or may demonstrate a rash (ie, petechia, hives). Fingernails may be clubbed or show splinter hemorrhages. The eyes may reveal abnormal pupils or jaundice. The conjunctiva may be pale, indicating an anemia. The patient may be alert, agitated, somnolent, asleep, or obtunded.

Palpation of the abdomen is an essential, but often overlooked, part of the examination of the critically ill patient. Areas of abdominal tenderness and palpable masses must be identified. The size of the liver and spleen must be noted as well as any associated tenderness. It is important to assess the abdomen for rigidity, distension, or rebound tenderness. Auscultation may reveal a vascular bruit or the absence of bowel sounds. Intrauterine or ectopic pregnancy must be considered in all women of childbearing age. The flanks and back must be examined, if possible.

The Glasgow Coma Scale score should be recorded during the initial assessment of central nervous system function and limb movement (**Chapter 8**). Pupillary size and reaction should be documented, and a more detailed assessment of central and peripheral sensory and motor functions should be undertaken when time permits.

C. Chart Review and Documentation

Critically ill patients have abnormal physiology that must be documented and tracked. Physiological monitoring provides parameters that are useful only when they are accurate and interpreted by trained personnel (**Chapter 6**). The values and trends of these data provide key information for the assessment of the patient's status and guidance for treatment. Data must be charted frequently and correctly to ensure good patient care. Particular attention must be paid to the accuracy and reliability of the data. For example, a true and reproducible central venous pressure measurement depends upon patient position, equipment calibration, and proper zeroing of the instrument, as well as on heart rate and valvular function. The source of the data should also be noted. Is the recorded temperature a rectal measurement or an oral measurement? Was the blood pressure measured with a manual cuff or with a pressure transducer in an arterial line? The medication record is an invaluable source of information about prescribed and administered drugs.

Routine monitoring and charting should include heart rate, heart rhythm, respiratory rate, blood pressure, core temperature, fluid balance, and Glasgow Coma Scale score. The fluid balance should include loss from all tubes and drains. The inspired oxygen concentration should be recorded for any patient receiving oxygen, and oxygen saturation should be charted if measured with pulse oximetry. Patients in the ICU setting may have central venous catheters or pulmonary artery catheters in place. These catheters can measure central venous pressure, various cardiac pressures, cardiac output, and mixed venous saturation. These complex monitoring devices require specific operational expertise. Likewise, the data must be interpreted by someone with clinical experience and expertise in critical care.

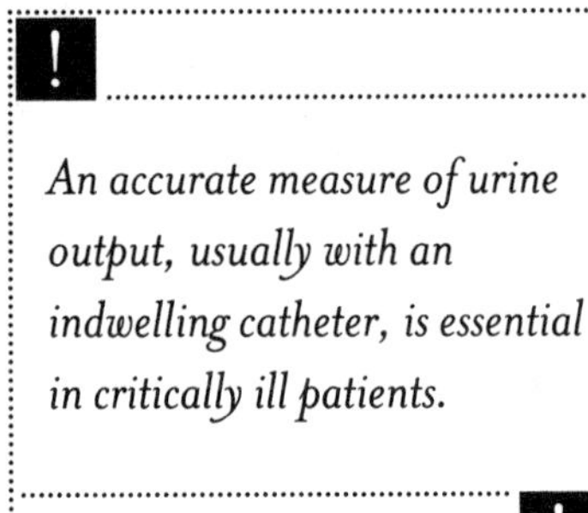

D. Investigations

Additional investigative tests should be based on the patient's history and physical examination as well as on previous test results. Standard biochemistry, hematology, microbiology, and radiology tests should be performed as indicated. *The presence of a metabolic acidosis is one of the most important indicators of critical illness.* When evaluating electrolyte results, decreasing total serum carbon dioxide and/or an increased anion gap are evidence of metabolic acidosis. An arterial blood gas analysis is often the most useful test in an acutely ill patient, providing information about blood pH, arterial oxygen tension, and arterial carbon dioxide tension. Additional tests, such as lactate, blood glucose, serum electrolytes, and renal function, can often be obtained from the same blood sample. The presence of lactic acidosis following cardiorespiratory resuscitation is usually an ominous sign that should be closely monitored.

IV. TRANSLATING INFORMATION INTO EFFECTIVE ACTION

The framework in **Table 1-1** lays out a course of action based on first ensuring physiological safety and then proceeding to treatment of the underlying cause. The basic principles are summarized as the ABCs of resuscitating the severely ill patient: airway—ensuring a patent airway; breathing—providing supplemental oxygen and adequate ventilation; and circulation—restoring circulating volume. These early interventions should proceed regardless of the situation, while the context of the clinical presentation (ie, trauma, postoperative situation, presence of chronic illness, advanced age) directs attention to the differential diagnosis and potential treatments. The clinical history, physical examination, and laboratory tests should aid in clarifying the diagnosis and determining the patient's degree of physiological reserve. Because the external features of critical illness may be more effectively disguised in young and previously fit patients than in elderly or chronically ill ones, an acute deterioration may seem to occur more abruptly in younger individuals. Thus, it is particularly important to assess trends in vital signs and physiological parameters as the patient undergoes treatment. These trends can help determine a patient's response and clarify the diagnosis.

More experienced help must be obtained if a patient's condition is deteriorating and there is uncertainty about the diagnosis or treatment. Transfer to the most appropriate site for care is influenced by resources and local configurations, but transfer to a high-dependency unit or ICU must be considered.

Key Points

Recognition and Assessment of the Seriously Ill Patient

- Early identification of a patient at risk is essential for preventing or minimizing critical illness.
- The clinical manifestations of impending critical illness are often nonspecific. Tachypnea is one of the most important predictors of risk and signals the need for more detailed monitoring and investigation.
- Resuscitation and physiological stabilization will often precede a definitive diagnosis and treatment of the underlying cause.
- A detailed history is essential for making an accurate diagnosis, determining a patient's physiological reserve, and establishing a patient's treatment preferences.
- Clinical and laboratory monitoring of a patient's response to treatment is essential.

Suggested Readings

1. Cooper DJ, Buist MD. Vitalness of vital signs, and medical emergency teams. *Med J Aust.* 2008;188:630-631.

2. Cretikkos, MA, Bellomo R, Hillman K, et al. Respiratory rate: the neglected vital sign. *Med J Aust.* 2008;188:657-659.

3. Goldhill DR, White SA, Sumner A. Physiological values and procedures in the 24 h before ICU admission from the ward. *Anaesthesia.* 1999;54:529-534.

4. Hillman KM, Bristow PJ, Chey T, et al. Duration of life-threatening antecedents prior to intensive care admission. *Intensive Care Med.* 2002;28:1629-1634.

5. Harrison GA, Jacques TC, Kilborn G, et al. The prevalence of recordings of the signs of critical conditions and emergency responses in hospital wards: the SOCCER study. *Resuscitation.* 2005;65:149-157.

6. Hodgetts TJ, Kenward G, Vlachonikolis IG, et al. The identification of risk factors for cardiac arrest and formulation of activation criteria to alert a medical emergency team. *Resuscitation.* 2002;54:125-131.

7. O'Grady NP, Barie PS, Bartlett JG, et al. Guidelines for evaluation of new fever in critically ill adult patients: 2008 update from the American College of Critical Care Medicine and Infectious Diseases Society of America. *Crit Care Med.* 2008;36:1330-1349.

Chapter 2

AIRWAY MANAGEMENT

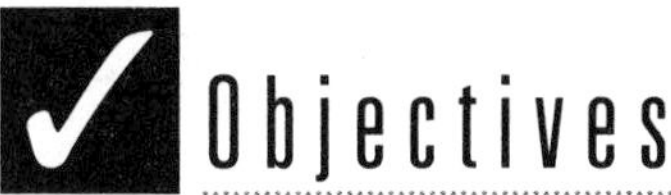

Objectives

- Recognize signs of a threatened airway.
- Describe manual techniques for establishing an airway and for mask ventilation.
- Explain proper application of airway adjuncts.
- Describe preparation for endotracheal intubation, including the recognition of a potentially difficult intubation.
- Describe alternative methods for establishing an airway when endotracheal intubation cannot be accomplished.

Case Study

A 40-year-old, morbidly obese man has arrived in the emergency department with severe respiratory distress. His respiratory rate is 40/min, pulse oximetry reveals hemoglobin saturation of 88% with high-flow oxygen supplementation, and he is actively using his accessory muscles of respiration. He is confused.

- Should this patient be intubated?
- What airway management issues might you anticipate?
- Should you call for help?

I. INTRODUCTION

The focus of this chapter is on ensuring that the airway is open and able to support gas exchange — the *A* in the ABCs of resuscitation. Secondary goals include the preservation of cardiovascular stability and the prevention of aspiration of gastric contents during airway management. Endotracheal intubation will often be required, but establishing and maintaining a patent airway instead of, or prior to, intubation is equally important and often more difficult. Healthcare providers must be skilled in manually supporting the airway and providing the essential processes of oxygenation and ventilation. Securing an artificial airway via orotracheal or nasotracheal intubation, cricothyrotomy, or tracheostomy is an extension of, not a substitute for, the ability to provide that primary response.

II. ASSESSMENT

Assessment of airway patency and spontaneous breathing effort is the crucial first step. The clinician must look, listen, and feel for diminished or absent air movement.

- Observe the patient's level of consciousness and determine if apnea is present. If respiratory efforts are absent and an immediate remedy is not available, proceed to manual support and assisted ventilation while preparing to establish an artificial airway.

- Identify injury to the airway or other conditions (eg, cervical spine injury) that will affect assessment and manipulation of the airway; see below).

- Observe chest expansion. Ventilation may be adequate with minimal thoracic excursion, but respiratory muscle activity and even vigorous chest movement do not ensure that tidal volume is adequate.

- Observe for suprasternal, supraclavicular, or intercostal retractions; laryngeal displacement toward the chest during inspiration (a tracheal tug); or nasal flaring. These often represent respiratory distress with or without airway obstruction.

- Auscultate over the neck and chest for breath sounds. Complete airway obstruction is likely when chest movement is visible but breath sounds are absent. Airway narrowing due to soft tissue, liquid, or a foreign body in the airway may be associated with snoring, stridor, gurgling, or noisy breathing.

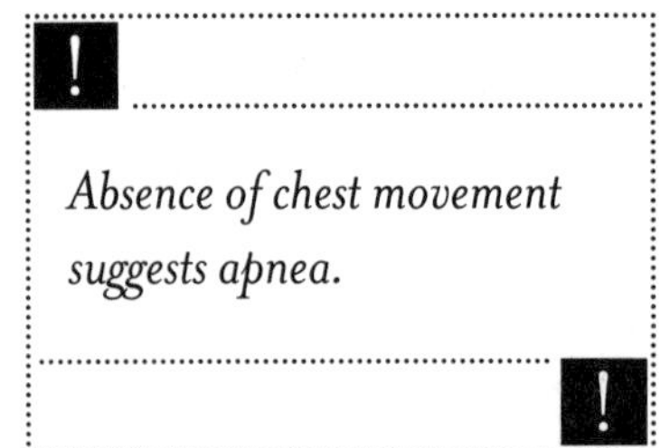

- Assess protective airway reflexes (ie, cough and gag).
  Although the reflexes are not necessarily associated with obstruction, this action is part of the initial survey of the airway. However, overly aggressive stimulation of the posterior pharynx while assessing these reflexes may precipitate emesis and aspiration of gastric contents. The absence of protective reflexes generally implies a need for advanced airway support if the cause cannot be immediately reversed.

III. MANUAL METHODS TO ESTABLISH AN AIRWAY

Initial interventions to ensure a patent airway in a spontaneously breathing patient with no possible injury to the cervical spine include the triple airway maneuver (**Figure 2-1**):

1. Slight neck extension
2. Elevation of the mandible (jaw thrust maneuver)
3. Opening of the mouth

If a cervical spine injury is suspected, neck extension is eliminated. After the cervical spine is immobilized, manual elevation of the mandible and opening of the mouth are performed.

Figure 2-1. Triple Airway Maneuver

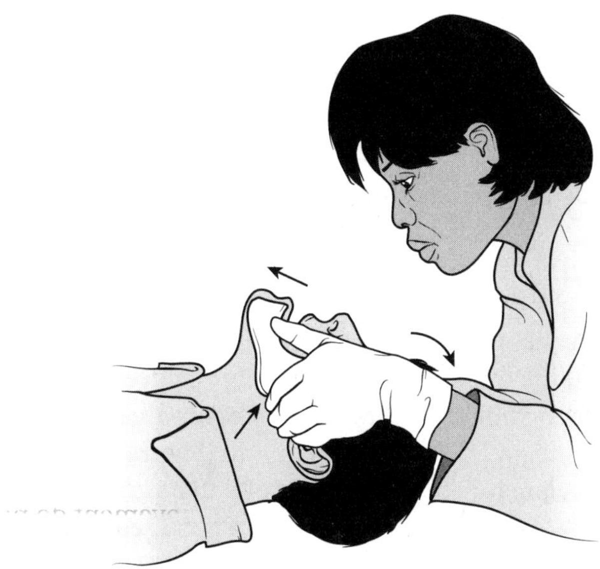

The operator extends the neck and maintains extension with his/her hands on both sides of the mandible. The mandible is elevated with the fingers of both hands to lift the base of the tongue, and the thumbs or forefingers are used to open the mouth.

Adjunctive devices such as properly sized oropharyngeal or nasopharyngeal airways may be useful. The oropharyngeal airway is intended to hold the base of the tongue forward toward the teeth and away from the glottic opening. The plastic flange should rest against the outer surface of the teeth while the distal end curves around the base of the tongue. If the oropharyngeal airway is too small, it may push the tongue back over the glottic opening; if it is too large, it may stimulate gagging and emesis. In fact, oropharyngeal airways should not be inserted if airway reflexes are intact, as gagging, laryngospasm, and emesis will be provoked. The diameter of a nasopharyngeal airway should be the largest that will easily pass through the nostril into the nasopharynx. Its length should extend to the nasopharynx, but it should not be so long as to obstruct gas flow through the mouth or touch the epiglottis. A nasopharyngeal airway

> **!** *The patient's tongue is the most common cause of airway obstruction.* **!**

is contraindicated in patients with suspected basilar skull fracture or coagulopathy. The correct length for each airway may be estimated by placing the device against the face in the correct anatomic position.

During manual support of the airway, supplemental oxygen should be supplied with a device providing a high concentration of oxygen (100%) at a high flow rate. Such devices include a face mask or a bag-mask resuscitation unit, possibly with a positive end-expiratory pressure (PEEP) valve.

IV. MANUAL MASK VENTILATION

Manual assisted ventilation by means of a bag-mask resuscitation unit is indicated:

- if the patient is apneic.
- if spontaneous tidal volumes are determined to be inadequate based on physical examination or arterial blood gas analysis.
- to reduce the work of breathing by assisting spontaneous inspiration.
- if hypoxemia is associated with poor spontaneous ventilation.

Successful manual mask ventilation depends upon: (1) maintaining an open airway, (2) establishing a seal between the patient's face and the mask, and (3) delivering an adequate minute ventilation from the resuscitation bag to distal lung units. The first two elements are achieved through the correct placement of the mask over the patient's nose and mouth (**Figure 2-2**) and completion of the triple airway maneuver as previously described. It is useful to have masks of different sizes available in the event that the initial selection does not achieve a good seal with the face.

Figure 2-2. Application of Face Masks

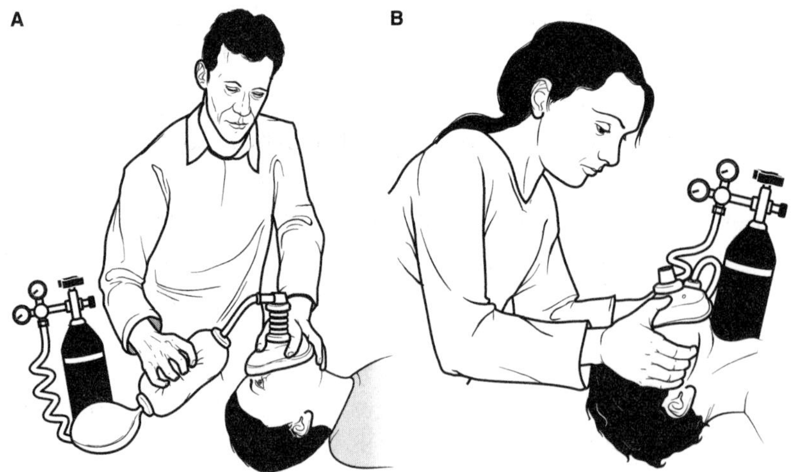

Single-handed (**A**) and two-handed (**B**) techniques for placement of a face mask.

A. When No Cervical Spine Injury Is Suspected

1. If needed and tolerated by the patient, an oropharyngeal or nasopharyngeal airway may be placed to maintain a patent airway. A small pad or folded towel may be positioned under the occiput.

2. The operator stands above and behind the head of the supine patient. The height of the bed should be quickly adjusted for the comfort of the operator.

3. The base of the mask is first placed into the skin crease between the lower lips and the chin, and the mouth is gently opened.

4. The apex of the mask is placed over the nose, using care to avoid pressure on the eyes.

5. As most operators are right-handed, the mask is stabilized on the face with the left hand by holding the superior aspect of the mask apex between the thumb and first finger, adjacent to its connection to the bag. This allows gentle downward pressure on the mask over the face.

6. The fifth, fourth, and perhaps third fingers of the left hand are then placed along the left side of the mandible. It is helpful to gently encircle the left side of the mask with the soft tissues of that cheek to reinforce the seal along that edge. This further secures the mask to the patient's face while allowing the mandible to be partially elevated.

7. The operator gently rotates the left wrist to cause slight neck extension and contracts the fingers around the mandible to raise it slightly. The composite motions of the left hand, therefore, produce slight neck extension, mandibular elevation, and gentle downward pressure on the face mask.

B. When a Cervical Spine Injury Is Suspected

1. The operator stands in the same position, and an oropharyngeal or nasopharyngeal airway is inserted, if possible.

2. Successful manual ventilation occasionally can be accomplished while the neck is stabilized in a cervical collar. Most often, however, an assistant is required to stand to the side, facing the patient. The anterior portion of the collar is removed, and the assistant places one hand or arm along each side of the neck to limit movement of the neck during manipulation of the airway. Linear traction is not applied.

3. The operator then proceeds with the steps described above, *except no rotation is applied by the left wrist to produce neck extension.* Alternatively, the operator may choose the two-handed method for mask placement, which further assures that no neck movement occurs. This method is discussed below.

C. Alternative Two-Handed Method to Ensure Airway Patency and Mask Application

The alternative two-handed method is useful if the patient has a large face or a beard, after neck injury, or in any other situation when a mask seal is difficult to secure.

1. The operator stands at the head of the bed as before, and adjunctive airway devices are used as previously suggested.

2. The base and apex of the mask are placed in the manner previously described.

3. The operator places the third, fourth, and fifth fingers of both hands along the mandible on each side of the face while the thumbs rest over the apex of the mask and first fingers rest over the base of the mask.

4. Soft tissues of the cheek are brought upward along the side edges of the mask and held in place by each hand to reinforce the mask's seal.

5. In the absence of possible cervical spine injury, the neck is slightly extended as the operator gently elevates the mandible from both sides and provides gentle pressure on the mask over the face.

6. An assistant provides ventilation, as needed, by compressing the resuscitation bag.

D. Compression of the Resuscitation Bag to Provide Assisted Manual Mask Ventilation

The goal of manual mask ventilation is to provide adequate minute ventilation, the product of the tidal volume delivered during each compression of the resuscitation bag and the number of compressions per minute. Overzealous bag compressions at a rapid rate may produce dangerous hyperventilation and respiratory alkalemia as well as gastric distension.

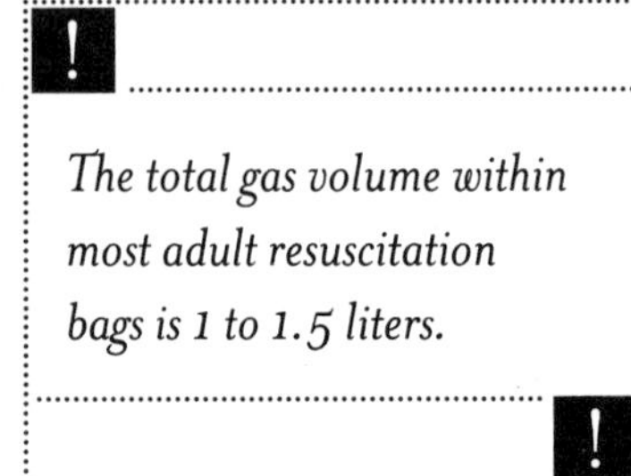

1. If a single-handed method of mask placement is used, the resuscitation bag is compressed over 1 second by the operator's right hand.

2. The delivered tidal volume must be estimated from the observed chest expansion and auscultated breath sounds.

3. During bag compression, the operator should listen carefully for any gas leaks around the mask. When a good seal is achieved, the feel of the bag during lung inflation

reflects some resistance caused by the normal airway anatomy. If gas is moving from the bag too easily, a leak is likely to be present.

4. If the patient is apneic but has a pulse, one-handed bag compressions should be delivered 10 to 12 times per minute. If spontaneous breathing is present, bag compression should be synchronized with the patient's inspiratory efforts. If the patient is breathing easily and inhaling adequate tidal volumes frequently enough to produce sufficient minute ventilation, the bag need not be compressed at all.

5. Oxygen (100%) is delivered to the resuscitation bag, usually at a flow rate of 15 L/min.

6. If the mask-to-face seal is not adequate and a leak is detected, the operator should consider the following interventions:

   - Reposition the mask and hands.
   - Adjust the inflation of the facial cushion of the face mask, if possible, to improve the seal or change to a larger or smaller mask.
   - Apply slightly more downward pressure to the face or displace the mandible in an upward fashion, provided cervical spine manipulation is not contraindicated.
   - Convert to the two-handed technique described earlier.
   - Reposition any orogastric or nasogastric tube present to a different part of the mask. Leaks are common when a tube is present, but rarely will it need to be removed.
   - Consider compensating for a small leak by increasing the frequency of bag compressions or the volume of gas delivered in each compression.
   - If the resuscitation bag has a pressure-relief (pop-off) valve designed to prevent transmission of high pressures to the lungs, adjust the pop-off valve to ensure adequate tidal volumes in patients with stiff lungs or high airway resistance.

Manual assisted ventilation should be continued in preparation for intubation or until the cause of inadequate ventilation is reversed. An assistant should prepare medications and equipment for intubation while the primary operator maintains ventilation. Pulse oximetry and cardiac monitoring are valuable adjuncts throughout assisted ventilation. The patient should be evaluated continuously for evidence of cyanosis, although this is a late finding in the setting of hypoxemia.

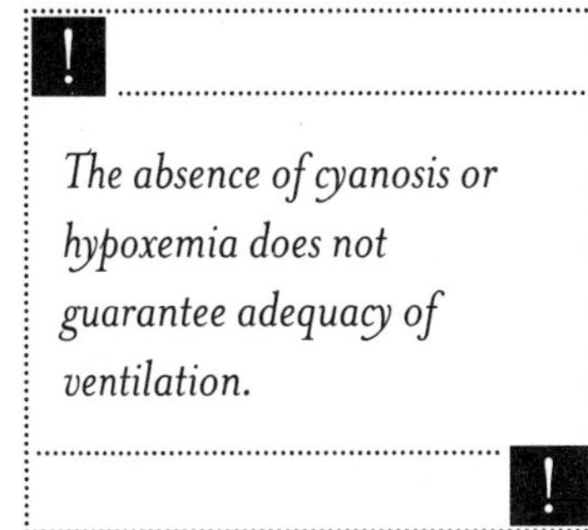

The absence of cyanosis or hypoxemia does not guarantee adequacy of ventilation.

E. Cricoid Pressure

Cricoid pressure (Sellick maneuver) is the application of downward (posterior) pressure on the anterior neck overlying the cricoid cartilage. The downward movement of the cricoid ring will physically occlude the esophagus and may decrease the risk of gastric distension during manual mask ventilation and reduce the risk of passive reflux of gastric contents into the lungs. If the patient lacks protective airway reflexes, cricoid pressure should be applied during mask ventilation and during attempts at tracheal intubation; it should be discontinued only after tracheal intubation has been confirmed. Proper application of cricoid pressure may improve visualization of the vocal cords, similar to the backward, upward, and rightward pressure maneuver (BURP maneuver) described in **Appendix 2**. Guidelines for managing the difficult airway, whether identified or unrecognized, are presented in **Figure 2-3**.

Figure 2-3. Management of the Difficult Airway

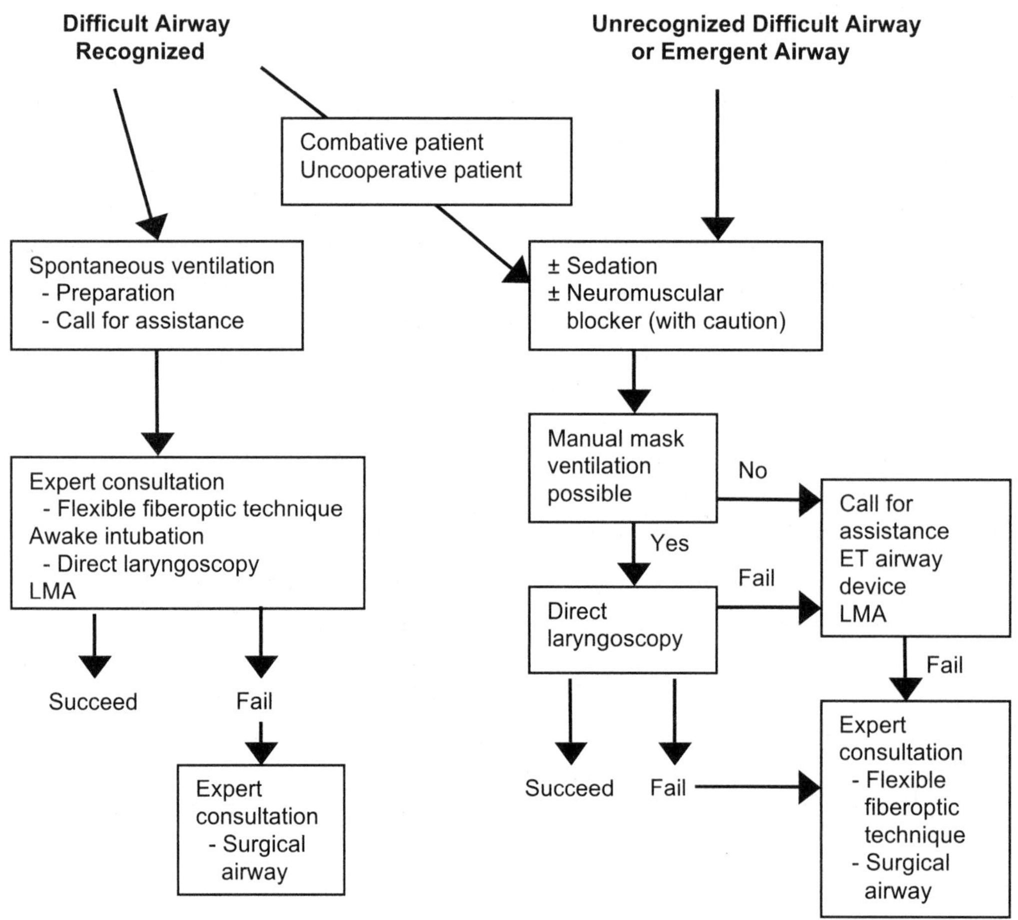

Abbreviations: LMA, laryngeal mask airway; ET, esophageal-tracheal

V. AIRWAY ADJUNCTS

In approximately 5% of the general population, manual mask ventilation is difficult or impossible to achieve. Predictors of difficulty are presence of a beard, absence of teeth, history consistent with obstructive sleep apnea, body mass index greater than 26 kg/m^2, and age greater than 55 years. The presence of two predictors indicates a high probability of difficulty in manual mask ventilation. Intubation via direct laryngoscopy is difficult in approximately 5% of the general population and impossible in 0.2% to 0.5%. A crisis situation occurs when manual mask ventilation and intubation are impossible. The laryngeal mask airway and esophageal-tracheal double-lumen airway device are useful adjuncts to provide an open airway and permit gas exchange in such situations. These devices are blindly inserted, cuffed pharyngeal ventilation devices employed when mask ventilation is difficult or impossible. Their use buys time after failed intubation. The choice of device depends on the operator's experience, equipment availability, and specific clinical circumstances.

A. Laryngeal Mask Airway

A laryngeal mask airway is a tube attached to a bowl-shaped cuff that fits in the pharynx behind the tongue. The standard type is reusable, but a single-use device is also available. A laryngeal mask airway may be used to ventilate the lungs when mask ventilation is difficult, provided that the patient does not have periglottal abnormalities. It may also serve as a conduit for intubation when a bronchoscope is used or as a rescue technique after failure to intubate. Less sedation is required with a laryngeal mask airway than with direct laryngoscopy because stimulation to the airway (eg, gagging, laryngospasm, sympathetic stimulation) in passing the device is only moderate. It is effective in ventilating patients ranging from neonates to adults, but it does not provide definitive airway protection. For specific details regarding use of a laryngeal mask airway, see **Appendix 3**.

B. Esophageal-Tracheal Double-Lumen Airway Device

Another tool for providing an emergency airway is a double-lumen device with two inflatable balloon cuffs. Although this item was designed primarily for blind intubation during cardiorespiratory arrest, it can provide ventilation if the distal cuffed portion of the tube device is inserted in the esophagus or trachea. Its use is contraindicated for patients with central airway obstruction, intact laryngeal or pharyngeal reflexes, known esophageal pathology, or ingestion of caustic substances. Adequate training is required to ensure appropriate use. (For information about inserting an esophageal-tracheal double-lumen airway device, see **Appendix 3**.)

VI. ENDOTRACHEAL INTUBATION

Direct laryngoscopy with orotracheal intubation is the principal method for tracheal intubation because of its speed, success rate, and availability of equipment. Blind nasotracheal intubation may be useful for selected patients. The indications for tracheal intubation are summarized in **Table 2-1**, and the techniques for orotracheal and nasotracheal intubation are discussed and illustrated in **Appendix 2**.

Table 2-1 Indications for Tracheal Intubation
Airway protection
Relief of obstruction
Provision of mechanical ventilation and oxygen therapy
Respiratory failure
Shock
Hyperventilation for intracranial hypertension
Reduction of the work of breathing
Facilitation of suctioning/pulmonary toilet

In preparation for intubation, important issues include:

- Assessment of airway anatomy and function to estimate degree of difficulty for intubation (discussed later)
- Assurance of optimal ventilation and oxygenation. Preoxygenation with 100% oxygen, using a bag-mask resuscitation device, occurs during periods of apnea and prior to intubation attempts.
- Decompression of the stomach with an existing orogastric or nasogastric tube. However, the insertion of such tube to decompress the stomach prior to intubation is often counterproductive, as it may elicit emesis and promote passive reflux of gastric contents.
- Provision of appropriate analgesia, sedation, amnesia, and neuromuscular blockade as required for a safe procedure (discussed later)

Although emergent intubation leaves little time for evaluation and optimization of conditions, elective and urgent intubation allows for assessment of factors that promote safe airway management. The patient's clinical situation, intravascular volume status, hemodynamics, and airway evaluation (degree of difficulty) should be assessed as a plan for airway management is formulated. Airway evaluation includes assessment of physical characteristics that together determine if visualization of the vocal cords will be difficult or impossible. This evaluation will suggest whether alternative techniques to direct laryngoscopy (eg, awake intubation, flexible fiberoptic intubation, surgical airway) are likely to be necessary and whether a more experienced individual should be summoned immediately. Keep in mind that many of these physical characteristics also cause difficulty with mask ventilation and the ability to perform an emergent cricothyrotomy. These characteristics are easy to remember if they are considered in the same order as the steps used in oral intubation — that is, head position, mouth opening, displacement of the tongue and jaw, visualization, and insertion of endotracheal tube:

- *Neck mobility.* The presence of possible cervical spine injury, short neck, or limited neck mobility due to prior surgery or arthritis will restrict the ability to position adequately.
- *External face.* The patient should be examined for evidence of micrognathia or the presence of surgical scars, facial trauma, small nares, or nasal, oral, or pharyngeal bleeding.
- *Mouth.* Mouth opening may be limited due to temporomandibular joint disease or facial scarring. An opening of less than three finger breadths (approximately 6 cm) is associated with an increased risk of difficult intubation.
- *Tongue and pharynx.* Tongue size relative to the posterior pharynx estimates the relative amount of room in the pharynx to visualize glottic structures.
- *Jaw.* Thyromental distance — the distance in finger breadths between the anterior prominence of the thyroid cartilage (Adam's apple) and the tip of the mandible (chin) —estimates the length of the mandible and the available space anterior to the larynx. A distance of less than three finger breadths (approximately 6 cm) indicates that the larynx may appear more anterior and be more difficult to visualize and enter during laryngoscopy. A more acute angulation of the stylet in the endotracheal tube may be helpful. See Section IV for discussion on head positioning.

> !
>
> *Failed intubation attempts can result in periglottic edema and create subsequent difficulty with mask ventilation, leading to a "can't intubate and can't ventilate" situation.*
>
> !

If one or a combination of these physical characteristics indicates the possibility of difficult intubation and if time allows, other options for obtaining a secure airway and calling in someone with additional airway expertise should be considered.

When difficulty in mask ventilation or intubation is anticipated, care is advised before suppressing spontaneous ventilation with neuromuscular blocking drugs or sedatives that cannot be reversed. Options for safe airway management include the following, all of which preserve spontaneous ventilation:

- Awake intubation by direct laryngoscopy or blind nasotracheal intubation
- Flexible fiberoptic intubation (expert consultation required)
- Awake tracheostomy (expert consultation required)

In the event that visualization of the glottis and mask ventilation are both impossible and there is no spontaneous ventilation, options include:

- Laryngeal mask airway or esophageal-tracheal double-lumen airway device
- Needle cricothyrotomy (expert consultation required)
- Surgical cricothyrotomy/tracheostomy (expert consultation required)
- Percutaneous tracheostomy (expert consultation required)

Recall that an algorithm for managing a potential or confirmed difficult airway is shown in **Figure 2-3**.

After tracheal intubation, significant alterations in hemodynamics should be anticipated. Hypertension and tachycardia may result from sympathetic stimulation, and some patients may require therapy with antihypertensive medications or sedatives. Hypotension is common, and decreased cardiac output, due to reduced venous return with positive pressure ventilation, can precipitate arrhythmias or cardiac arrest. The effects of sedative agents on the vasculature or myocardium, hypovolemia, and a possible postintubation pneumothorax may also contribute to hypotension. Other complications associated with positive pressure ventilation are discussed in **Chapter 5**.

VII. PHARMACOLOGIC PREPARATION FOR INTUBATION

During the process of airway management, both parasympathetic and sympathetic responses are common and may require control with proper pharmacologic therapy. The pharmacologic goal before intubation is to provide the patient with optimal analgesia/anesthesia, amnesia, and sedation without altering cardiorespiratory stability. At times, preservation of spontaneous ventilatory drive is necessary. Obviously, the selection of particular methods or drugs depends upon the clinical circumstances and the patient's status, patient allergies, and the experience and preferences of the operator.

A. Analgesia/Anesthesia

- A variety of topical anesthetic sprays are available, or lidocaine may be delivered via aerosol. Anatomic areas for special emphasis include the base of the tongue, directly on the posterior wall of the pharynx, and bilaterally in the tonsillar fossae. Care should be taken not to exceed 4 mg/kg of lidocaine (maximum dose 300 mg), as it is easily absorbed from the airway mucosa.

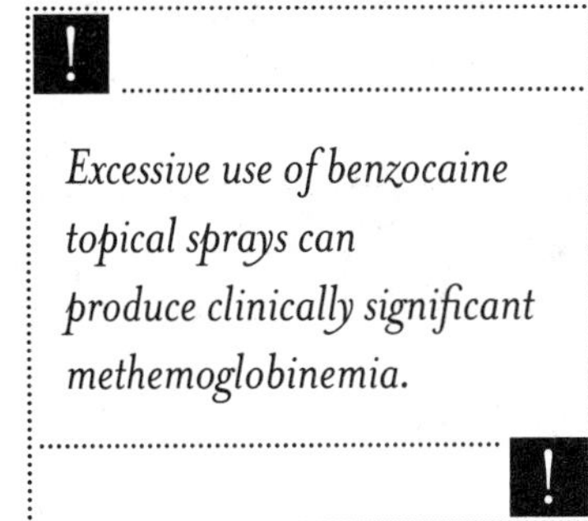

- Administration of nerve blocks and transcricoid membrane lidocaine requires special expertise outside the scope of this course.

- Analgesia is also provided by some sedative agents.

B. Sedation/Amnesia

Rapid-acting, short-lived, and potentially reversible agents are preferred for sedation. No single agent has every desirable feature, and often more than one agent may be considered to provide a balanced technique. The status of the patient's intravascular volume and cardiac function must be carefully considered during the selection of an agent and its dosage. Most may induce hypotension when heart failure or hypovolemia is present. Examples of commonly used medications are listed in **Table 2-2**. Be prepared to manage hypotension following induction (**Chapters 5** and **7**).

C. Neuromuscular Blockers

Often, intubation can be safely and easily performed after topical anesthesia (ie, an awake intubation), or with sedation alone. Therefore, neuromuscular blockade is not always required prior to endotracheal intubation. Obviously, if the operator cannot intubate the patient after neuromuscular blockers have been given, effective manual mask ventilation must be continued while a more experienced person is sought, an alternative plan to secure the airway is developed, or the agent is metabolized with return of spontaneous ventilation. Hence, a short-acting agent is advantageous. The following are examples of neuromuscular blockers:

- Succinylcholine, 1 to 1.5 mg/kg intravenous bolus: rapid onset; shortest duration, which provides an element of safety; may cause muscle fasciculations because this agent depolarizes skeletal muscle; emesis may occur if abdominal muscle fasciculations are severe; contraindicated when ocular injury is present; relatively contraindicated when head injury or hyperkalemia is present (potassium release of 0.5-1 mmol/L will occur routinely, and massive potassium release may occur in burn and crush injury, upper motor neuron lesions, or primary muscle disease); may precipitate malignant hyperthermia. Effects are prolonged in patients with atypical cholinesterase or decreased pseudocholinesterase levels.

- Vecuronium, 0.1 to 0.3 mg/kg; rocuronium, 0.6 to 1 mg/kg; or cisatracurium, 0.1 to 0.2 mg/kg intravenous bolus: no fasciculations because these are nondepolarizing agents; slower onset of muscle paralysis; significantly longer duration of effects than with succinylcholine.

Table 2-2 Drugs Used to Facilitate Tracheal Intubation[a]

Agent	Dosing	Benefits	Cautions
Fentanyl	0.5-2 μg/kg IV bolus every several minutes titrated to sedative effect	Rapid onset of action Short acting Reversible with naloxone	Chest wall rigidity with rapid administration Respiratory depression Does not inhibit patient awareness of procedure
Midazolam	0.1-0.3 mg/kg bolus titrated to sedative effect every several minutes	Provides amnesia Rapid onset of action Short acting Reversible with flumazenil	Additive respiratory depression when combined with narcotic Does not provide analgesia
Etomidate	0.1-0.3 mg/kg single IV bolus	Provides hypnosis May be preferred in head injury No adverse cardiovascular effects	May induce myoclonus, including mild trismus (consider premedication with 50 μg fentanyl) No reversal agent Transient adrenal suppression
Lidocaine	1-1.5 mg/kg IV bolus 2-3 minutes before laryngoscopy	Blunts hemodynamic and tracheal response to intubation *May* reduce elevations of intracranial pressure during laryngoscopy	Should not exceed 4 mg/kg total dose due to neurotoxicity (seizures)
Ketamine	1-4 mg/kg IV bolus	Rapid onset No adverse cardiovascular effects (except in severe congestive heart failure) Short acting	May increase intracranial pressure May result in hallucinations upon emergence Consider small dose of benzodiazepine (midazolam 0.5-1 mg IV) as an adjunct
Propofol	1-2 mg/kg IV bolus	Rapid onset Short acting Provides amnesia	Severe hypotension in volume-depleted patients Does not provide analgesia Respiratory depression

[a]The medications and doses listed are for induction in intubation in adult patients and are not intended for ongoing sedation or pain control.

D. Rapid Sequence Intubation

Rapid sequence intubation is the simultaneous administration of a sedative agent and a neuromuscular blocker along with cricoid pressure, designed to facilitate intubation and reduce the risk of gastric aspiration. It is the technique of choice when there is an increased risk of aspiration (eg, full stomach, pain, gastroesophageal reflux) and examination does not suggest a difficult intubation. Patients for whom intubation is likely to be difficult should not have rapid sequence intubation. The emergency methods described earlier will be necessary if the patient cannot be intubated and is impossible to ventilate, because the ability to ventilate via mask is not tested before administration of the neuromuscular blocker.

E. Intracranial Pressure

Intracranial pressure may rise during laryngoscopy and intubation, and this may be harmful in patients with preexisting intracranial hypertension. Intravenous lidocaine (1-1.5 mg/kg) has been shown to blunt this response and should be administered prior to laryngoscopy when intracranial pathology is suspected.

Key Points

Airway Management

- Assessment of the patient's level of consciousness, airway protective reflexes, respiratory drive, obstruction(s) to gas flow into the airway, and work of breathing will determine the steps necessary to ensure appropriate respiratory support.
- Every primary care provider must be skilled in manual methods to secure and maintain a patent airway.
- Manual assisted ventilation performed with a bag-mask resuscitation unit is a skill expected of every healthcare provider. The goal is to optimize oxygenation and CO_2 removal before, or in lieu of, intubation of the patient.
- Proper application of cricoid pressure may reduce the risk of gastric distension and passive aspiration.
- The laryngeal mask airway and the esophageal-tracheal double-lumen airway device are useful airway adjuncts when expertise in intubation is lacking or intubation is unsuccessful.
- Before intubation, further patient evaluation is necessary to assess the degree of intubation difficulty and determine the appropriateness of analgesia, sedation, amnesia, and possible neuromuscular blockade.
- A plan for managing a potentially difficult intubation includes maintenance of spontaneous ventilation, alternatives to endotracheal intubation, and requests for expert assistance. When manual mask ventilation is impossible after failed intubation, proper use of adjunct devices, cricothyrotomy, or percutaneous tracheostomy may be lifesaving.

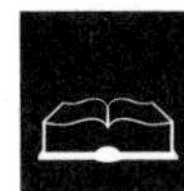

Suggested Readings

1. Agro F, Frass M, Benumof J, et al. The esophageal tracheal combitube as a noninvasive alternative to endotracheal intubation: A review. *Minerva Anestesiol.* 2001;67:863-874.

2. American Society of Anesthesiologists Task Force on Management of the Difficult Airway. Practice guidelines for management of the difficult airway: An updated report by the American Society of Anesthesiologists Task Force on Management of the Difficult Airway [published correction appears in Anesthesiology. 2004; 101:565]. *Anesthesiology.* 2003;98:1269-1277.

3. Danks RR, Danks B. Laryngeal mask airway: Review of indications and use. *J Emerg Nurs.* 2004;30:30-35.

4. Dunham CM, Barraco RD, Clark DE, et al; for the EAST Practice Management Guidelines Work Group. Guidelines for emergency tracheal intubation immediately after traumatic injury. *J Trauma.* 2003;55:162-179.

5. Henderson JJ, Popat MT, Latto IP, et al. Difficult Airway Society guidelines for management of unanticipated difficult intubation. *Anaesthesia.* 2004;59:675-694.

6. Langeron O, Masso E, Huraux C, et al. Prediction of difficult mask ventilation. *Anesthesiology.* 2000;92:1229-1236.

7. Rosenblatt WH. Preoperative planning of airway management in critical care patients. *Crit Care Med.* 2004;32:S186-S192.

8. Murray MJ, Cowen J, DeBlock H, et al. Clinical practice guidelines for sustained neuromuscular blockade in the critically ill adult patient. *Crit Care Med.* 2002;30: 142-156.

9. Nasraway SA Jr., Jacobi J, Murray MJ, et al. Sedatives, analgesia, and neuromuscular blockade of the critically ill adult: Revised clinical practice guidelines for 2002. *Crit Care Med.* 2002;30:117-118.

10. Walz JM, Zayaruzny M, Heard SO. Airway management in critical illness. *Chest.* 2007;131:608-620.

Chapter 3

Cardiopulmonary/Cerebral Resuscitation

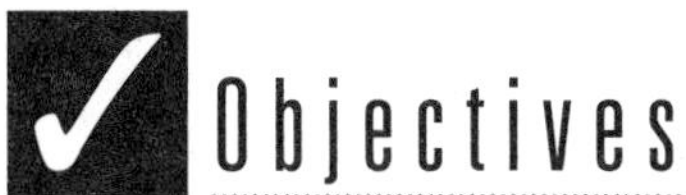

Objectives

- Identify patients who are likely to benefit from cardiopulmonary resuscitation.
- Propose a process for delegating responsibilities during a resuscitation process.
- Discuss important treatment issues in cardiopulmonary arrest.
- Emphasize goals and interventions for brain protection and recovery, including use of therapeutic hypothermia.
- Review specific cardiorespiratory events that occur in critically ill, ventilated patients.

Case Study

The hospital paging operator announces the cardiac arrest of a 54-year-old man on the general floor. On arrival at the scene, you note that one nurse is applying an oxygen mask and another nurse is attempting to measure the patient's blood pressure.

- Assuming the patient should be resuscitated, what are your immediate actions?
- What are the next steps if you are the team leader?
- What tasks are delegated to team members during the resuscitation?

I. INTRODUCTION

The immediate response to an in-hospital cardiac arrest is frequently the responsibility of primary care providers, hospitalists, nurses, house staff, and other members of the healthcare team. The Society of Critical Care Medicine and the Fundamental Critical Care Support program recognize the valuable training provided by the American Heart Association's Basic Life Support (BLS), Advanced Cardiovascular Life Support (ACLS), and Pediatric Advanced Life Support (PALS) curricula. All healthcare practitioners are encouraged to successfully complete the appropriate course in that series. Algorithms from the 2010 International Consensus Conference and recommended by the American Heart Association are reproduced in **Appendix 4**.

II. ETHICAL ISSUES

A. Who Should Be Resuscitated?

The purpose of cardiopulmonary resuscitation (CPR) and advanced life support in the critical care setting is to reverse sudden, unexpected death resulting from reversible disease processes or iatrogenic complications. If possible, resuscitation status should always be discussed with the patient, the patient's family, or the surrogate decision maker before a cardiac arrest event (**Chapter 15**). Resuscitation is unlikely to benefit patients experiencing an arrest despite maximal medical therapy for progressive cardiogenic or septic shock. Out-of-hospital arrest can carry a very high mortality rate in conjunction with prolonged CPR. Several other underlying conditions (eg, pneumonia, congestive heart failure, renal failure, and sepsis) make survival from cardiac arrest exceedingly unlikely but not unprecedented. No set of variables is sensitive enough to accurately predict a poor outcome.

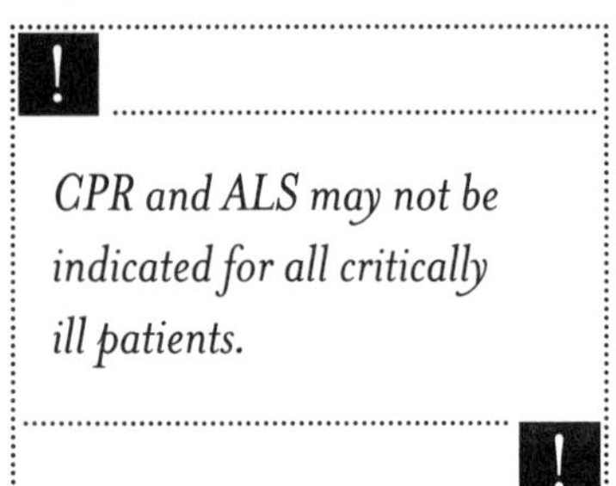

B. Level of Therapeutic Support

CPR is instituted based on implied consent, without a physician's order, whereas limitation of resuscitation requires an order. Do-not-attempt-resuscitation (DNAR) orders should be documented in the chart with an explanation of the rationale. Such orders do not and should not indicate that the patient is not to be treated. Patients and their families should not be abandoned emotionally because of such orders. "No resuscitation" does not mean "no care." Intermediate resuscitative plans suited to a patient's particular wishes and condition should be clearly delineated in the chart by the attending physician and should be respected by the hospital staff. "Slow codes" that give the illusion of resuscitation are not appropriate. Pain and anxiety should be treated in all cases regardless of a patient's resuscitation status.

C. Documentation

The level of therapeutic support should be documented in the patient's chart so that the staff knows exactly how to proceed should cardiorespiratory arrest occur unexpectedly. If this level of support were addressed only in the sickest patients, no instructions would exist for many patients who experience arrest. The staff should follow valid DNAR orders. Information about advance directives, living wills, durable powers of attorney, and related forms also should be documented and respected.

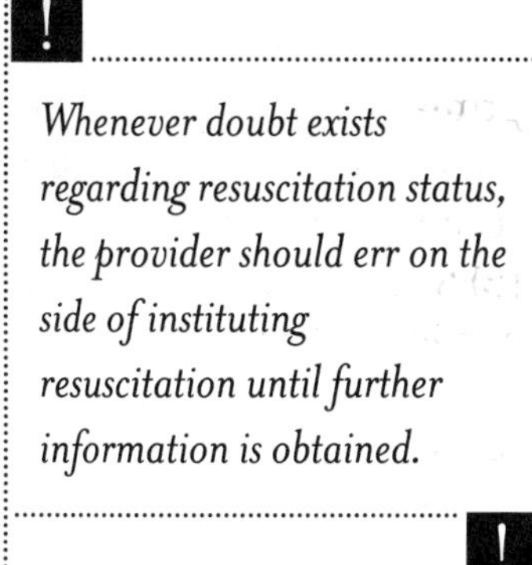

III. PRIMARY RESPONSE

Responders will usually have resuscitation resources available for cardiorespiratory arrests that occur within the hospital. Often, however, the most important aspects of a successful resuscitation relate to the interactions, knowledge, and skills of the responders and the ability to delegate and accept responsibility for components of the resuscitation effort. A suggested approach to resuscitation is outlined below and further information is presented in **Appendix 4**.

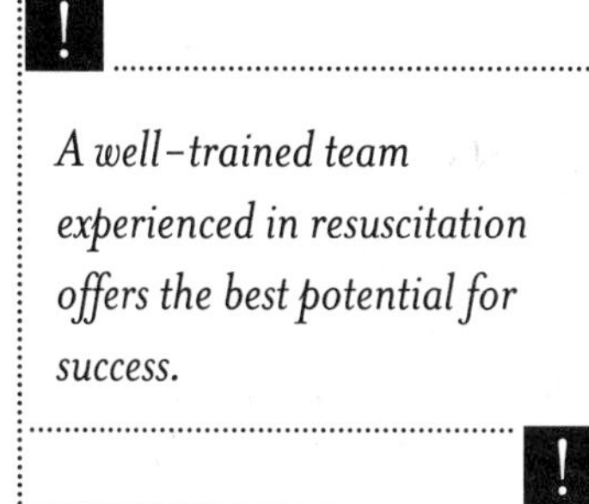

A. Assessment of the Immediate Situation

Has an appropriate individual assumed the leadership role?

- If so, how can you assist? Identify yourself and offer help. Be ready to accept a delegated role and to focus your efforts upon that role while remaining aware of other evolving resuscitation activities.

- If not, you may be required to assume the leadership role until a more qualified individual or the designated team member arrives.

B. The Leader's Role

Proceed with primary assessment and intervention, and delegate appropriate activities to others.

1. Evaluation and Initial Cardiac Resuscitation

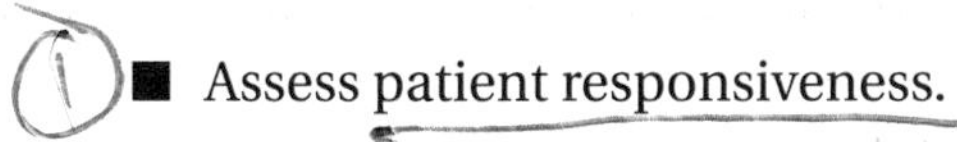

- Assess patient responsiveness.

- If the patient is unresponsive, assess respiratory effort, pulse, or any body movement that is evidence of circulation. If absent, activate your emergency response system, obtain an automated external defibrillator (AED) or monitor/defibrillator, and start chest compressions (CPR) immediately at a rate of at least 100/minute, and at a depth of at least 2 inches in adults. *Push hard, push fast.* Healthcare providers should provide 2 breaths over 1 second each during each 2-minute cycle of CPR. The breaths should be of sufficient volume to see the chest rise and contain the maximum oxygen concentration available. Compressions-only CPR is acceptable for non-healthcare providers. The "Look, Listen, and Feel" step found in previous CPR algorithms has been eliminated.

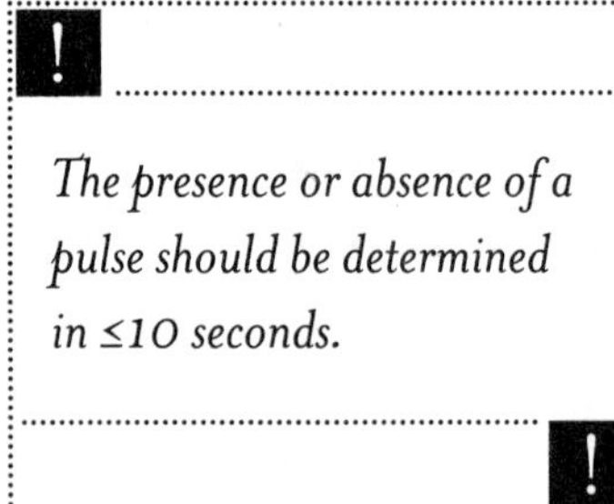

- Defibrillation should be initiated as soon as possible if monitoring (eg, quick-look paddles) indicates ventricular fibrillation or pulseless ventricular tachycardia (**Appendix 5**). A single shock should be delivered at the energy level appropriate for the defibrillator (360 joules with a monophasic defibrillator and manufacturer's recommended energy level if known, or 200 joules with a biphasic defibrillator). Chest compressions should be resumed immediately after the shock is delivered without checking the pulse or rhythm. Rhythm analysis should usually occur after 2 minutes of compressions, but this sequence may be modified in the hospital setting with continuous electrocardiographic (ECG) monitoring.

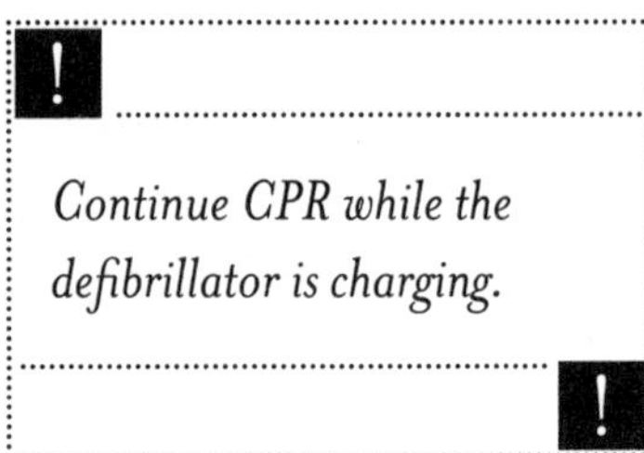

- If intubated and connected to a mechanical ventilator, the patient must be disconnected and changed to manual bag-mask ventilation.

2. Delegation

- Delegate tasks to the most appropriate personnel available whenever possible. This allows the resuscitation leader to maintain an overall perspective, monitor cardiac rhythm, direct assessments and interventions, and prescribe medications. The leader may need to perform some of these tasks or reassign them if the primary designee is unsuccessful. Obviously, if the number of responders is not sufficient, team members must establish priorities for performance. Delegated duties should include the following:

  a. Manage the airway (**Chapter 2**). Establish a patent airway, provide manual bag-mask ventilation, utilize available airway adjuncts, and/or perform endotracheal intubation. Ventilations should not exceed the recommended 8 to 10 breaths/min to optimize coronary artery perfusion pressure by decreasing the percentage of time in positive intrathoracic pressure. Avoid hyperventilation.

b. Perform chest compressions. The resuscitation leader should designate a second person for relief and instruct the rescuers to exchange responsibilities every 2 minutes. Evidence shows that a compression rate of at least 100/min results in maximal blood flow for the patient. The ratio of compression to ventilation is 30:2 without an advanced airway in place, and the depth of compressions for adults is at least 2 inches (5 cm). The chest should recoil completely between compressions. If the patient has an advanced airway in place, compressions are continuous, and asynchronous ventilation is provided at a rate of 8 to 10 breaths/min. The person on relief should monitor the effectiveness of compressions by checking the carotid or femoral pulse. Although the results of such checks do not correlate highly with intravascular flow, they constitute a minimal monitoring method. Chest compressions are interrupted only for shock delivery and rhythm checks once the airway is secured. Pulse checks are performed only if an organized rhythm is noted.

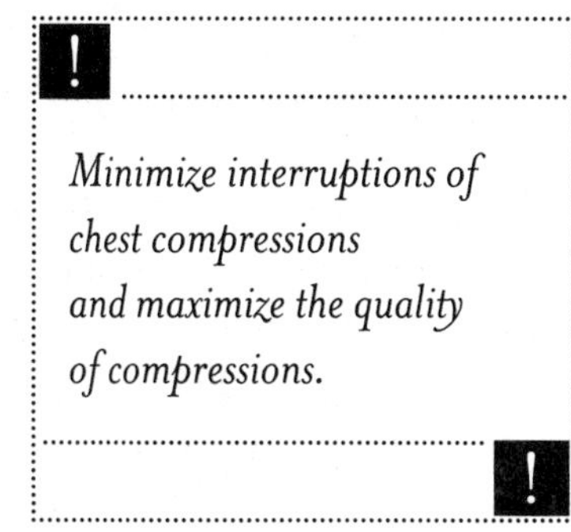
Minimize interruptions of chest compressions and maximize the quality of compressions.

c. Attach ECG monitor/machine.

d. Obtain intravenous access and assume primary responsibility for administering medications. Peripheral venous access with a large catheter is preferred because it does not require interruption of chest compressions. The intraosseous route can be used as a temporary measure when other vascular sites are not immediately available in children or adults (**Appendix 6**).

e. Provide medications as requested (eg, to manage the code cart, defibrillator/pacer, and so forth).

f. Maintain record of resuscitation interventions and patient assessments.

g. Obtain medical record and/or provide pertinent patient information.

h. Notify the patient's personal attending physician of the cardiopulmonary event and obtain further guidance. Discuss the patient's status, medical history, existence of advance directives, and related topics.

i. Remove furniture, unnecessary equipment, and extra personnel from the resuscitation area.

IV. CONTINUING RESUSCITATION

Once the primary response and assigned tasks have been successfully initiated, each team member continues an appropriate role as the resuscitation interventions are implemented.

- Critical laboratory data should be obtained to assist with decisions during the resuscitation and, perhaps, to reveal a cause for the cardiac arrest. Important data include levels of glucose, arterial blood gases, potassium, ionized calcium, and magnesium. Suspected abnormalities or those documented in recent laboratory values may be treated empirically. Repetitive blood testing must be expedited by a team member, and the laboratory must be notified of the ongoing resuscitation.

- The patient's chart should be reviewed for history and any possible medication reaction that could lead to cardiac arrest, arrhythmia, or decreased ventilatory drive. Notify the primary physician immediately.

- It is appropriate to assume that the initial cardiopulmonary arrest would not have been announced if a DNAR or similar directive had been ordered by a physician – but this should be confirmed as other patient information and data are obtained. Whenever doubt exists about a resuscitation status, full resuscitative measures should be initiated and continued until clarified with the patient's attending physician and/or family.

- The point at which family members are notified of the cardiopulmonary arrest will vary. If family is present, a team member should provide information periodically during the resuscitation. The presence of family during resuscitation should be carefully considered and planned for if this practice is accepted by the institution and the resuscitation team.

- Arrangements for patient transfer to an ICU should be considered, usually by a nursing supervisor. A transport cart, emergency drugs, external pacer (**Appendix 7**), portable monitors, oxygen, and other crucial supplies should be available to facilitate immediate transfer as the patient stabilizes. The ICU will need to prepare, so additional patient needs (eg, arterial or central line transducer setups, ECG, chest radiograph, mechanical ventilator) should be communicated.

V. OTHER CONSIDERATIONS IN CARDIOPULMONARY/ CEREBRAL RESUSCITATION

- The method that best produces blood flow to the coronary arteries, brain, and other organs during a cardiopulmonary arrest has not yet been determined. At present, closed-chest compressions remain the standard technique for circulatory support. Interposed abdominal compression CPR and active compression-decompression CPR (device not available in the United States) may be considered acceptable alternatives whenever personnel trained in the techniques are available. The invasive alternative of open-chest cardiac massage requires a team with special expertise and early institution for optimal outcome. Immediate cardiopulmonary bypass may be effective in improving the success of resuscitation but is not available in most hospitals.

> ! *Closed-chest compressions produce approximately one-third of normal cardiac output.* !

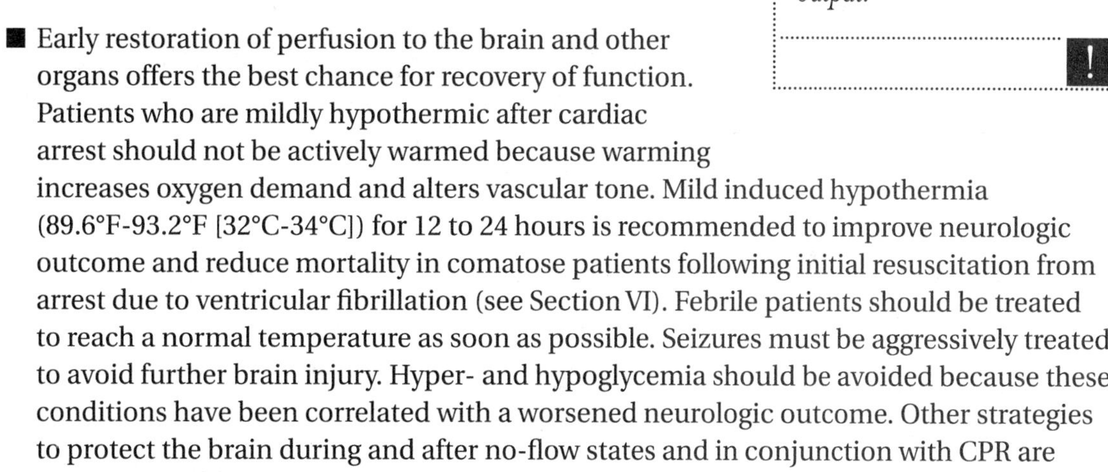

- Early restoration of perfusion to the brain and other organs offers the best chance for recovery of function. Patients who are mildly hypothermic after cardiac arrest should not be actively warmed because warming increases oxygen demand and alters vascular tone. Mild induced hypothermia (89.6°F-93.2°F [32°C-34°C]) for 12 to 24 hours is recommended to improve neurologic outcome and reduce mortality in comatose patients following initial resuscitation from arrest due to ventricular fibrillation (see Section VI). Febrile patients should be treated to reach a normal temperature as soon as possible. Seizures must be aggressively treated to avoid further brain injury. Hyper- and hypoglycemia should be avoided because these conditions have been correlated with a worsened neurologic outcome. Other strategies to protect the brain during and after no-flow states and in conjunction with CPR are under investigation.

- Quantitative end-tidal CO_2 measurement with waveform display is recommended for the intra- and post-resuscitation management of cardiac arrest. Detection of or a rapid quantum increase in end-tidal CO_2 is often the earliest indication of return of spontaneous circulation (ROSC). Normocapnia (PCO_2 38-42 mm Hg) is the goal.

VI. TARGETED TEMPERATURE MANAGEMENT

Targeted temperature management (TTM), or therapeutic hypothermia, is a critical part of the cardio-cerebral resuscitation process. Early restoration of perfusion to the brain and other organs offers the best chance for functional recovery. Avoidance of hyperthermia in the post-cardiac arrest period is essential. TTM as low as 89.6°F to 93.2°F (32°C to 34°C) core body temperature is recommended for patients with out-of-hospital cardiac arrest due to ventricular fibrillation or pulseless ventricular tachycardia who remain unconscious after ROSC (**Figure 3-1**). TTM is associated with both reduced mortality rates and improved neurological recovery after cardiac arrest. The improvement in neurologic outcome appears to be mediated by reduction of inflammation in the brain. Data exist on a select group of comatose cardiac arrest survivors (**Table 3-1**). Many centers now apply this strategy to all patients (out-of-hospital or inpatient) who have ROSC irrespective of the initial rhythm resulting in cardiac arrest.

Figure 3-1. Example of Targeted Temperature Management Algorithm[a]

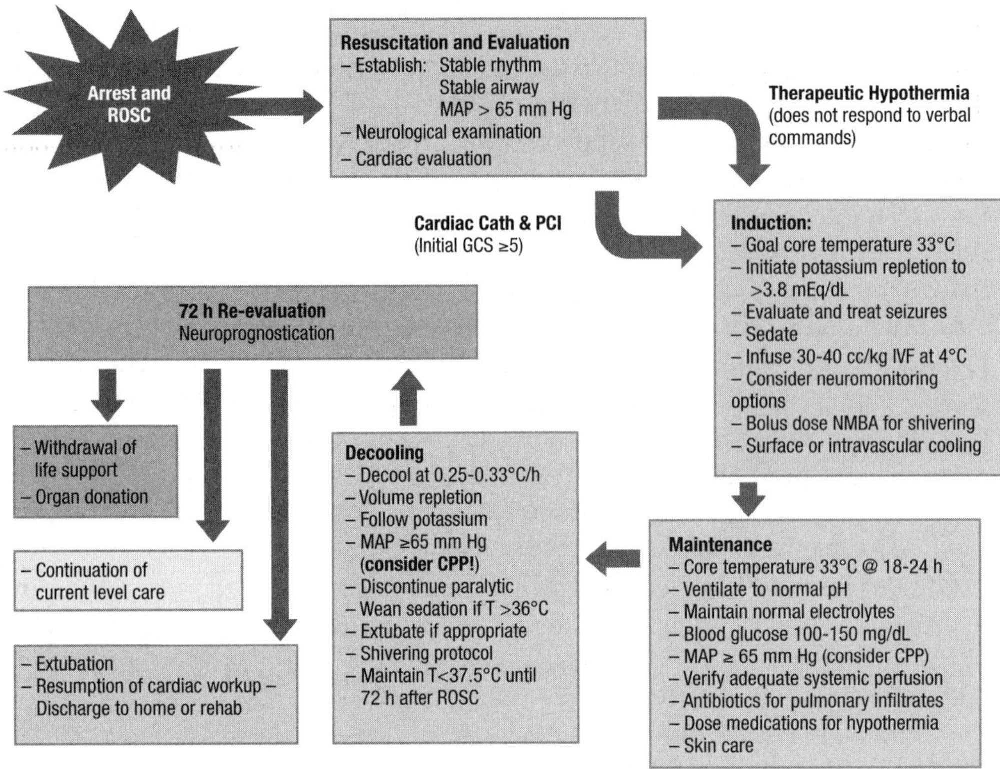

Abbreviations: ROSC, return of spontaneous circulation; MAP, mean arterial pressure; Cath, catheter; PCI, percutaneous coronary intervention; GCS, Glasgow Coma Scale score; IVF, intravenous fluid; NMBA, neuromuscular blocking agent; CPP, cerebral perfusion pressure; T, temperature

[a]Reproduced with permission from Lippincott, Williams & Wilkins. Seder DB, Van der Kloot TE. Methods of cooling: Practical aspects of therapeutic temperature management. *Crit Care Med.* 2009; 37:S211–S222.[11]

Table 3-1 Considerations for Targeted Temperature Management

Patients for whom therapeutic hypothermia should be considered:

- Adult patients who remain comatose (ie, patients with a Glasgow Coma Scale Score less than 8 and/or patients who do not obey any verbal command after restoration of spontaneous circulation, but before the initiation of cooling) following successful resuscitation from a witnessed out-of-hospital cardiac arrest of presumed cardiac cause; in-hospital cardiac arrest survivors may also benefit.
- Patients with an initial rhythm of ventricular fibrillation or pulseless ventricular tachycardia; patients with initial rhythms of asystole or pulseless electrical activity may also benefit.
- Patients with hemodynamic stability. Retrospective data suggest that patients in cardiogenic shock also may safely undergo therapeutic hypothermia treatment.

Patients for whom therapeutic hypothermia should not be considered:

- Patients with tympanic-membrane temperature below 86°F (30°C) on admission
- Patients who were comatose before the cardiac arrest
- Pregnant patients
- Patients who are terminally ill or for whom intensive care does not seem to be appropriate
- Patients with inherited blood coagulation disorders
- Bleeding patients or those at risk for hemorrhage

No specific time frame has been established to start TTM after cardiac arrest. However, it is generally recommended that the induction phase of cooling begin as soon as possible after cardiac arrest if the patient remains in a comatose state. Although target temperature should be reached within the first several hours after ROSC, lifesaving cardiac procedures should not be delayed to initiate TTM. Improved outcomes have been associated with 12 to 24 hours of TTM. Active temperature modulation during rewarming is favored over passive rewarming. Avoid rebound fever. Warming should be performed slowly over 12 hours.

A. Temperature Management Devices

Invasive and external devices are available for TTM, but no one strategy has proven superior. In the absence of specific temperature management devices, the use of iced saline and ice packs can be effective, although hypervolemia from excessive administration of iced saline should be avoided.

B. Potential Organ System Effects of TTM

- Neurologic: shivering
- Cardiac: dysrhythmias
- Renal: diuresis and potassium shifts
- Liver: coagulopathy
- Skin: frostbite
- Altered drug metabolism

C. Sedation and Pain Protocol

There are no specific pain or sedation protocols for TTM. Drug pharmacokinetics and pharmacodynamics are altered during therapeutic hypothermia. Aggressive attention to shivering is important; neuromuscular blockade may be necessary if conventional management fails.

VII. RESPIRATORY ARREST

Case Study

You are asked to evaluate a patient with difficulty breathing. The patient is intubated and transferred to the ICU, where mechanical ventilation is instituted. One hour later, the patient's oxygen saturation decreases and the heart rate decreases to 40/min with loss of pulse.

- What are possible etiologies for the patient's deterioration?
- What steps should you take to optimize the patient's respiratory status?

A. Respiratory Arrest in the Nonintubated Patient

1. Immediate Concerns

One of the most common catastrophic events in nonintubated patients is respiratory arrest. These patients are typically found in asystole or pulseless electrical activity (PEA) but may be in ventricular fibrillation. The first responders should institute immediate basic life support, including bag-mask ventilation. Early endotracheal intubation allows for the most effective ventilation and oxygenation. Manual bag-mask ventilation with 100% oxygen until a provider experienced in endotracheal intubation arrives is preferable to prolonged, unsuccessful attempts at intubation.

2. Patient Assessment

In many instances, careful assessment of vital signs (including pulse oximetry), air movement, and work of breathing will indicate that respiratory impairment is present. Tachypnea progressing to bradypnea, paradoxical abdominal breathing, and progressively decreasing alertness may herald imminent respiratory arrest. Noninvasive respiratory monitoring may identify patients who are decompensating. Normal arterial blood gas measurements do not rule out the need for mechanical ventilatory support since decompensation can occur precipitously once respiratory muscle fatigue becomes manifest. Moreover, certain acute conditions (eg, asthma or pulmonary embolus) cause a tachypnea. A normal P_{CO_2} in these instances portends advanced respiratory failure and fatigue. Quantitative end-tidal CO_2 monitoring is recommended.

B. Special Management Issues

1. Cardiac Arrest in Patients Receiving Mechanical Ventilation

If a patient suffers cardiac arrest while receiving mechanical ventilation, some mishap related to ventilation must be suspected, especially if the initial cardiac rhythm is bradycardia or asystole. Etiologic possibilities include tension pneumothorax, ventilator failure or disconnection, or displacement or obstruction of the endotracheal tube. Patients should be disconnected from the ventilator immediately, and manual ventilation with 100% oxygen should be initiated while further assessment is undertaken. If high resistance to airflow is present, the endotracheal tube should be unsecured and checked for kinks, and attempts should be made to pass a suction catheter. Verification of tube placement with expired CO_2 monitoring is recommended as an adjunct to physical assessment. If tube position or patency is in question, the tube should be removed and the patient reintubated after being adequately oxygenated and ventilated by means of a bag-mask device. Tension pneumothorax also should be considered as a cause of high airway resistance. In instances of cardiac arrest, there is not sufficient time to obtain a chest radiograph to check for this possibility. The chest should be decompressed urgently with a needle placed at the level of the second intercostal space in the mid-clavicular position if breath sounds are absent or subcutaneous crepitus is noted.

2. Tension Pneumothorax

Patients with tension pneumothorax typically have hypotension and/or PEA with narrow complex tachycardia. Physical assessment may reveal jugular venous distension and ipsilateral decreased or absent breath sounds. Ipsilateral tympanitic percussion or subcutaneous emphysema may be noted as well. In mechanically ventilated patients, airway pressures for normal tidal volume values will be high, and the ventilator high-pressure alarm limit may be exceeded. Resistance to bag-mask ventilation should increase as well. For patients with severe hypotension or PEA and findings consistent with tension pneumothorax, treatment should be instituted at once, without waiting for radiologic confirmation. Needle thoracostomy can be accomplished on the affected side by sterile placement of a 16- or 18-gauge catheter (a 23-gauge butterfly needle may be used in infants) through the anterior chest wall in the second intercostal space, at the midclavicular line (**Appendix 8**). Successful decompression is associated with a rush of air, restoration of pulses, and a decrease in airway pressures in response to bag-mask or mechanical ventilation. *All* needle thoracostomy procedures should be followed by standard tube thoracostomy because this procedure can result in: 1) temporary relief of a tension pneumothorax; 2) creation of a pneumothorax if the presumption of a tension pneumothorax was wrong; or 3) no change in the patient's condition if the needle does not decompress the pleural space. Endotracheal tube obstruction (from a patient biting the tube or buildup of secretions) can mimic some of the findings described but does not usually cause severe hypotension or PEA.

VIII. ADVANCED LIFE SUPPORT IN THE CRITICAL CARE UNIT

A. General Issues

To be prepared for critical events such as cardiorespiratory arrest, professionals should know the clinical background and status of patients in the critical care unit. They should review each patient's record during checkout rounds for signs of potential problems, such as electrolyte abnormalities. In addition, the clinical history and course may give clues to the etiology of a potential mishap. For instance, a ventilated patient who is known to have a large emphysematous bulla and who suddenly develops PEA has a high likelihood of developing a tension pneumothorax secondary to bleb rupture. Making rounds at the beginning of each tour of duty also gives the staff an opportunity to clarify the resuscitation or code status of each patient.

B. Principal Concerns

Airway management and oxygenation/ventilation are important issues in the initial approach to acute decompensation of an ICU patient. Adequate oxygenation/ventilation should be evaluated by physical assessment as well as expired CO_2 monitoring (if intubation is performed). Patients who are mechanically ventilated at the time of the arrest should be disconnected from the ventilator immediately and should receive 100% oxygen by bag-mask ventilation. Early endotracheal intubation should be performed for those who are not intubated already; tube placement should be verified by physical assessment, chest radiograph, and exhaled CO_2 detection. Pulselessness can be verified by observing the arterial waveform if a functioning arterial line is in place or by carotid or femoral pulse checks. Chest compressions should be performed and early defibrillation for ventricular fibrillation should be undertaken as recommended by ACLS guidelines.

Key Points

Cardiopulmonary/Cerebral Resuscitation

- The patient's resuscitation status should be in accordance with documented directives.
- Familiarity with recommendations for cardiopulmonary resuscitation (**Appendix 4**) is encouraged for all members of the resuscitation team.
- The person assuming the leadership role during resuscitation must effectively delegate specific duties and supervise the process of resuscitation.
- Resuscitation team members must accept delegation and remain focused upon those duties.
- Chest compressions should be optimized by ensuring a rate of at least 100/min, changing compressors every 2 minutes, continuing compressions before and after shock delivery, and minimizing interruptions.
- A mishap related to mechanical ventilation should be suspected in patients who sustain an arrest while receiving ventilation, especially if the initial dysrhythmia is bradycardia or asystole.
- In patients with hypotension and/or PEA and findings consistent with tension pneumothorax, needle thoracostomy should be instituted without delay.
- Critically ill patients, or patients at risk of becoming critically ill, should be monitored for early signs of physiologic deterioration, and appropriate intervention should be instituted to avoid cardiopulmonary arrest.

Suggested Readings

1. Abella BS, Alvarado JP, Myklebust H, et al. Quality of cardiopulmonary resuscitation during in-hospital cardiac arrest. *JAMA.* 2005;293:305-310.

2. American Heart Association. 2010 American Heart Association guidelines for cardiopulmonary resuscitation and emergency cardiovascular care science. *Circulation.* 2010;122(suppl 3):S639-S946.

3. Bernard SA, Gray TW, Buist MD, et al. Treatment of comatose survivors of out-of hospital cardiac arrest with induced hypothermia. *N Engl J Med.* 2002;346:557-563.

4. Holzer M. Targeted temperature management for comatose survivors of cardiac arrest. *N Engl J Med.* 2010;363:1256-1264.

5. Holzer M, Bernard SA, Hachimi-Idrissi S, et al. Hypothermia for neuroprotection after cardiac arrest: Systematic review and individual patient data meta-analysis. *Crit Care Med.* 2005;33:414-418.

6. Hypothermia After Cardiac Arrest Study Group. Mild therapeutic hypothermia to improve the neurologic outcome after cardiac arrest. *N Engl J Med.* 2002;346:549-556.

7. Kellum MJ, Kennedy KW, Barney R, et al. Cardiocerebral resuscitation improves neurologically intact survival of patients with out-of-hospital cardiac arrest. *Ann Emerg Med.* 2008;52:244-252.

8. Nadkarni VM, Larkin GL, Peberdy MA, et al. First documented rhythm and clinical outcome from in-hospital cardiac arrest among children and adults. *JAMA.* 2006;295: 50-57.

9. Nolan JP, Soar J, Zideman DA, et al. European Resuscitation Council Guidelines for Resuscitation 2010 Section 1. Executive summary. *Resuscitation.* 2010;81:1219-1276.

10. Nunnally ME, Jaeschke R, Belligan GJ, et al. Targeted temperature management in critical care: A report and recommendations from five professional societies. *Crit Care Med.* 2011;39:1113-1125.

11. Seder DB, Van der Kloot TE. Methods of cooling: Practical aspects of therapeutic temperature management. *Crit Care Med.* 2009;37:S211–S222.

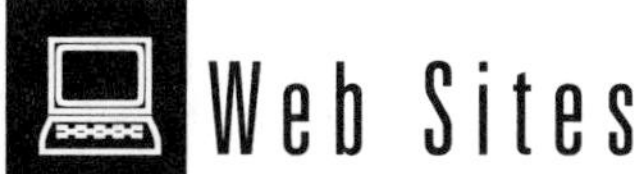

Web Sites

1. American Heart Association. http://www.americanheart.org. *This Web site allows access to the 2010 AHA guidelines for CPR and emergency cardiovascular care and provides other information on resuscitation and cardiac issues.*

2. Circulation. http://www.circulationaha.org. *This Web site allows access to the 2010 AHA guidelines for CPR and emergency cardiovascular care and provides guidelines for cardiac conditions.*

3. European Resuscitation Council. http://www.erc.edu. *This Web site provides the ERC 2010 guidelines for resuscitation and other educational information and material.*

Chapter 4

Diagnosis and Management of Acute Respiratory Failure

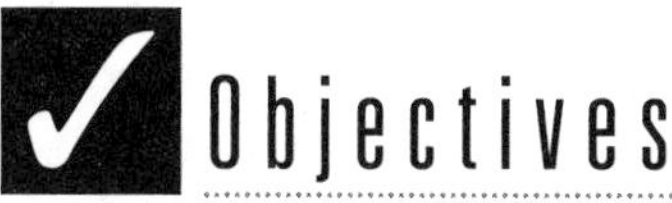

Objectives

- Define and classify acute respiratory failure.
- Describe the pathophysiology and manifestations of acute respiratory failure.
- Review oxygen supplementation strategies in acute respiratory failure.

Case Study

A 75-year-old man with a long history of smoking, chronic lung disease, and treatment noncompliance is brought to the emergency department by his daughter, who says that he complained of progressive dyspnea overnight. The patient is awake, alert, and in moderate respiratory distress, with evident use of accessory muscles during inspiration and expiration and a respiratory rate of 30/min. There are audible expiratory wheezes. You are called to assess the patient and initiate treatment.

- What tests would be useful to evaluate the severity of the patient's condition?
- Which oxygen supplementation device should be used?
- What pharmacologic treatment should be initiated?

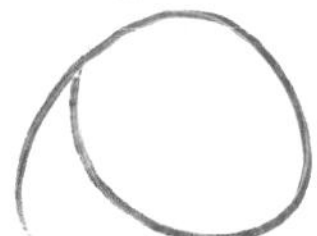

I. INTRODUCTION

Acute respiratory failure (ARF) is one of the leading causes of admission to the ICU. Acute respiratory failure is defined as the inability of the respiratory system to meet the oxygenation, ventilation, or metabolic requirements of the patient. The pulmonary system is involved in two crucial functions: elimination of carbon dioxide (CO_2) and oxygenation of the blood. There are three types of respiratory failure: hypoxemic, hypercapnic, and mixed. Hypoxemic respiratory failure is defined by a room air partial pressure of arterial oxygen (Pao_2) of ≤50 to 60 mm Hg (≤6.7-8 kPa) or an abnormal ratio of Pao_2 to fraction of inspired oxygen (Pao_2:Fio_2, or P:F ratio; see Section III). This abnormality of Pao_2 should exist in the absence of intracardiac right-to-left shunting. Hypercapnic respiratory failure is defined by a partial pressure of arterial CO_2 ($Paco_2$) ≥50 mm Hg (≥6.7 kPa) that is not due to respiratory compensation for metabolic alkalosis. Mixed respiratory failure has features of both hypercapnia and hypoxemia and is a common form of respiratory failure in critically ill patients. Respiratory failure is considered chronic once the renal system begins to compensate by retaining bicarbonate. This usually occurs within a few days of persistent hypercapnia and the resulting respiratory acidosis. Frequently, in patients with chronic lung disease, ARF may be superimposed on chronic respiratory insufficiency. The acute component in such circumstances is distinguishable from the chronic component by the degree of respiratory acidosis in relation to $Paco_2$ and knowledge of baseline oxygen requirements, $Paco_2$ levels, and bicarbonate values.

II. CAUSES OF ACUTE RESPIRATORY FAILURE

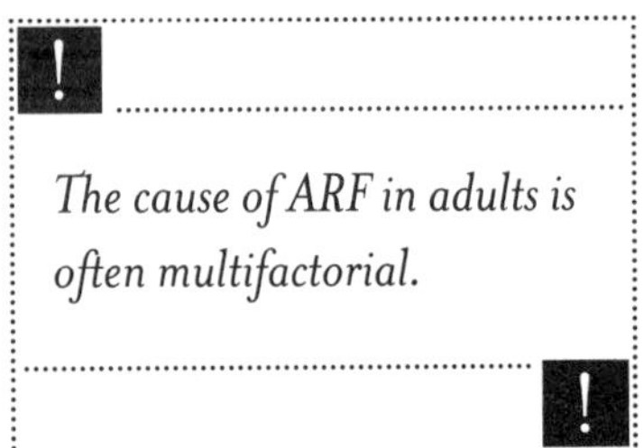

Acute respiratory failure develops in a variety of clinical settings. Respiratory failure may result from primary pulmonary insults or from other systemic nonpulmonary disorders, as summarized in **Table 4-1**. Diseases of the central nervous system, neuromuscular system, upper and lower airways, pulmonary parenchyma, pulmonary vasculature, thoracoabdominal cavity, and cardiovascular system may all give rise to ARF.

Hypoxemic respiratory failure is often seen in patients with severe pneumonia, acute lung injury, or acute pulmonary edema, disorders that interfere primarily with adequate oxygenation of the blood as it circulates through the alveolar capillaries. Hypercapnic respiratory failure is seen in patients with severe airflow obstruction, central respiratory failure, or neuromuscular respiratory failure. Hypercapnia most often results from inadequate alveolar ventilation, which causes ineffective CO_2 clearance.

Table 4-1 Causes of Respiratory Failure

DISORDERS ASSOCIATED WITH ABNORMAL OXYGEN ONLOADING (HYPOXEMIC RESPIRATORY FAILURE)

Lower Airway and Parenchyma

NEOPLASM	TRAUMA	Acute respiratory distress syndrome
INFECTIONS	Pulmonary contusion	Interstitial lung disease
Viral	Pulmonary laceration	Pulmonary emboli
Bacterial	OTHER	Atelectasis
Fungal	Bronchospasm	Cystic fibrosis
Mycoplasma	Heart failure	
Other		

DISORDERS ASSOCIATED WITH INADEQUATE CARBON DIOXIDE OFFLOADING (HYPERCAPNIC RESPIRATORY FAILURE)

Brain

DRUGS	METABOLIC	INFECTION
Opioids	Hyponatremia	Meningitis
Benzodiazepines	Hypocalcemia	Encephalitis
Propofol	Alkalosis	Abscess
Barbiturates	Myxedema	Polio
General anesthetics	NEOPLASM	West Nile myelitis
Poisons		INCREASED INTRACRANIAL PRESSURE
		OTHER
		Central alveolar hypoventilation
		Central sleep apnea

Nerves and Muscles

TRAUMA	METABOLIC	OTHER
Spinal cord injury	Hypokalemia, hyperkalemia	Motor neuron disease
Diaphragmatic injury	Hypophosphatemia	Myasthenia gravis
DRUGS/POISONS	Hypomagnesemia	Multiple sclerosis
Neuromuscular blocking agents	NEOPLASM	Muscular dystrophy
	INFECTIONS	Guillain-Barré syndrome
Aminoglycoside antibiotics	Tetanus	Botulism
Arsenic	West Nile myelitis	
Strychnine		
Botulism		

Upper Airway

TISSUE ENLARGEMENT	INFECTIONS	OTHER
Tonsil and adenoid hyperplasia	Epiglottitis	Bilateral vocal-cord paralysis
	Laryngotracheitis	Laryngeal edema
Malignant neoplasm	TRAUMA	Tracheomalacia
Polyps		Cricoarytenoid arthritis
Goiter		Obstructive sleep apnea

Chest Bellows

TRAUMA	OTHER CONTRIBUTING FACTORS	Fibrothorax
Rib fractures	Kyphoscoliosis	Supine position
Flail chest	Scleroderma	Obesity
Burn eschar	Spondylitis	Pain
	Pneumothorax	Ascites
	Pleural effusion	

The following are common ICU scenarios that lead to ARF:

- Exacerbations of chronic obstructive pulmonary disease (COPD), characterized by thick mucopurulent secretions as well as bronchospasm, are often associated with both hypoxemic and hypercapnic acute respiratory failure (ie, mixed ARF).

- Pneumonia is most commonly associated with hypoxemic respiratory failure, although it also can be associated with hypercapnic respiratory failure, especially in the setting of other diseases such as COPD.

- Acute respiratory distress syndrome (ARDS) is a manifestation of a systemic inflammatory response caused by pulmonary or nonpulmonary injury or disease. The predominantly hypoxemic respiratory failure is caused primarily by an increased shunt fraction due to alveolar filling.

- Traumatic brain injury is associated with predominantly hypercapnic respiratory failure, although it can be complicated by hypoxemic respiratory failure in the setting of concurrent aspiration, pulmonary contusions, neurogenic pulmonary edema, or chronic pulmonary disease.

- Overdose with central nervous system-depressing agents, such as benzodiazepines, opioids, or barbiturates, presents with alveolar hypoventilation and thus acute hypercapnic respiratory failure.

- Decompensated congestive heart failure is associated with predominantly hypoxemic failure (secondary to alveolar filling and increased shunt); however, hypercapnic respiratory failure may also occur in severe exacerbations or in the presence of pulmonary disease.

III. PATHOPHYSIOLOGY OF ACUTE RESPIRATORY FAILURE

A. Hypoxemia

The most common underlying physiologic abnormality in hypoxemic respiratory failure is a mismatch of alveolar ventilation $\dot{V}$ and pulmonary perfusion $\dot{Q}$, as illustrated in **Figure 4-1**. The mismatch of ventilation and perfusion, where ventilation is decreased relative to perfusion, is called low $\dot{V}/\dot{Q}$.

Figure 4-1. Ventilation and Perfusion Matching in the Lung

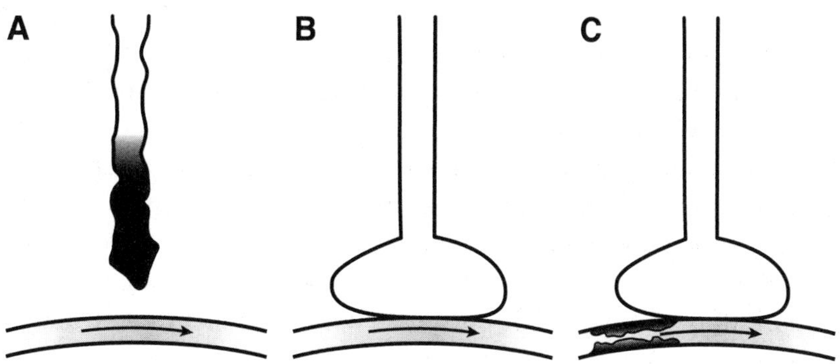

A, At one end of the pathologic continuum, areas of limited ventilation relative to perfusion produce shunt effect and hypoxemia. **B**, Ventilation and perfusion are matched in the normal lung. **C**, At the opposite end of the continuum, areas of better ventilation than perfusion produce dead space effect.

$\dot{V}/\dot{Q}$ matching is of particular importance to oxygenation of blood as opposed to elimination of CO_2 (discussed in Section IV) because of the kinetics of the hemoglobin oxygen dissociation curve. Lung areas with high $\dot{V}/\dot{Q}$ ratios, which provide a high Pao_2, cannot compensate for areas with a low $\dot{V}/\dot{Q}$ ratio (providing low Pao_2) as the hemoglobin molecule is already about 90% saturated at a Pao_2 of about 60 mm Hg. The admixture of poorly oxygenated blood returning from abnormal alveoli dilutes oxygenated blood from more normal lung units, resulting in systemic hypoxemia. The hypoxemia caused by $\dot{V}/\dot{Q}$ mismatch is usually easily corrected by supplemental O_2.

Disease processes that cause progressive obstruction of distal airways, alveolar filling, or atelectasis (eg, pneumonia, aspiration, pulmonary edema) result in a decrease in the amount of oxygen available in distal airways for uptake through the pulmonary capillaries. Through hypoxic pulmonary vasoconstriction, blood flow to such abnormal lung units decreases, but this decline is of lesser magnitude than the decrease in oxygen availability. This allows for a greater proportion of deoxygenated blood (venous admixture) to return to the left side of the heart.

One extreme of $\dot{V}/\dot{Q}$ mismatch is shunt, as there is perfusion of the unventilated lung. In diseases that cause diffuse alveolar flooding (eg, ARDS), there may be refractory hypoxemia due to shunt physiology. Treatment of hypoxemia due to $\dot{V}/\dot{Q}$ mismatch should be directed towards treating the underlying cause such as infections, reversing airway obstruction, reopening (recruiting) atelectatic lung zones, and preventing closure (de-recruitment) of the affected lung units. Oxygen therapy and/or mechanical ventilation are cornerstones in providing support until such time that the cause of $\dot{V}/\dot{Q}$ mismatch has been reversed.

Other, less common causes of hypoxemia include:

- Decreased diffusion of oxygen across the alveolocapillary membrane complex because of interstitial edema, inflammation, fibrosis, etc.

- Alveolar hypoventilation

- High altitude with low inspired partial pressure of oxygen
- Low mixed venous oxygen saturation

Diffusion abnormality is rarely the primary cause for hypoxemia as O_2 transport across alveolocapillary membrane is generally perfusion limited and not diffusion limited; however, in cases such as increased cardiac output and tachycardia, diffusion may be limited when the transit time across pulmonary capillaries is reduced. Therapy for diffusion abnormalities, in addition to maintaining adequate circulating volume, includes treatment of the cause of interstitial pathology (ie, diuretics for cardiogenic pulmonary edema, corticosteroids for inflammatory disorders). Ensuring adequate minute ventilation will correct hypoxemia that is solely due to hypoventilation. High altitude is a rare cause of acute hypoxemia in patients. As a compensatory strategy, increasing oxygen supplementation (F_{IO_2}) while the cause of the hypoxemia is sought and corrected may improve oxygenation.

The gradient between the partial pressure of oxygen in the alveolus (P_{AO_2}) and in the arterial circulation (Pa_{O_2}), the $P(A\text{–}a)O_2$ gradient, can be used to determine whether hypoxemia is caused only by hypoventilation. The Pa_{O_2} is obtained from arterial blood gas analysis while the patient breathes room air. The P_{AO_2} is estimated from the modified alveolar air equation:

$$P_{AO_2} = [F_{IO_2} \times (PB - 47)] - (1.25 \times Pa_{CO_2})$$

In the above equation, F_{IO_2} is expressed as a fraction (not a percentage), PB is barometric pressure, 47 represents water vapor pressure, and Pa_{CO_2} is obtained from the same arterial blood gas analysis.

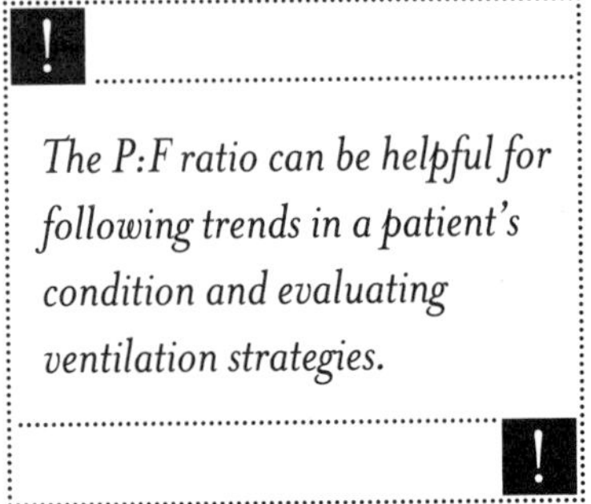

The $P(A\text{–}a)O_2$ gradient should be <10 mm Hg (<1.3 kPa) in young adults and <20 mm Hg (<2.7 kPa) in all patients. A normal gradient suggests that hypoxemia is likely due to hypoventilation alone; whereas, an increased gradient suggests that other causes (eg, $\dot{V}/\dot{Q}$ mismatch) are responsible for the hypoxemia. Another utility of calculating A–a gradient is when the Pa_{O_2} is low normal in the presence of significant hypocapnia, thus indicating a widened A–a gradient and, therefore, an incipient abnormality in $\dot{V}/\dot{Q}$ matching. The usefulness of this assessment is limited because supplemental oxygen without an accurate measure of F_{IO_2} greatly distorts its interpretation. As most hypoxic patients should not be stressed by breathing room air, measurements are usually made while the patient receives oxygen. Therefore, the $P(A\text{–}a)O_2$ gradient has significant limitations. In the absence of hypercarbia, all hypoxemic patients except those with low inspired partial pressure of oxygen will have a widened A–a gradient. The use of this value gives no information about the cause of hypoxemia, but should prompt the physician to search for one.

Numerous methods for quantifying hypoxemia have been proposed to provide a means of following the degree of hypoxemia and to communicate this information to other providers. The P:F ratio (where Pa_{O_2} is measured as mm Hg and F_{IO_2} is the fraction of inspired oxygen) is commonly used for quantifying the degree of patient hypoxemia. It requires accurate assessment of FIO_2, which is difficult in the nonintubated patient. Calculating the P:F ratio is a simple method both to assess the degree of hypoxemia and follow it over time. Lower ratios indicate more severe hypoxemia. However, one must be cognizant of the fact that PaO_2 — hence, the P:F ratio — can be greatly modified by the application of positive end-expiratory pressure and other recruitment maneuvers. Thus, different P:F ratios may be obtained for the same amount of FIO_2.

B. Hypercapnia

Hypercapnic respiratory failure is caused by either excess CO_2 production (VCO_2) or decreased effective alveolar ventilation (V_A) as is evident from the equation:

$$PCO_2 = K \cdot VCO_2 / V_A.$$

Therefore, for a constant VCO_2, one or more factors described in the equation for alveolar minute ventilation given below must be present to cause hypercapnia:

$$V_A = (V_T - V_D)f$$

where V_A is minute alveolar ventilation, V_T is tidal volume, V_D is dead space, and f is respiratory frequency.

Hypercapnia, resulting from either decreased V_T or f, occurs with drug ingestion, anesthesia, depression of the medullary center for respiration, and fatigue, for example. An elevated $PaCO_2$ normally increases ventilatory drive. Therefore, hypercapnic respiratory failure implies that the patient is unable to sustain minute ventilation ($f \times V_T$).

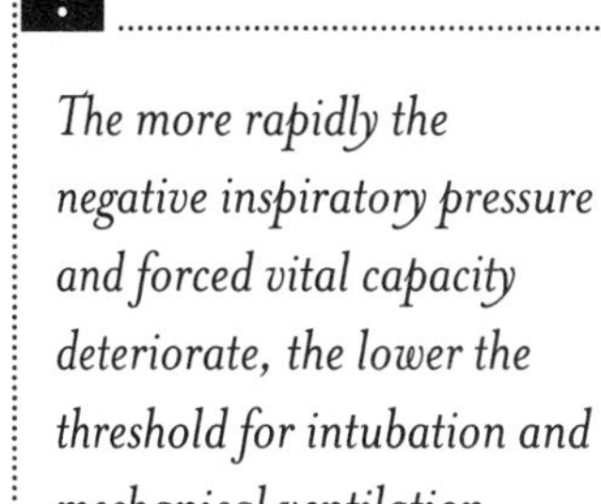

Treatment of decreased V_T or respiratory rate may require reversal of sedation or other drugs, intubation/mechanical ventilation to rest fatigued muscles, nutrition, respiratory stimulants, or treatment of other possible primary causes. Measures of ventilatory mechanics, such as peak negative inspiratory pressure and forced vital capacity (FVC), monitor a patient's course and may signal when endotracheal intubation and mechanical ventilation are warranted, especially in neuromuscular disorders such as myasthenia gravis and Guillain-Barré syndrome. A single measurement is less useful than measurements made over time. Negative inspiratory pressures below –20 to 25 cm H_2O or an FVC <10 mL/kg, or both, should raise concern that a patient's ventilatory mechanics may be sufficiently impaired to warrant tracheal intubation and mechanical ventilation.

Increased physiologic dead space (V_D) may also produce hypercapnia and is another type of mismatch illustrated in **Figure 4-1**. When gas flow to and from airways remains adequate but blood flow is absolutely or relatively diminished, CO_2 does not have the opportunity to diffuse out of the pulmonary circulation, and CO_2-rich blood is returned to the left atrium. Increased dead space ventilation may occur in respiratory muscle fatigue from any cause, leading to rapid shallow breathing. Increased V_D may also be seen in hypovolemia, pulmonary embolism, poor cardiac output, or when the regional airway pressure is relatively higher than the regional perfusion pressure, reducing pulmonary blood flow in that area.

Strategies to reduce dead space may include reduction in peak or mean airway pressures, if the patient is receiving mechanical ventilation, augmentation of intravascular volume and/or cardiac output, or treatment of other causes for limited pulmonary blood flow. It may be possible to compensate for hypercapnia due to high V_D by modifying parameters to increase minute ventilation during mechanical ventilation while the cause of hypercapnia is sought and corrected. Because of the high solubility of CO_2, a diffusion barrier rarely ever occurs. Increased CO_2 production may contribute to hypercapnia secondary to either excess carbohydrate nutritional calories or extreme hypercatabolic conditions (eg, burns, hyperthyroidism, persistent fever).

C. Mixed Respiratory Failure

Patients commonly demonstrate characteristics of both pathophysiologic categories of ARF during the course of illness. An understanding of the underlying pathophysiology of each, therefore, is necessary for planning therapeutic support. Several related disease processes often act in concert or synergistically to compound respiratory failure. For example, the patient with chronic pulmonary disease and a large dead space often has associated heart failure, which increases $\dot{V}/\dot{Q}$ mismatching and worsens hypoxemia.

IV. MANIFESTATIONS OF ACUTE RESPIRATORY FAILURE

A. Clinical Presentation of Respiratory Distress

Clinical manifestations of respiratory distress commonly include signs and symptoms of hypoxemia, hypercapnia, or both. These include:

- Altered mental status ranging from agitation to somnolence
- Evidence of increased work of breathing, such as nasal flaring in infants, use of accessory respiratory muscles, intercostal/suprasternal/supraclavicular muscle retraction, tachypnea, hyperpnea, or a paradoxical or dysynchronous breathing pattern (**Figure 4-2**)

Figure 4-2. Normal Versus Abnormal Respiration

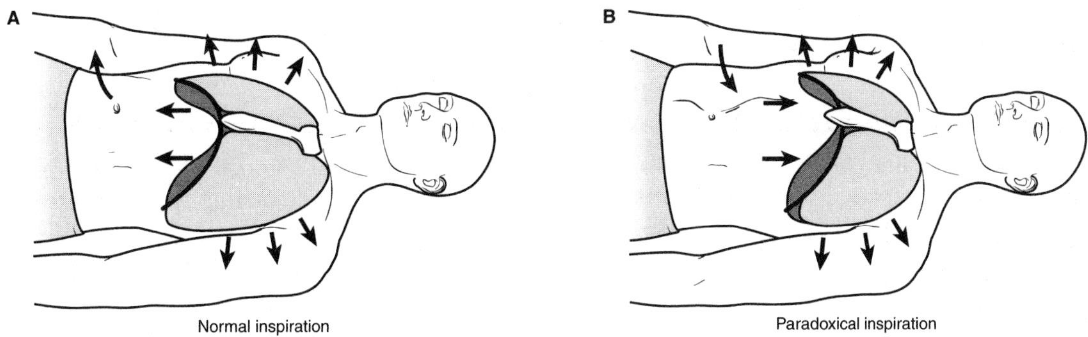

A, The abdominal wall moves outward as the diaphragm moves downward in normal inspiration.
B, With respiratory muscle fatigue, the diaphragm becomes flaccid and moves upward during inspiration resulting in inward movement of the abdominal wall.

- Bradypnea
- Cyanosis of mucosal membranes (eg, tongue, mouth) or nail beds
- Diaphoresis, tachycardia, hypertension, and other signs of catecholamine release

B. Diagnostic Tests

Pulse oximetry can be used to rapidly evaluate oxygenation in a patient with respiratory distress by estimating the arterial oxyhemoglobin saturation (**Chapter 6**). However, pulse oximetry provides no assessment for hypercapnia. Arterial blood gas analysis is commonly used in severely ill patients to determine the two primary measures of respiratory failure, the Pa_{O_2} and Pa_{CO_2}, as well as pH. Additional tests such as electrolytes, hematocrit, and drug levels may provide clues to the underlying etiology of ARF. Chest radiography in combination with these laboratory tests is invaluable in suggesting the underlying pathophysiology of ARF.

V. MANAGEMENT CONSIDERATIONS

A. Oxygen Supplementation

Most patients with ARF require supplemental oxygen. Oxygen transfer from alveolar gas to capillary blood occurs by diffusion across the alveolar-capillary membrane and is driven by the oxygen partial-pressure gradient between the P_{AO_2} and the P_{O_2} of the pulmonary capillary blood. In most cases of ARF, the P_{AO_2} can be substantially increased by use of supplemental oxygen, thus increasing the gradient across the membrane and improving the Pa_{O_2}.

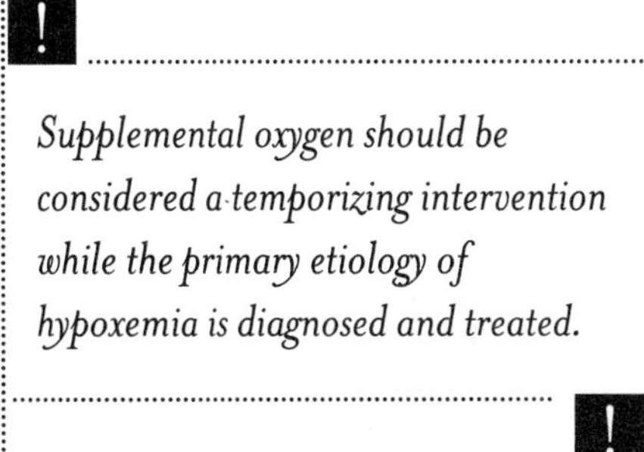

Supplemental oxygen should be considered a temporizing intervention while the primary etiology of hypoxemia is diagnosed and treated.

Supplemental oxygen can be provided by a variety of devices (**Figure 4-3**). The effectiveness of each is determined by its capacity to deliver sufficient oxygen at a high enough flow rate to match the patient's spontaneous inspiratory flow rate. Matching between the flow capacity of the oxygen device and the patient's inspiratory flow demand determines how much room air is entrained by the nonintubated patient breathing in an open system. Any entrained room air (F_{IO_2} = 0.21) will dilute (decrease) the F_{IO_2} of the delivered gas in such a way that the tracheal F_{IO_2}, and hence P_{AO_2}, may be considerably lower than the F_{IO_2} delivered from the oxygen source. Therefore, oxygen-supplement systems are usually classified as high oxygen (capable of delivering up to 100% oxygen), controlled oxygen (set oxygen percentage), or low oxygen. Similarly, the devices are also categorized as either high flow, moderate flow, or low flow, reflecting the flow-delivery capacity of the gas at the preset F_{IO_2} level.

Figure 4-3. Oxygen Supplementation Devices

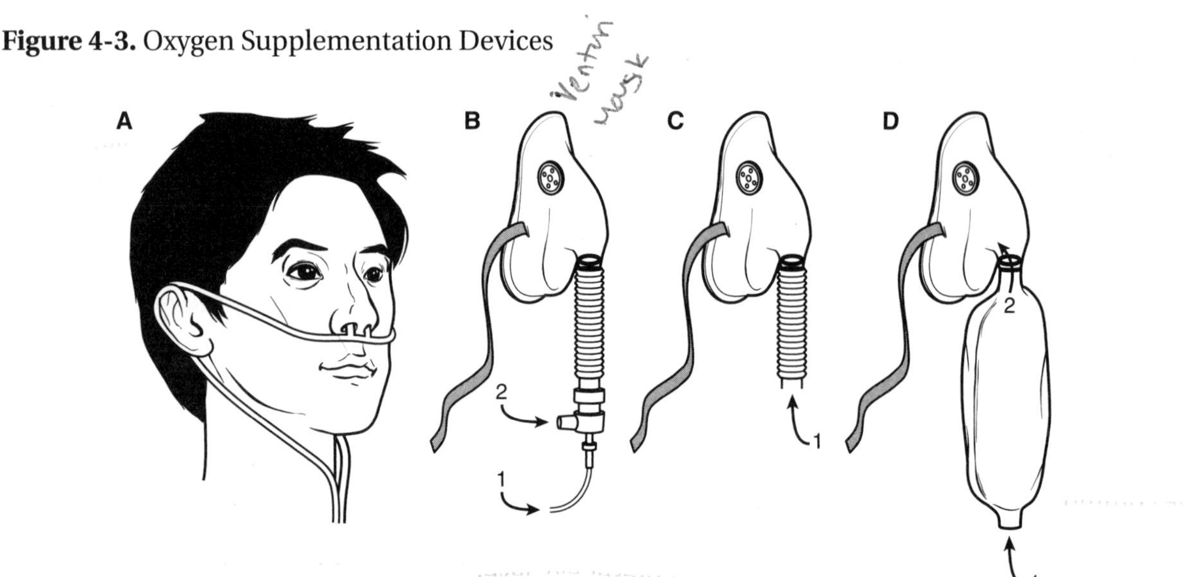

A, Nasal cannula. **B**, Air-entrainment face mask with 100% oxygen source gas (1) and a changeable nozzle (2), which controls entrainment of room air through an opening. **C**, Aerosol face mask with blended preset F_{IO_2} (1) from a nebulizer. **D**, Reservoir face mask with high oxygen concentration (1) supplied to a reservoir, where a one-way valve (2) directs inhaled and exhaled gas.

For example, a tachypneic and hyperpneic patient will have a high inspiratory flow rate during each breath. In such cases, hypoxemia is not likely to respond well to oxygen supplementation by nasal cannula because it is a low-oxygen, low-flow system and cannot match the patient's high inspiratory flow rate. Room air will be entrained during inspiration, and the tracheal F_{IO_2} will be reduced. A high-oxygen, high-flow system should be selected for this type of patient.

1. Low-Flow Nasal Cannula

Short prongs of the nasal cannula are inserted into the nares. Oxygen (100%) is delivered through the cannula, but at a rate between 0.5 and 5 L/min. The resulting F_{IO_2} depends on the patient's minute ventilation and, therefore, cannot be precisely controlled, but the maximal tracheal F_{IO_2} is not likely to exceed 0.4 to 0.5 (40% to 50%). Higher flow rates do not result in much higher F_{IO_2} levels and have a drying and irritating effect on nasal mucosa. The nasal cannula is comfortable and well tolerated by many patients with ARF in whom precise control of F_{IO_2} is not necessary. It is a low-flow, low-oxygen device.

2. High-Flow Nasal Cannula

In contrast to the low-flow cannulas, high-flow nasal cannula systems involve delivery of heated and humidified oxygen via special devices (eg, Vapotherm®, Optiflow™) at rates up to 50 L/min in adults. These devices may be better tolerated than face masks in terms of comfort. They also provide higher amounts of F_{IO_2} in patients with high minute ventilation requirements by matching the patients' inspiratory demands and minimizing air dilution. These devices may generate positive end-expiratory pressure that is difficult to measure and have the potential for causing barotrauma.

3. Air-Entrainment Face Mask

Air-entrainment masks (also called Venturi masks) deliver oxygen through a jet-mixing device that increases the velocity of oxygen and causes a controlled entrainment. The F_{IO_2} can be more precisely controlled from 0.24 to 0.5 (24% to 50%) at high-flow rates simply by selecting the interchangeable jet nozzle and adjusting the oxygen flow rate. It is a high-flow, controlled-oxygen device.

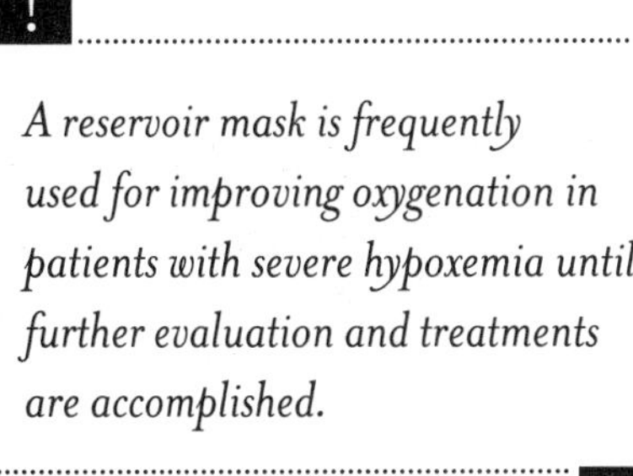
A reservoir mask is frequently used for improving oxygenation in patients with severe hypoxemia until further evaluation and treatments are accomplished.

4. Aerosol Face Mask

The commonly used aerosol face mask combines a variable oxygen setting and moderate flows. The mask, which has large side holes, is attached by large-bore tubing to a nebulizer that blends 100% oxygen and room air to deliver gas at a preset F_{IO_2} level. Flow matching can be evaluated by observing the patient during spontaneous breathing. If the entire aerosol mist disappears from the mask during inhalation, the patient's inspiratory flow demands are probably exceeding the capacity of the nebulizer and room air is being entrained. The aerosol face mask is a variable oxygen, moderate-flow device.

5. Reservoir Face Mask

The reservoir face mask incorporates a reservoir bag from which the patient breathes. This bag is filled with 100% oxygen from a supply source. The flow rate is adjusted so that the bag remains completely or partially distended throughout the respiratory cycle. When the mask is properly applied, oxygen delivery to the nonintubated patient can be maximized but rarely exceeds an F_{IO_2} of 0.6 to 0.9. The reservoir face mask is a high-oxygen, high-flow device.

6. Resuscitation Bag-Mask Unit

Although not commonly considered an oxygen-supplement device, bag-mask units are usually included with other emergency equipment and, therefore, are readily accessible. When the mask is held firmly over the patient's face, room air entrainment is largely excluded. If the oxygen flow to the bag is kept high (≥15 L/min), a high-oxygen supply is provided at sufficient flow. The resuscitation bag need not be compressed to supply oxygen. It is a high-oxygen, high-flow device.

B. Pharmacologic Adjuncts

Many diseases that cause ARF produce similar anatomic and physiologic derangements, including bronchial inflammation, mucosal edema, smooth muscle contraction, and increased mucus production and viscosity. Each of these processes may contribute to obstruction of airway gas flow, increased airway resistance, mismatch, and elevated V_D. Some pharmacologic agents may be helpful in the care of such patients and may directly alter shunt or dead-space effects.

1. β_2-Agonists

Inhaled β_2-agonists are important therapy in patients with ARF secondary to many causes. Stimulation of β_2-adrenergic receptors causes bronchial and vascular smooth-muscle relaxation. These agents are typically administered by metered-dose inhaler or by intermittent or continuous nebulization (**Table 4-2**). On rare occasions, in very critically ill patients with obstructive airway disease, β_2-agonists are administered by both inhalation and subcutaneous injection. Long-acting inhaled agents do not have a role in the management of patients with acute respiratory deterioration. Racemic epinephrine aerosol is an established therapy for upper airway obstruction in children with croup and is also used for laryngeal edema in adults.

2. Anticholinergic Agents

Ipratropium bromide competes with acetylcholine at the bronchial receptor site, resulting in bronchial smooth-muscle relaxation. This agent is delivered by metered-dose inhaler or nebulization (**Table 4-2**). Ipratropium has a more delayed onset of action than β_2-agonists and has more consistent bronchodilatory effects in COPD than in asthma. The addition of ipratropium to albuterol appears to have an additive benefit in approximately 30% of asthma patients. Tiotropium is a long-acting anticholinergic bronchodilator that has sustained bronchodilator effects in COPD patients, but its use in acute exacerbations is not recommended.

3. Corticosteroids

The central role of inflammation in obstructive airway disease is well established, and the benefit from aggressive corticosteroid use in asthmatic patients with ARF is well documented. In addition, corticosteroids may decrease β-receptor tachyphylaxis. Limited consensus exists on dosing schedules in asthma. Doses of methylprednisolone of 80 mg/24 h have been as effective as >360 mg/24 h. Some clinicians use doses equivalent to those given for asthma when treating COPD, whereas others begin with doses equivalent to 1 mg/kg/24 h, adjusting as patient response dictates. The intravenous and oral routes are equally effective. Careful monitoring of corticosteroid side effects is warranted. Acute myopathies have been described after moderate to high dosages of corticosteroids in patients with COPD and/or asthma. After the acute exacerbation, inhaled corticosteroids are often useful adjuncts to therapy and may allow reduction in systemic corticosteroid dosage. However, routine use of inhalational agents is not recommended in the setting of acute severe bronchospasm.

Table 4-2 Pharmacologic Agents for Obstructive Airway Disease

Drug	Preparation	Route of Administration	Dosage
Albuterol	0.05% solution	Inhaled (aerosol)	*Adult:* 2.5–5 mg q 2–4 h[a] *Pediatric:* 0.05–0.15 mg/kg q 4–6 h[a]
	MDI (90 μg/puff)	Inhaled	*Adult:* 1–2 puffs q 2–4 h[a] *Pediatric:* 1–2 puffs q 4–6 h[a]
Levalbuterol	0.31, 0.63, or 1.25 mg/unit dose solution	Inhaled (aerosol)	*Adult and children ≥ 12 y:* 0.63–1.25 mg q 6–8 h *Pediatric (6–11 y):* 0.31–0.63 mg q 6–8 h; more aggressive dosing may be used in acute exacerbations
	MDI (45 μg/puff)	Inhaled	*Adult:* 1–2 puffs q 4–6 h *Pediatric (age ≥4 y):* 1–2 puffs q 4–6 h
Metaproterenol Sulfate	5% solution	Inhaled (aerosol)	*Adult:* 0.3 mL q 2–4 h[a] *Pediatric:* 0.25–0.5 mg/kg q 2–4 h[a]
	MDI (0.65 μg/puff)	Inhaled	*Adult:* 2–3 puffs q 4–6 h[a] *Pediatric:* 1–3 puffs q 4–6 h[a]
Terbutaline	MDI (0.2 μg/puff)	Inhaled	*Adult:* 1–2 puffs q 4–6 h[a] *Pediatric:* 1–2 puffs q 4–6 h[a]
	0.1% solution	Subcutaneous	*Adult:* 0.2–0.4 mL; repeat in 15–30 min *Pediatric:* 0.2 mg/kg; maximum 6 mg
Epinephrine	1 mg/mL (1:1000)	Subcutaneous	*Adult:* 0.1–0.5 mg; repeat in 20–30 min *Pediatric:* 0.01 mg/kg
Racemic Epinephrine	2.25% solution	Inhaled	*Adult:* 0.3–1 mL *Pediatric:* 0.05 mL/kg/dose; maximum 0.5 mL/dose diluted to 3 mL with NS
Ipratropium	0.025% solution	Inhaled (aerosol)	*Adult:* 500 μg q 6–8 h *Pediatric:* Infant and child: 250 μg q 6–8 h >12 y: 250–500 μg q 6–8 h
	MDI (18 μg/puff)	Inhaled	*Adult:* 2–4 puffs q 6 h *Pediatric:* 1–2 puffs q 8 h

Abbreviations: q, every; MDI, metered-dose inhaler; NS, normal saline
[a]In patients with severe asthma, frequency of administration of inhaled β-agonists should be guided by response to therapy and risk for side effects. Therapy is routinely initiated with three treatments every 20 minutes. Further therapy adjustments are then based on response. Continuous nebulization may also be employed. Caution should be exercised when considering use of continuous nebulized β_2-agonists, particularly in older patients and those with underlying cardiac disease.

4. Antibiotics

Bacterial infection (bronchitis/pneumonia) frequently precipitates ARF. Antibiotics should be used when there is clinical suspicion that bacterial pulmonary infection is present (eg, change in sputum characteristics, pulmonary infiltrates on the chest radiograph, fever, leukocytosis), and they should be chosen to effectively treat usual pathogens (**Chapter 11**). Therapy should be subsequently adjusted when culture and sensitivity data become available.

E. Miscellaneous Agents and Treatments

Agents to hydrate or otherwise alter the composition, elasticity, or viscosity of mucus have been used, although their efficacy has not been demonstrated except in selected patient groups (eg, patients with cystic fibrosis). Examples of these agents include mucolytics such as acetylcysteine or propylene glycol, bronchorrheic agents such as saturated solution of potassium iodide or glycerol guaiacolate, and alkalinizing agents such as aerosolized sodium bicarbonate.

Postural drainage, chest physical therapy, nasotracheal suctioning, incentive spirometry, intermittent positive pressure breathing, and cough/deep-breathing exercises have long been used. Also available are newer measures such as positive expiratory pressure therapy, vest devices (high-frequency chest oscillator), and mattress percussion devices. Many of these modalities may be applied to treat specific symptoms of ARF or the cause of respiratory failure. The effectiveness and positive impact of the contributions of the bedside nurse or the respiratory care practitioner and the avoidance of intubation/mechanical ventilation should not be underestimated.

Key Points

Diagnosis and Management of Acute Respiratory Failure

- Acute respiratory failure is classified as hypoxemic, hypercapnic, or mixed. Arterial blood gas measurements are the primary assessment tool for determining this classification.
- The most common pathophysiologic mechanism for hypoxemic acute respiratory failure is ventilation/perfusion mismatch.
- Hypercapnic acute respiratory failure is primarily the result of a change in one or more determinants of the alveolar minute ventilation equation: tidal volume, respiratory frequency, and physiologic dead space.
- Oxygen supplementation is commonly used to treat hypoxemia. The oxygen supply device that is chosen must be capable of matching the oxygen and respiratory flow demands of the patient.
- Pharmacologic and therapeutic adjuncts should be considered when treating patients with acute respiratory failure.

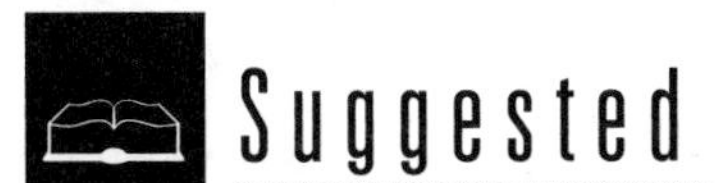

Suggested Readings

1. Dolovich MB, Ahrens RC, Hess DR, et al. Device selection and outcomes of aerosol therapy: Evidence-based guidelines: American College of Chest Physicians/American College of Asthma, Allergy and Immunology. *Chest.* 2005;127:335-371.

2. Manser R, Reid D, Abramson M. Corticosteroids for acute severe asthma in hospitalised patients. *Cochrane Database Syst Rev.* 2001;(1):CD001740. doi:10.1002/14651858.CD001740.

3. Pontoppidan H, Geffin B, Lowenstein E. Acute respiratory failure in the adult: 3. *N Engl J Med.* 1972;287:799-806.

4. Pontoppidan H, Geffin B, Lowenstein E. Acute respiratory failure in the adult: 2. *N Engl J Med.* 1972;287:743-752.

5. Pontoppidan H, Geffin B, Lowenstein E. Acute respiratory failure in the adult: 1. *N Engl J Med.* 1972;287:690-698.

Chapter 5

MECHANICAL VENTILATION

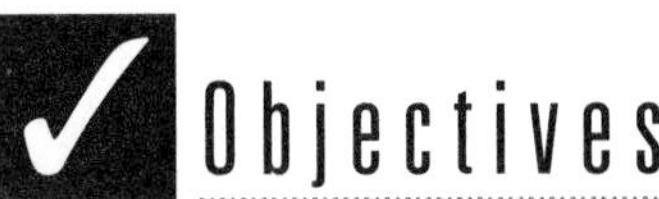

Objectives

- Discuss the indications and techniques for noninvasive positive pressure ventilation.
- Describe the characteristics of different types of breaths and modes of mechanical ventilation.
- Outline ventilator settings and monitoring needs for the initiation of mechanical ventilation.
- Describe interactions between ventilatory parameters and modifications needed to avoid harmful effects of mechanical ventilation.
- Review the guidelines for initial ventilator management that apply to specific clinical situations.

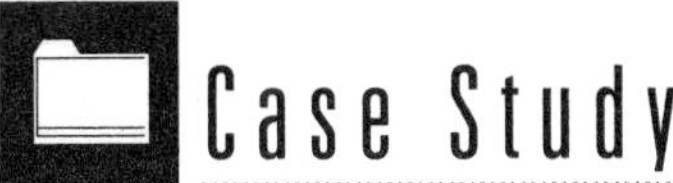

Case Study

A 65-year-old woman with an exacerbation of chronic obstructive pulmonary disease is admitted to the hospital. She is receiving oxygen at 3 L/min by nasal cannula. She continues to have significant respiratory distress after receiving two bronchodilator nebulizer treatments. Her vital signs are blood pressure 160/110 mm Hg, heart rate 110/min, respirations 30/min, and temperature 99.0°F (37.2°C). Physical examination is remarkable for use of accessory muscles of respiration and diffuse wheezing bilaterally. An arterial blood gas analysis demonstrates a pH 7.24, Pco_2 60 mm Hg (8 kPa), and Po_2 65 mm Hg (8.7 kPa).

- What type of respiratory support should be initiated?
- What settings should be selected for respiratory support?
- What are the goals of respiratory support?

I. INTRODUCTION

When hypoxic or hypercapnic respiratory failure cannot be treated by other means, as discussed in **Chapter 4**, advanced support with positive pressure ventilation may be needed. A ventilator is a device used to assist or replace the work of the respiratory system. Positive pressure ventilation can be delivered noninvasively via a mask or helmet or invasively via an endotracheal tube. Generally accepted indications for initiating positive pressure ventilatory support are summarized in **Table 5-1**.

Table 5-1 Indications for Positive Pressure Ventilatory Support

Ventilation abnormalities	Respiratory muscle dysfunction • Respiratory muscle fatigue • Chest wall abnormalities • Neuromuscular disease Decreased ventilatory drive Increased airway resistance and/or obstruction
Oxygenation abnormalities	Refractory hypoxemia Need for positive end-expiratory pressure Excessive work of breathing
Need for sedation and/or neuromuscular blockade	
Need to decrease systemic or myocardial oxygen consumption	
Use of hyperventilation to reduce intracranial pressure	
Facilitation of alveolar recruitment and prevention of atelectasis	

The choice between noninvasive or invasive positive pressure ventilation is dependent on patient characteristics, the type and severity of the respiratory and/or systemic condition, anticipated clinical course, availability of resources, as well as the experience and training of the clinician and healthcare team.

II. NONINVASIVE POSITIVE PRESSURE VENTILATION

A. What Is Noninvasive Positive Pressure Ventilation?

Noninvasive positive pressure ventilation (NPPV) refers to a form of mechanical ventilation that provides respiratory assistance without an invasive artificial airway. The potential beneficial effects of NPPV are similar to those of invasive mechanical ventilation and include decreased work of breathing, improved oxygenation, and improved gas exchange. In addition, this type of ventilation avoids many of the complications associated with intubation and invasive mechanical ventilation. Potential advantages and disadvantages of NPPV are listed in **Table 5-2**.

Table 5-2 Advantages and Disadvantages of NPPV

Advantages	Disadvantages
• Reduced need for sedation • Preservation of airway-protective reflexes • Avoidance of upper airway trauma • Decreased incidence of nosocomial sinusitis and pneumonia • Improved patient comfort • Shorter length of stays in ICU and hospital • Improved survival	• Claustrophobia • Increased workload for respiratory practitioner • Facial/nasal pressure lesions • Unprotected airway • Inability to suction deep airway • Gastric distension with use of face mask or helmet • Possible upper-extremity edema, axillary vein thrombosis, tympanic dysfunction, and intrahelmet noise with use of helmet • Delay in intubation

B. How Does NPPV Work?

NPPV utilizes two levels of positive airway pressure, combining the modalities of pressure support ventilation (PSV) and continuous positive airway pressure (CPAP) (see Section III). By convention, the PSV modality is referred to as *IPAP* (inspiratory positive airway pressure), and the CPAP modality is referred to as *EPAP* (expiratory positive airway pressure). CPAP alone can also be delivered noninvasively but does not provide support of ventilation. CPAP allows spontaneous breathing from a gas source at an elevated baseline system pressure (higher than atmospheric pressure) and is functionally equivalent to positive end-expiratory pressure (PEEP). The difference between these two pressure levels ($\triangle P$) determines tidal volume generated. NPPV can be delivered using a standard ICU ventilator or a portable device. The benefits of using an ICU ventilator include delivery of a more precise and higher concentration of oxygen, the separation of inspiratory and expiratory tubing to prevent rebreathing CO_2, better monitoring and alarm features, and improved detection of air leaks. Alarm setups may need to be altered on standard ventilators because the alarms are typically triggered by exhalation, and noninvasive ventilation inherently has more gas leakage compared to ventilation via an endotracheal tube. Ventilators specifically designed to provide patient-triggered noninvasive pressure support or patient-triggered volume-cycled breaths are optimal.

C. What Types of Interfaces Are Available?

The ventilator connects to a tightly fitted face mask, nasal mask, nasal plugs, or a helmet (**Figure 5-1**). Many patients with acute respiratory failure are mouth breathers, thus the face mask is preferred as it is associated with smaller leaks than the nasal plugs and nasal mask. The nasal passages may offer significant resistance to airflow, limiting the benefits of NPPV. Some gas leakage is anticipated with both masks and can be compensated for by increasing pressure settings or increasing the set tidal volume (VT) level. When a nasal mask is used, the patient's mouth should be kept closed or chin straps should be employed to reduce leakage.

Figure 5-1. Devices for Delivery of NPPV

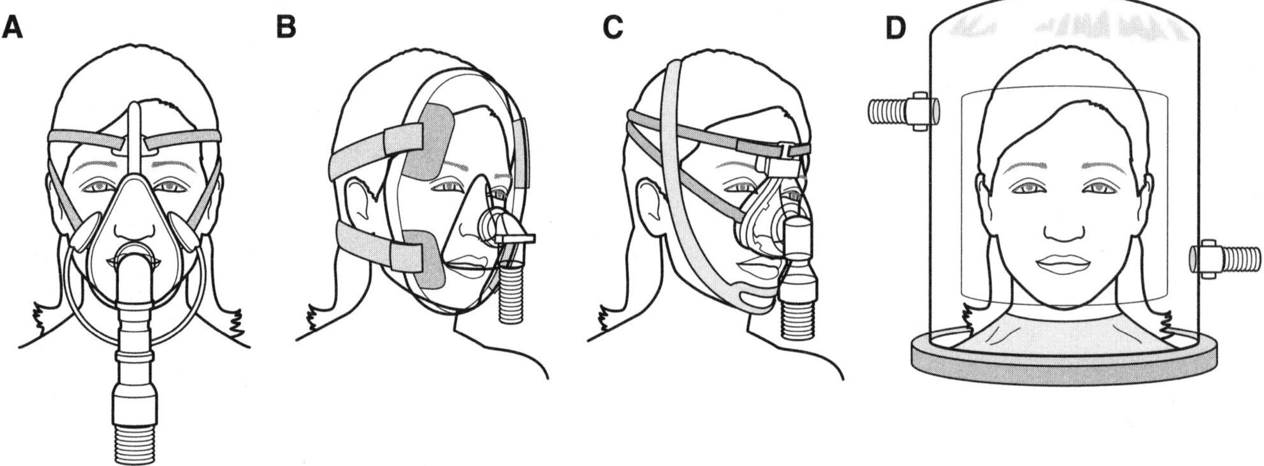

Examples of NPPV delivery devices: **A**, face mask; **B**, total face mask; **C**, nasal mask with chin strap; and **D**, helmet.

D. Which Patients Benefit From NPPV?

Before NPPV is initiated, patient characteristics and the potential for successfully treating the underlying respiratory condition should be evaluated. **Table 5-3** lists conditions leading to respiratory failure that are likely to improve with use of NPPV. Of these, acute exacerbations of chronic obstructive pulmonary disease and cardiogenic pulmonary edema are the two best studied and accepted indications for the application of NPPV. An approach to initiating NPPV after appropriate patient evaluation is outlined in **Table 5-4**. NPPV is best utilized in the alert, cooperative patient whose respiratory condition is expected to improve in 48 to 72 hours. Potential candidates should be hemodynamically stable, able to control airway secretions, and able to synchronize with the ventilator. If a provider skilled in the application of NPPV is not available, if the patient is too sick for this support, or if NPPV has failed to benefit the patient, it is critical to move quickly to invasive mechanical ventilation.

Table 5-3 Respiratory Conditions Likely to Respond to NPPV

Hypoxemic Respiratory Failure

- Cardiogenic pulmonary edema without hemodynamic instability
- Respiratory failure in patients with *Pneumocystis* pneumonia
- Respiratory failure in immunocompromised patients (especially in hematologic malignancies and transplant patients)

Hypercapnic Respiratory Failure

- Acute exacerbation of chronic obstructive pulmonary disease
- Acute exacerbation of asthma
- Respiratory failure in patients with cystic fibrosis

Abbreviation: NPPV, noninvasive positive-pressure ventilation

Table 5-4 Initiation of NPPV

- Do not delay intubation if needed and keep in mind the patient's resuscitation status.
- Consider ABG analysis prior to initiation.
- Explain the procedure.
- Keep head of bed at ≥45°.
- Ensure appropriate mask or helmet size.
- Assess the patient's tolerance of the mask by applying it by hand before securing the harness.
- Use the following initial ventilator settings:
    - Mode: Spontaneous
    - Trigger: Maximum sensitivity
    - FIO_2: 1.00
    - EPAP: 4-5 cm H_2O (higher levels are poorly tolerated initially)
    - IPAP: 10-15 cm H_2O
    - Backup rate: Start at 6/min
- Adjust the difference between EPAP and IPAP to achieve an effective V_T and CO_2 clearance. Adjust EPAP for alveolar recruitment in increments of 2 cm H_2O per step to improve oxygenation. Depending on the ventilator, a similar increase in IPAP may be required to maintain the same V_T.
- If assist-control volume ventilation is used, begin with a V_T of 6 to 8 mL/kg (depending on the underlying pulmonary condition).
- Titrate pressures, volume, and FIO_2 to achieve appropriate pH, PaO_2, and $PaCO_2$ levels. Ventilator changes can be made every 15 to 30 minutes.
- Follow vital signs, pulse oximetry, mental status, clinical appearance, and ABG (if indicated).
- Remember that goals of NPPV may include a respiratory rate <30/min, V_T >7 mL/kg of predicted body weight, improved gas exchange, and patient comfort.

Abbreviations: NPPV, noninvasive positive-pressure ventilation; ABG, arterial blood gas; EPAP, expiratory positive airway pressure; IPAP, inspiratory positive airway pressure; V_T, tidal volume

E. Which Patients Should Not Receive Noninvasive Mechanical Ventilation?

In general, NPPV should not be initiated in the following circumstances: uncooperative patients; patients with difficulty clearing secretions, recurrent emesis, or post-cardiac or respiratory arrest; and patients with hemodynamic instability. A more detailed list of contraindications for the use of NPPV is presented in **Table 5-5**.

Table 5-5 Contraindications to Use of NPPV

- Cardiac or respiratory arrest
- Hemodynamic instability
- Myocardial ischemia or arrhythmias
- Patient who is unable to cooperate
- Inability to protect the airway
- High risk for aspiration
- Active upper gastrointestinal hemorrhage
- Severe hypoxemia
- Severe encephalopathy
- Facial trauma, recent surgery, and/or burns
- Significant agitation

F. How Are Patients Monitored on NPPV?

Patients receiving NPPV must be monitored closely in a proper setting, and continuous pulse oximetry and cardiac monitoring are suggested. Close clinical follow-up assessments are required, including evaluations of the pH, $Pa{O_2}$, and $Pa{CO_2}$. Consider transition to invasive ventilation when a clear trend toward improvement has not been observed over the first 1 or 2 hours, or when the therapeutic goals have not been achieved within the first 4 to 6 hours. Sedation should be used cautiously and with adequate monitoring as NPPV is initiated. Additional measures that may be considered include application of a protective nose patch when using a nasal mask and gastric decompression if a face mask or helmet is used. Oral intake should be restricted until the patient has stabilized and intubation is no longer a consideration. An algorithm for assessing NPPV is presented in **Figure 5-2**.

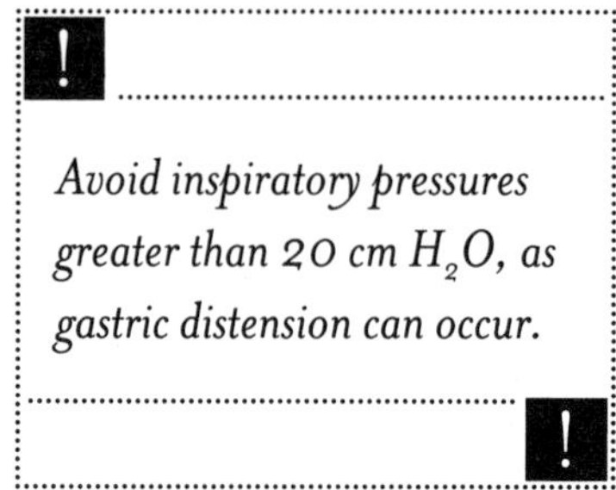

Figure 5-2. Assessment of NPPV

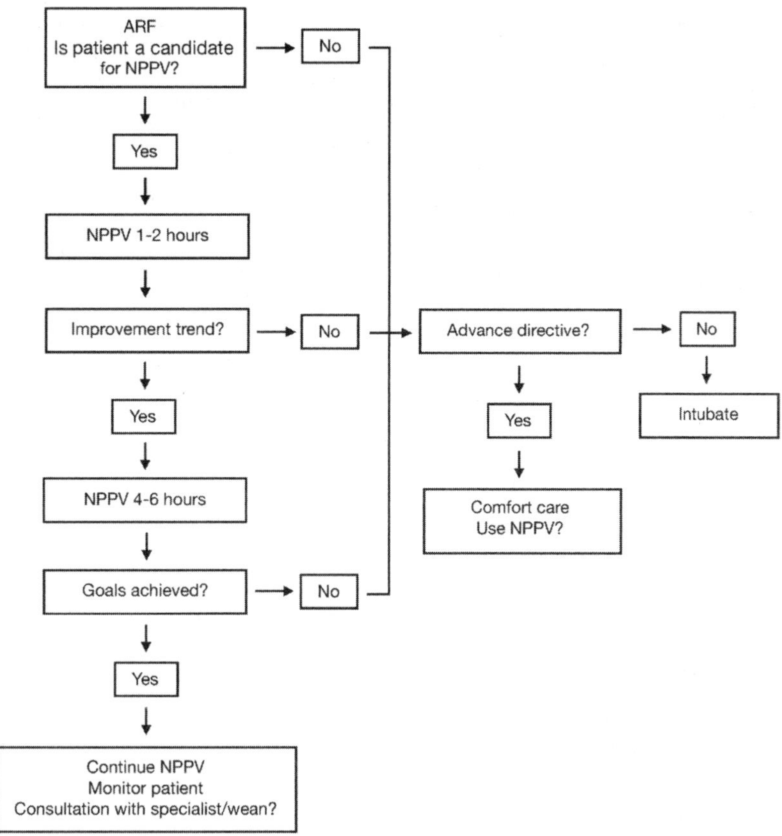

Abbreviations: NPPV, noninvasive positive pressure ventilation; ARF, acute respiratory failure

III. INVASIVE MECHANICAL VENTILATION

Mechanical ventilation via an endotracheal tube is commonly used to support critically ill patients. It is a definitive intervention to ensure acceptable oxygenation and ventilation with a secure airway.

Each mechanical ventilation respiratory cycle can be divided into two phases: inspiration and expiration (**Figure 5-3**). *Inspiration* is the point at which the exhalation valve closes and fresh gas under pressure from the ventilator enters the chest. The amount of gas delivered during inspiration is determined by three targets that can be set on the ventilator: volume, pressure, and/or flow. *Cycling* is the changeover from the end of inspiration to the expiratory phase, and occurs in response to one of three parameters: elapsed time, delivered volume, or a decrease in flow rate. During expiration, the ventilator gas flow is stopped and the exhalation circuit is opened to allow gas to escape passively from the lungs. Expiration continues until the next inspiration begins. *Triggering* is the changeover from expiration to inspiration. All mechanical ventilators require some signal from the patient (except when the patient does not interact with the ventilator) to

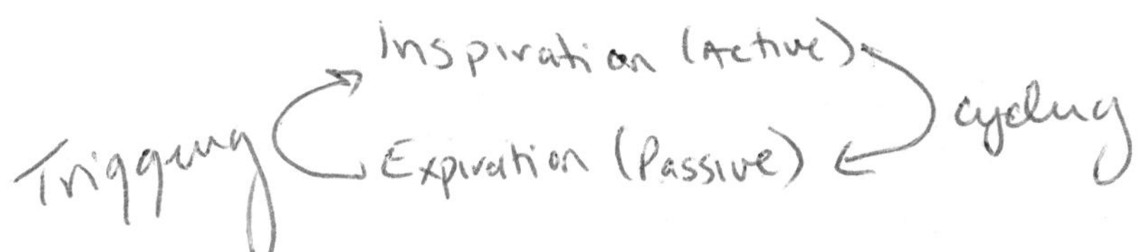

determine when inspiration should begin. When the patient initiates a breath, it is called an *assisted breath,* and a triggering signal results when the patient's inspiratory effort produces a drop in airway pressure or a diversion of constant gas flow in the ventilator circuitry. In the absence of patient interaction with the ventilator, breaths are delivered based on elapsed time (eg, at a set rate of 10 breaths/minute and no detection of patient effort, the ventilator will be triggered every 6 seconds). This is called an *unassisted* or *mandatory breath.* Using these definitions, two ventilator breath types are possible: full ventilator control (mandatory or unassisted) and partial ventilator control (assisted). Spontaneous breaths (no ventilator assist) are also possible in modes such as synchronized intermittent mandatory ventilation (SIMV) and bi-level ventilation. The most common ventilator breaths are further described later. CPAP allows spontaneous breathing but is not a mode of ventilation.

Figure 5-3. Respiratory Cycle During Mechanical Ventilation

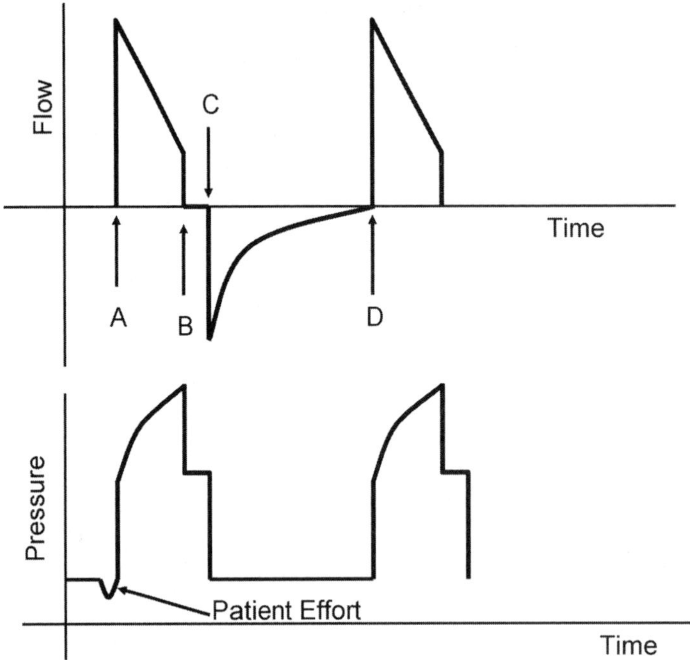

The respiratory cycle is the time from the initiation of one breath until the initiation of the next breath. Triggering (**A**) signals the transition from expiration to inspiration; cycling (**C**) indicates the transition from inspiration to expiration. Inspiratory pause (**BC**), total respiratory cycle (**ABCD**), inspiration (**ABC**), and expiration (**CD**).

A. Volume-Cycled Breath

A volume-cycled breath, often called *volume assist-control breath,* ensures the delivery of a preset tidal volume (unless the peak pressure limit is exceeded). On most ventilators, the setting of peak inspiratory flow rate and the choice of inspiratory flow waveform (square, sine, or decelerating) determine the length of inspiration. Some ventilators change the peak inspiratory flow rate to maintain constant inspiratory time on switching between a constant flow (square) and decelerating flow (ramp) waveforms. With volume-cycled breaths, worsening airway resistance or lung/chest-wall compliance results in increases in peak inspiratory pressure with continued delivery of the set tidal volume (unless the peak pressure limit is exceeded).

B. Time-Cycled Breath

A time-cycled breath, often called *pressure assist-control breath,* applies a constant pressure for a preset time. The application of constant pressure throughout inspiration results in a square pressure-over-time waveform during inspiration and a decelerating inspiratory flow waveform as the pressure gradient falls between the ventilator (pressure remains constant) and the patient (pressure rises as the lung fills). Flow in this breath format is variable and this leads to variable tidal volumes. Flow depends on the resistance of the lung, the compliance of the lung, and patient effort. With this type of breath, changes in airway resistance or lung/chest-wall compliance will alter tidal volume (ie, worsening of airway resistance or lung compliance results in a decrease in tidal volume). This disadvantage of time-cycled (pressure assist-control) breaths may be overcome by delivering pressure-regulated volume-control breaths, in which the ventilator adjusts the pressure up or down in response to a fall or rise of the tidal volume. Each delivered breath is a pressure-targeted and time-cycled breath, with the ventilator adjusting the amount of pressure applied to the airway to maintain a constant tidal volume. However, in this dual control mode of mechanical ventilation, abnormally increased patient efforts may lead to a pressure decrease due to the ventilator algorithm, resulting in under-support of the acutely ill patient.

C. Flow-Cycled Breath

A flow-cycled breath, usually called a *pressure support breath,* is very similar to a time-cycled breath in that a set pressure is applied constantly throughout the patient's triggered inspiration and the inspiratory flow waveform is decelerating. Pressure support breaths are terminated when the flow rate decreases to a predetermined percentage of the initial peak flow rate (typically 25%). As the patient's inspiratory effort decreases, the flow decreases, marking the proximity of the end of inspiration.

IV. MODES OF MECHANICAL VENTILATION

The mode of ventilation describes how one or more types of ventilator breaths interface with the patient to provide ventilatory support. When mechanical ventilation is initiated, the optimum ventilatory support for a given clinical circumstance and the specific needs of the patient must be determined. CPAP is seldom used as initial support for acute respiratory failure in an intubated patient. It is not considered a mode of mechanical ventilation because positive pressure is not applied during inspiration. The respiratory rate and V_T are dependent on the patient's inspiratory effort as the patient inspires against the resistance of the endotracheal tube. It is mainly used in the final stages of invasive ventilation, when patients are being assessed for their potential readiness for extubation.

Commonly used modes of ventilation include assist-control (AC) ventilation, SIMV, and PSV. The various modes are achieved by using some combination of the three types of ventilator breaths (described earlier) and may be combined with the application of PEEP. Airway pressure and flow tracings of spontaneous respiration, CPAP, and the different modes of mechanical ventilation are illustrated in **Figure 5-4**. Each has advantages and disadvantages, as summarized in **Table 5-6**. In choosing a mode of ventilation, it is important to consider specific goals, the most important of which are adequacy of ventilation and oxygenation, reduction in the work of breathing, and the assurance of patient comfort and synchrony with the ventilator.

Figure 5-4. Airway Pressure and Flow Tracings

A. Assist-control ventilation (volume format)

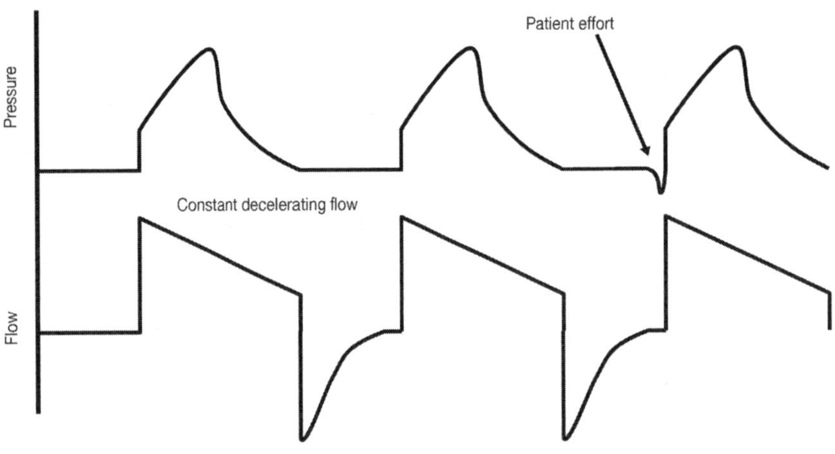

B. Assist-control ventilation (pressure format)

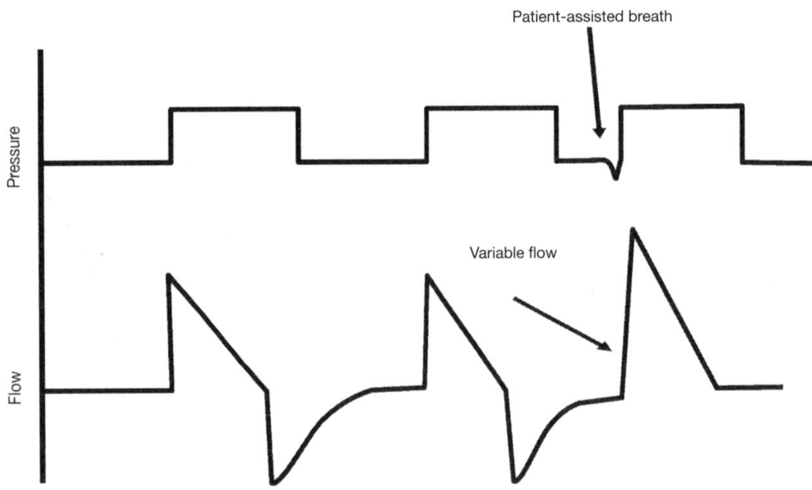

Figure 5-4. Airway Pressure and Flow Tracings (continued)

C. Synchronized intermittent mandatory ventilation (SIMV)

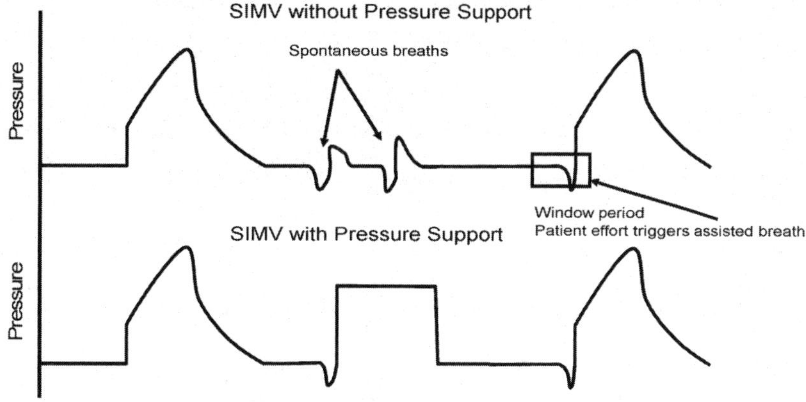

D. Pressure support ventilation

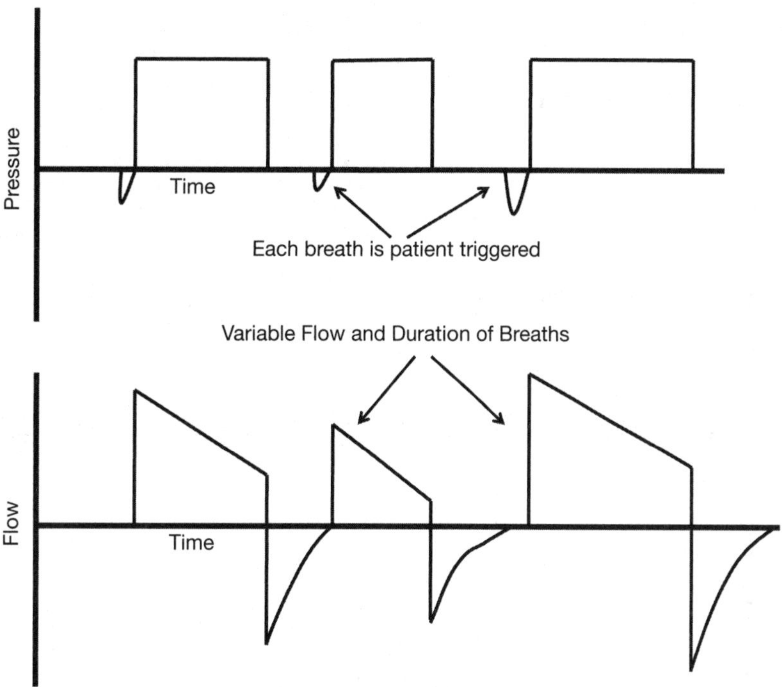

Figure 5-4. Airway Pressure and Flow Tracings (continued)

E. Pressure control inverse ratio ventilation

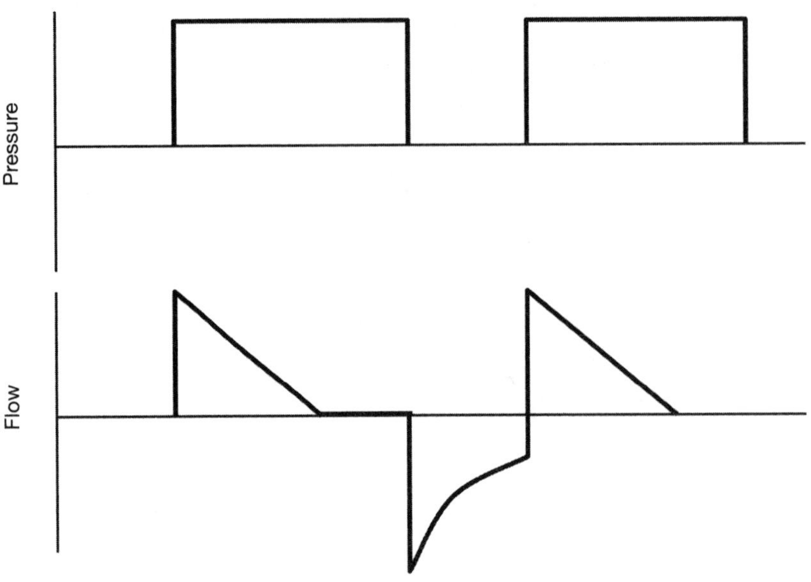

F. Spontaneous breathing

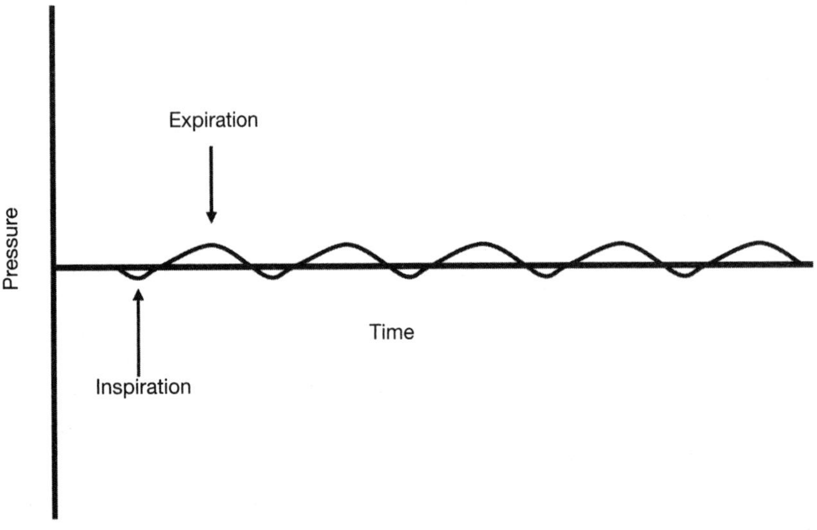

Airway pressure and flow tracings for spontaneous breathing, for CPAP, and for commonly used modes of mechanical ventilation. Time is represented on the horizontal axis and pressure or flow on the vertical axis.

Table 5-6 Potential Advantages and Disadvantages of Selected Modes of Mechanical Ventilation

Mode	Advantages	Disadvantages
Assist-control (AC) ventilation	Patient can increase ventilatory support; reduced work of breathing compared with spontaneous breathing	Adverse hemodynamic effects; inappropriate hyperventilation; increased work of breathing if V_T and/or flow do not meet patients demands
AC volume ventilation	Guarantees delivery of set V_T (unless peak pressure limit is exceeded)	Excessive inspiratory pressures
AC pressure ventilation	Limitation of peak inspiratory pressures; variable flow rates accommodate to patients' demands	V_T decreases or increases with lung resistance/compliance changes
Pressure support ventilation	Patient comfort; improved patient-ventilator interaction; decreased work of breathing	Apnea alarm may not trigger backup ventilation mode; variable patient tolerance
Synchronized intermittent mandatory ventilation	Less interference with normal cardiovascular function	Increased work of breathing compared with AC
Controlled mechanical ventilation (CoMV)	Rests muscles of respiration completely	Requires use of sedation/neuromuscular blockade; adverse hemodynamic effects

Abbreviations: V_T, tidal volume

A. Assist-Control Ventilation

AC ventilation is typically delivered with either volume-cycled or time-cycled (pressure assist-control) breaths. In volume AC, a preset V_T with a preset flow rate is delivered at a preset minimum rate. Similarly in pressure AC, a preset airway pressure is delivered for a preset length of inspiratory time. The patient receives the minimum number of ventilator breaths (set rate); however, the total number of breaths may be higher if the patient triggers the ventilator with additional inspiratory efforts. This mode of ventilation is commonly used when mechanical ventilation is initiated in patients with acute respiratory failure.

With proper use of AC, the work of breathing may be significantly decreased. If the ventilator and the patient are not in synchrony, or if the ventilator inspiratory flow rates are not matched to the patient's demand, however, this mode may result in an increase in the patient's work of breathing.

This mode has also been called *continuous mandatory ventilation* (CMV), which more accurately represents a situation in which the patient doesn't trigger additional breaths (ie, absent respiratory drive) (Section D).

B. Pressure Support Ventilation

PSV provides a preset level of inspiratory pressure assist with each ventilator-detected patient effort. This inspiratory assist is selected to overcome the increased work of breathing imposed by the disease process, endotracheal tube, inspiratory valves, and other mechanical aspects of ventilatory support. The set amount of pressure that is applied augments each patient-triggered breath. All breaths are flow cycled. With PSV, the patient controls the respiratory rate and exerts a strong influence on the duration of inspiration, inspiratory flow rate, and V_T. In addition, the delivered V_T is influenced by pulmonary compliance and resistance. Rapid changes in these parameters potentially alter the tidal volume and work of breathing. PSV may be coupled with SIMV, primarily as a means to diminish excess work of breathing for spontaneous breaths occurring between mandatory breaths (Section C).

> !
>
> *PSV augments the patient's own respiratory effort and is best adjusted by observing changes in the patient's respiratory rate, V_T, and comfort.*
>
> !

The amount of pressure support is titrated according to the patient's V_T measured by the ventilator during expiration. Suggested parameters include a setting that achieves one or more of the following goals:

- A V_T of 6 to 10 mL/kg, depending on patient needs
- A slowing of spontaneous breathing rate to an acceptable range
- The desired minute ventilation

Appropriate apnea alarms and a backup ventilation setting are essential. Potential benefits of PSV include the comfort and tolerance this ventilatory mode offers some patients. In addition, PSV may reduce the work of breathing by diminishing patient-ventilator asynchrony. Typically, as pressure support is increased in patients with lung disease, the patient's work of breathing and respiratory rate decrease and V_T increases. With PSV, an endotracheal tube cuff leak may interfere with appropriate cycling because flow may never drop to the preset threshold for cycling (typically 25% of the peak flow rate).

C. Synchronized Intermittent Mandatory Ventilation

SIMV delivers either volume-cycled or time-cycled breaths at a preset mandatory rate. Volume cycling is most commonly used for the mandatory breaths. Between mandatory breaths, the patient can breathe spontaneously through either a demand valve or a continuous flow of gas. The addition of pressure support to these patient-initiated breaths is recommended, using a value that offsets the resistance of the endotracheal tube. Typically, SIMV is initially set to deliver full ventilatory support, and support is then decreased as the patient tolerates spontaneous breathing. Synchronization allows for enhanced patient-ventilator interaction by delivering the preset machine breaths in conjunction with the patient's inspiratory effort before each mandatory breath. When no effort is detected, the ventilator delivers the preset VT.

The SIMV mode allows patients to contribute to and determine a portion of their ventilatory requirement. The negative inspiratory pressure generated by spontaneous breathing may lead to increased venous return to the right side of the heart, which may improve cardiac output and cardiovascular function. When no pressure support is added, potential increases in work of breathing and delays in weaning from mechanical ventilation may occur.

> **!** *It is recommended that PSV be used in conjunction with SIMV to decrease the patient's work of breathing during spontaneous breaths.*

D. Controlled Mechanical Ventilation

CMV delivers unassisted ventilator breaths at a preset rate. All breaths are mandatory and are either volume cycled or time cycled. No additional spontaneous assisted breaths are initiated beyond the set number of controlled breaths. Current ventilators do not allow direct setting of CMV, and this mode can be achieved only in patients who are not capable of spontaneous respiratory effort, such as those who are heavily sedated or receiving neuromuscular blockade. In this situation, AC and SIMV resemble CMV.

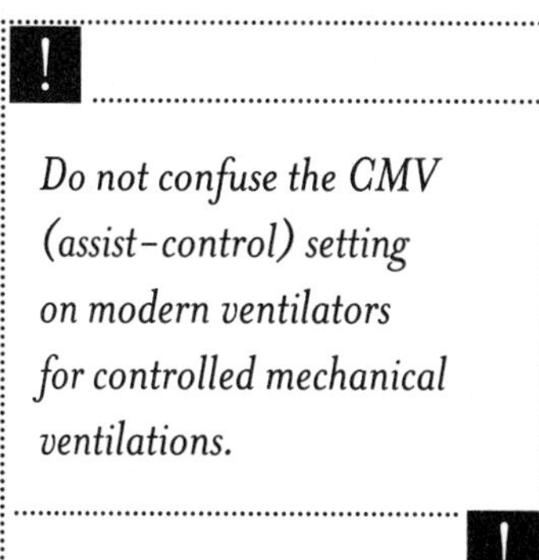

V. CHOOSING A MODE AND INITIAL VENTILATOR SETTINGS

The most important goals of mechanical ventilation are adequacy of ventilation and oxygenation, a reduction in the work of breathing, and the assurance of patient comfort and synchrony with the ventilator. Choosing a mode of mechanical ventilation depends on the reason it is required and the underlying disease process. In general, AC is used as the initial mode for a patient needing invasive mechanical ventilation. Each mode has both advantages and disadvantages, as summarized in **Table 5-6**. When initiating ventilatory support in adults, an FIO_2 of 1.0 is used to ensure maximal amount of available oxygen during the patient's adjustment to the ventilator and during the initial attempts to stabilize the patient's condition. In addition, the high level of oxygen offers support for complications that may have occurred before and during intubation. The usual recommended VT level is 8 to 10 mL/kg and should be calculated by using predicted body weight. Higher VT levels should be avoided to reduce the possibility of pulmonary injury. An appropriate respiratory rate should be set to achieve the desired minute ventilation. Normal minute ventilation (VT × respiratory rate) is approximately 7 to 8 L/min, but certain conditions may require levels that more than double this baseline. Minute ventilation should be adjusted to produce the $PaCO_2$ level that allows an acceptable acid-base (pH) status for the patient's clinical condition. As a general rule, F_{IO_2}, mean airway pressure, and PEEP affect the Pa_{O_2}, whereas the respiratory rate, V_D, and V_T affect alveolar minute ventilation and Pa_{CO_2}. One should be cognizant of the fact that in many circumstances (acute respiratory distress syndrome and severe obstructive lung disease), the goals of mechanical ventilation are not to normalize blood gases. Hypercapnia and respiratory acidosis are tolerated in such situations to achieve goals such as minimizing dynamic hyperinflation and avoiding ventilator-associated lung injury. Guidelines for the initiation of mechanical ventilation are listed in **Table 5-7.**

!

To Estimate Predicted Body Weight

- *Males:* 50 + 2.3 *(Height in Inches* – 60)
  50 + 0.91 *(Height in cm* – 152.4)
- *Females:* 45.5 + 2.3 *(Height in Inches* – 60)
  45.5 + 0.91 *(Height in cm* – 152.4)

!

Table 5-7 Guidelines For the Initiation of Mechanical Ventilation

1. Choose the ventilator mode with which you are most familiar. The primary goals of ventilatory support are adequate oxygenation/ventilation, reduced work of breathing, synchrony between patient and ventilator, and avoidance of high end-inspiration alveolar pressures.
2. The initial F_{IO_2} should be 1.0. The F_{IO_2} thereafter can be titrated downward to maintain the Sp_{O_2} at 92% to 94%. In severe acute respiratory distress syndrome, an Sp_{O_2} ≥88% may be acceptable to minimize complications of mechanical ventilation.
3. Initial V_T = 8 to 10 mL/kg in patients with relatively normal lung compliance. In patients with poor lung compliance (eg, ARDS), a target V_T of 6 mL/kg by PBW is recommended to avoid overdistension and to maintain an inspiratory plateau pressure ≤30 cm H_2O. (See Section VIII for more information.)
4. Choose a respiratory rate and minute ventilation appropriate for the particular clinical requirements. Target pH, not Pa_{CO_2}.
5. Use PEEP in diffuse lung injury to maintain open alveoli at end expiration. If volume is held constant, PEEP may increase peak inspiratory plateau pressure, a potentially undesirable effect in ARDS. PEEP levels >15 cm H_2O are rarely necessary.
6. Set the trigger sensitivity to allow minimal patient effort to initiate inspiration. Beware of auto-cycling if the trigger setting is too sensitive.
7. In patients at risk of obstructive airway disease, avoid choosing ventilator settings that limit expiratory time and cause or worsen auto-PEEP (see Section VI).
8. Call the critical care consultant or other appropriate consultant for assistance.

Abbreviations: V_T, tidal volume; Sp_{O_2}, oxyhemoglobin saturation as measured by pulse oximetry; ARDS, acute respiratory distress syndrome; PBW, predicted body weight; PEEP, positive end-expiratory pressure

VI. CONTINUING CARE DURING MECHANICAL VENTILATION

After mechanical ventilation has been initiated, the following parameters should be assessed and titrated to achieve the desired goals. Many important inter-relationships exist among ventilator settings, and the consequences of making any change must be appreciated. This interdependency of parameters may lead to beneficial or harmful effects in the respiratory and/or cardiovascular systems. Critical care consultation should be obtained for complex patients.

A. Inspiratory Pressures

During positive pressure volume assist-control ventilation, airway pressure rises progressively to a peak inspiratory pressure (Ppeak; **Figure 5-5**), which is reached at end inspiration. The Ppeak is the sum of the pressure required to overcome airway resistance and the pressure required to overcome the elastic properties of the lung and chest wall. Ppeak, sometimes referred to as peak airway pressure, is affected by many other variables, such as the flow rate, diameter of the endotracheal tube, secretions, and diminished bronchial diameter. When an inspiratory hold is applied at the end of inspiration, gas flow ceases, all dynamic factors are eliminated, and the pressure drops to a measurement called the *inspiratory plateau pressure* (Pplat). The Pplat reflects the pressure required to overcome the elastic recoil within the lung and chest wall and is, contrary to the Ppeak, a static pressure. The Pplat is the best estimate of peak alveolar pressure, which is an important indicator of alveolar distension. Accurate measurement of Pplat requires the absence of any patient effort, and an inspiratory hold for a minimum of 0.5 seconds.

Potential adverse effects from high inspiratory pressures include barotrauma, volutrauma, and reduced cardiac output. Barotrauma (pneumothorax, pneumomediastinum) and volutrauma (lung parenchymal injury due to overinflation), although linked to high Ppeak, correlate best with Pplat. As mentioned earlier, an example of the relationship of Ppeak and Pplat to alveolar distension is demonstrated by the effect of endotracheal tube size on Ppeak and Pplat. As the internal diameter of an endotracheal tube is decreased in a patient receiving volume ventilation, the same VT will result in higher Ppeak, yet Pplat and alveolar distension remain unchanged as the pressure is dissipated across the resistance of the endotracheal tube. The same VT, regardless of the type of breath, produces the same alveolar distension at end inspiration. To avoid injury in patients receiving mechanical ventilation, inspiratory plateau pressure should be maintained <30 cm H_2O. The relation of Ppeak and Pplat is illustrated in **Figure 5-5**.

Elevated Pplat may be reduced by the following interventions:

- Decrease PEEP, which may also decrease oxygenation and worsen alveolar collapse (if PEEP is used to improve oxygenation and alveolar stability).
- Decrease VT, which may lead to hypercapnia due to a reduction in minute ventilation.
- Decrease auto-PEEP (see next section) with interventions that prolong the expiratory time, understanding that this may lead to hypercapnia.

Figure 5-5. Relationship of Peak Inspiratory Pressure and Inspiratory Plateau Pressure

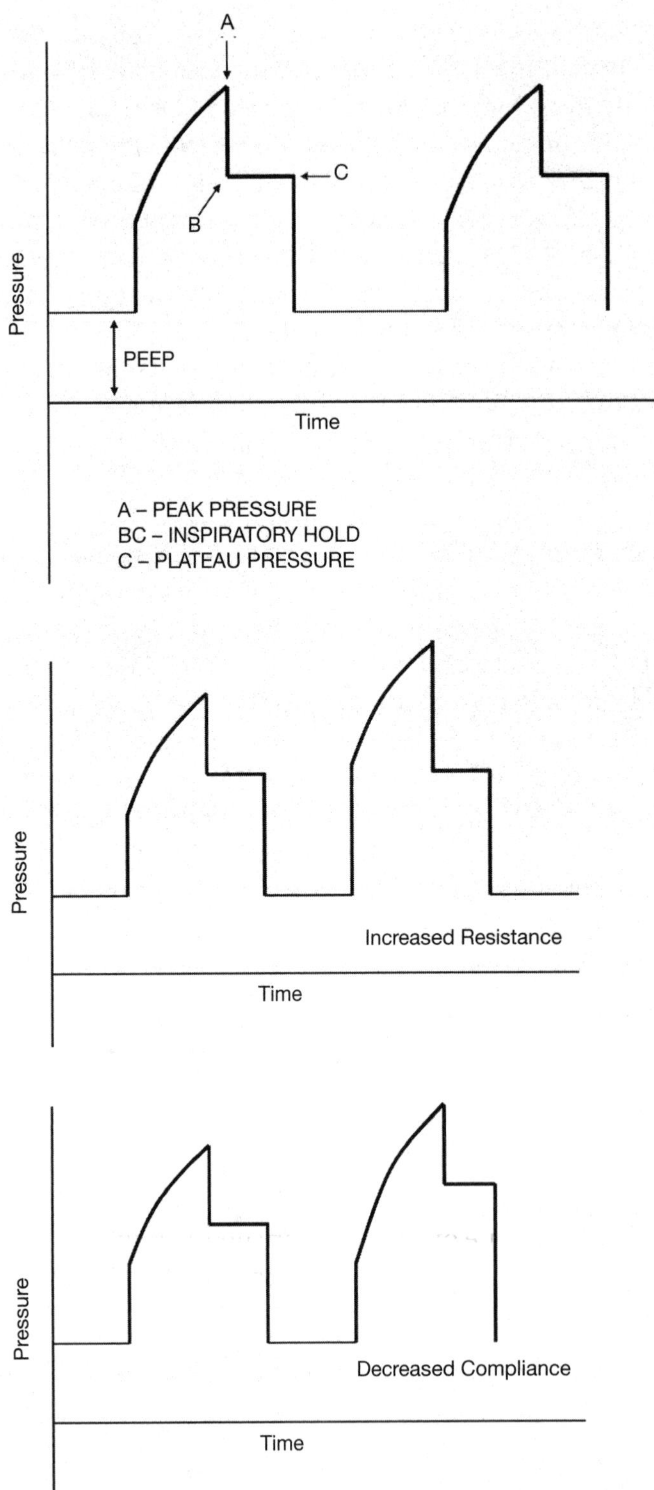

Abbreviation: PEEP, positive end-expiratory pressure

B. Relation of Inspiratory Time to Expiratory Time and Auto-PEEP

If the expiratory time is too short to allow full exhalation, the previously delivered breath is not completely expired and the next lung inflation is superimposed upon the residual gas in the lung. This results in lung hyperinflation and PEEP over and above the preset level on the ventilator. This increase in end-expiratory pressure is called *auto-PEEP,* or *intrinsic, inadvertent,* or *occult PEEP.* Auto-PEEP can be quantified by using manual methods or through electronic programs within some ventilators during an expiratory hold maneuver. However, it is most easily diagnosed qualitatively by viewing the flow-versus-time graphic waveform tracing available on most mechanical ventilators, as the expiratory flow fails to reach the zero flow level before the initiation of the next breath (**Figure 5-6**). The potentially harmful physiologic effects of auto-PEEP on peak, plateau, and mean airway pressures are the same as those of preset PEEP. In addition, high levels of PEEP may decrease venous return to the heart, resulting in hypotension and higher P_{CO_2} due to increased dead space, and adversely affect oxygenation (especially with asymmetric lung disease).

Figure 5-6. Flow-Versus-Time Waveform Demonstrating Auto-PEEP

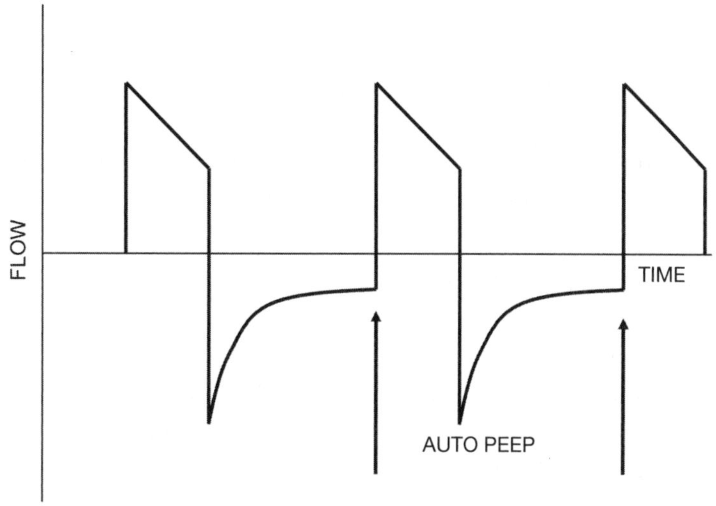

Abbreviation: PEEP, positive end-expiratory pressure

Auto-PEEP is demonstrated by the failure of the expiratory flow to return to zero before inspiratory flow is initiated. Auto-PEEP may be reduced by the following interventions:

- Decrease respiratory rate by changing the set rate or sedating the patient. These interventions result in fewer inspirations per minute and thus increase the total expiratory time available; this is the most effective way of decreasing auto-PEEP.
- Decrease V_T, which requires less time to deliver a smaller breath and allows more time for exhalation.
- Increase gas flow rate, delivering the V_T faster and allowing more time in the cycle for exhalation. This intervention has little impact unless the initial flow rate was set at an extremely low level.
- Changing the inspiratory waveform from decelerating (ramp) to constant (square).

The first two interventions, as discussed earlier, may lead to hypercapnia due to a reduction in minute ventilation; however, the benefits of a decrease in auto-PEEP despite the lower minute ventilation may lead to little change in $Paco_2$. When severe air trapping occurs, allowing sufficient expiratory time may improve ventilation and CO_2 removal. Hypercapnia and a controlled reduction in pH (permissive hypercapnia) may be acceptable in some clinical conditions but requires expert consultation. This approach may not be suitable for patients with intracranial hypertension because hypercapnia causes cerebral vasodilation and further increases in the intracranial pressure.

C. FIO_2

High levels of inspired oxygen may be harmful to lung parenchyma after prolonged exposure. Although the precise threshold for concern is not known, it is desirable to reduce the $FIO_2 \leq 0.5$ (50% oxygen) within the first 24 hours. However, hypoxemia is always considered a greater risk to the patient than high FIO_2 levels.

The primary determinants of oxygenation during mechanical ventilation are FIO_2 and mean airway pressure (Paw), V_T, I:E ratio, inspiratory flow rate, PEEP, auto-PEEP, use of inspiratory pause, and the inspiratory flow waveform pattern (volume breaths). In the patient with acute lung injury (ALI) and acute respiratory distress syndrome (ARDS), PEEP becomes a major determinant of mean airway pressure. The inter-relationships of these various parameters, as already demonstrated, often lead to complex adjustments within the plan for mechanical ventilation.

D. Minute Ventilation and Alveolar Minute Ventilation

Minute ventilation, defined as the amount of gas exchanged by an individual in 1 minute, is calculated as the respiratory rate multiplied by mean V_T. The primary determinant of CO_2 exchange during mechanical ventilation is the alveolar minute ventilation, calculated as:

$$VA = (V_T - V_D)f$$

where V_D is dead space and f is the respiratory rate (**Chapter 4**). The V_T, the respiratory rate, and their inter-relationships with other ventilatory parameters have already been discussed. Physiologic V_D represents, in general, lung units that are relatively well ventilated but underperfused. The physiologic effect of high amounts of V_D is hypercapnia. Dead space may result from the pathologic process in the lung or from mechanical ventilation complicated by high airway pressures, low intravascular volume, or low cardiac output. It may be necessary to use a low V_T to avoid high airway pressure and/or a low respiratory rate to avoid auto-PEEP, thus permitting hypoventilation and hypercapnia.

As previously discussed, adequate ventilation is assessed by consideration of both the $Paco_2$ and the pH. Hyperventilation resulting in a low $Paco_2$ level may be an appropriate short-term compensatory goal during metabolic acidosis while the primary etiology is corrected. Similarly, a patient with chronic hypercapnia has an increased baseline $Paco_2$ and maintains a near-normal pH by renal compensation (increased bicarbonate retention). Patients with chronic compensated hypercapnia should receive sufficient minute ventilation during mechanical ventilation to maintain the $Paco_2$ at their usual level, and utmost attention should be paid to the pH to avoid severe alkalemia and loss of retained bicarbonate.

E. Humidification

Gases delivered by mechanical ventilators are typically dry, and the upper respiratory tract is bypassed by artificial airways, resulting in loss of heat and moisture. Heating and humidification of gases are routinely provided during mechanical ventilation to prevent mucosal damage and minimize inspissation of secretions. Available systems include passive humidifiers (artificial nose) or active, microprocessor-controlled heat and humidifying systems (heated humidifiers). The passive humidifiers are contraindicated in the presence of copious secretions, minute ventilation >12 L/min, air leaks >15% of delivered tidal volume, or blood in the airway.

F. Use of Positive End-Expiratory Pressure (PEEP)

PEEP is the cornerstone strategy employed for disease states that cause alveolar collapse or airway closure (eg, ARDS). It causes alveolar recruitment and prevents repeated opening and closing of the alveoli (atelectrauma). Titration of PEEP for hypoxemic respiratory failure secondary to ARDS can be performed according to the PEEP/Fio_2 combinations given in **Table 5-8**.

Table 5-8 Suggested Combinations of PEEP and Fio_2 to Reach Goal Pao_2

Fio_2	PEEP (cm H_2O)
0.3	5–14
0.4	5–14
0.4	8–16
0.5	8–16
0.5	10–20
0.6	10–20
0.7	10–20
0.7	12–20
0.7	14–20
0.8	14–22
0.9	14–22
0.9	14–22
0.9	16–22
1.0	18–22
1.0	20–22
1.0	22
1.0	24

Abbreviations: PEEP, positive end-expiratory pressure

In cases of severe obstructive lung disease, applying external PEEP and setting it close to the auto-PEEP value can help offset the work of breathing to trigger the ventilator. Seeking expert consultation is prudent if higher levels of PEEP are required to maintain oxygenation.

G. Prophylactic Therapies

Mechanical intubation is a risk factor for venous thromboembolism, gastric stress ulceration, and nosocomial pneumonia. Measures to prevent venous thromboembolism include the prophylactic use of anticoagulation (unless contraindicated) and/or pneumatic compression devices. Using a proton pump inhibitor or histamine$_2$-receptor blocker is warranted for stress ulcer prevention. The risk of ventilator-associated pneumonia (ventilator bundle) is reduced by elevating the head of the bed to ≥30°, oral hygiene, and daily evaluations for liberation from mechanical ventilation. Please see **Chapter 13** for prophylactic therapies and **Chapter 11** for the ventilator bundle.

VII. SEDATION, ANALGESIA, AND NEUROMUSCULAR BLOCKADE

Endotracheal intubation and mechanical ventilation can be uncomfortable and anxiety provoking. To improve the patient's comfort and synchrony with the ventilator, anxiolytics, sedatives, and analgesics may be administered. Neuromuscular blocking agents should be used with caution, and expert consultation should be sought beforehand. Guidelines for the use of these agents are outlined in the Society of Critical Care Medicine's *Clinical Practice Guidelines for Sustained Neuromuscular Blockade in the Adult Critically Ill Patient.* Caution also should be taken with use of sedation in nonintubated patients with acute respiratory insufficiency or impending respiratory failure.

VIII. VENTILATORY GUIDELINES FOR SPECIFIC CLINICAL SITUATIONS

A. Acute Lung Injury/Acute Respiratory Distress Syndrome

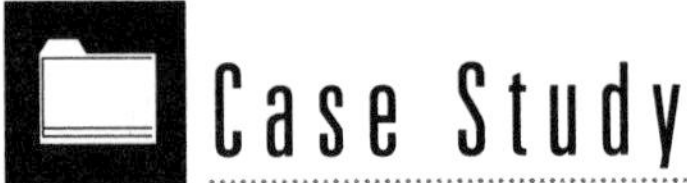

Case Study

An 18-year-old female patient is brought to the emergency department after being found unresponsive at a party where alcohol was consumed. The paramedics reported vomitus in the oral cavity and a difficult intubation due to copious foreign matter. In spite of bag-mask ventilation with 100% oxygen, her oxyhemoglobin saturation remained 87% to 88% during transport. The initial assessment reveals diffuse crackles, more prominent on the right hemithorax, and a chest radiograph shows diffuse bilateral infiltrates. The ventilator alarm is constantly warning of high pressure.

- What ventilator settings are recommended for this patient?
- What steps should be taken to avoid triggering the pressure alarm?
- What parameters should be measured and monitored?

ALI and ARDS cause a decrease in lung compliance, making the lungs stiff and difficult to inflate, and produce hypoxemic respiratory failure (**Chapter 4**). Guidelines for mechanical ventilation in ALI and ARDS are outlined in **Tables 5-8** and **5-9**. High Ppeak and Pplat complicate mechanical ventilation because of the low lung compliance or high airway resistance. Lower VT is required and the Pplat should be maintained at the desired level of ≤30 cm H_2O; permissive hypercapnia may be required to accomplish that goal. The FIO_2 is increased as necessary to prevent hypoxemia but reduced as soon as other ventilatory interventions are effective. Because of increased shunt in ARDS, hypoxemia may be severe. PEEP is the most effective way to improve oxygenation and is

Table 5-9 Mechanical Ventilation in ALI/ARDS

Goals

- PaO_2: 55-80 mm Hg (7.3-10.7 kPa)
- Pplat: ≤30 cm H_2O
- VT: 6 mL/kg PBW
- pH: <7.15 is acceptable

Start With Assist-Control With VT of 8 mL/kg PBW

- Decrease by 1 mL/kg at a time over the next 4 hours until VT of 6 mL/kg is reached.
- If Pplat is >30 cm H_2O, decrease VT by 1 mL/kg at a time until VT is 4 mL/kg or arterial pH reaches 7.15.
- If using VT of 4 mL/kg and Pplat is <25 cm H_2O, VT can be increased 1 mL/kg at a time until Pplat is 25 cm H_2O or VT is 6 mL/kg.
- If a Pplat of ≤30 cm H_2O has been achieved with a VT >6 mL/kg and a lower VT is clinically problematic (ie, need for increased sedation), it is acceptable to maintain the higher VT.

Initiation of PEEP in ARDS

- Initiate PEEP at 5 cm H_2O and titrate up in increments of 2-3 cm H_2O, according to **Table 5-8.**
- Full recruitment effect may not be apparent for several hours.
- Monitor blood pressure, heart rate, and PaO_2 or pulse oximetry during PEEP titration and at intervals while the patient is receiving PEEP therapy.
- Optimal PEEP settings are typically 8-15 cm H_2O.

NOTE: These guidelines are summarized to facilitate early intervention in critical patients. The physician should be familiar with these situations and seek appropriate specialist advice as soon as possible.

Abbreviations: ALI, acute lung injury; ARDS, acute respiratory distress syndrome; Pplat, inspiratory plateau pressure; PBW, predicted body weight; VT, tidal volume; PEEP, positive end-expiratory pressure typically applied in the range of 8 to 15 cm H_2O, based on the severity of hypoxemia. Higher PEEP levels may be indicated in severe lung injury. Although patients with ARDS are somewhat less likely to develop auto-PEEP because expiratory time requirements are reduced due to decreased lung compliance (stiffness), its presence should be monitored, especially at higher I:E ratios. **Table 5-9** outlines the recommended strategy for ventilating patients with ARDS. **Table 5-8** outlines the recommended F_{IO_2} and PEEP combinations.

B. Obstructive Airway Disease

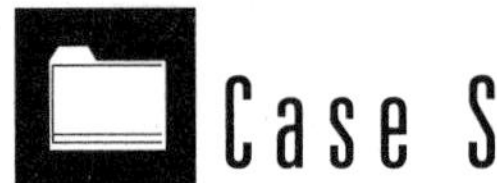

Case Study

A 70-year-old patient with a long history of smoking has been kept on an observation unit where a trial of NPPV has lasted 4 hours. The patient's breathing difficulty has progressively worsened, and he has become uncooperative and agitated. He was recently sedated, intubated, and placed on mechanical ventilation. A low blood pressure alarm is now sounding.

- What ventilator settings are recommended for this patient?
- What are the possible causes of this patient's hypotension?
- What immediate interventions should be performed?

Mechanical ventilation for patients with asthma and chronic obstructive pulmonary disease is designed to support oxygenation and assist ventilation until airway obstruction has improved. Mechanical ventilation in these patients may produce hyperinflation, auto-PEEP, and resultant hypotension. Therefore, careful attention is needed to balance cycle, inspiratory, and expiratory times.

The initial V_T should be ~6 to 8 mL/kg, and the minute ventilation should be adjusted to a low normal pH. With volume ventilation, the inspiratory flow rate should be set to optimize the I:E ratio and allow complete exhalation. Such management reduces breath stacking and the potential for auto-PEEP. As flow rate increases, Ppeak may rise but not be mirrored in the Pplat; this is a function of airways resistance and not an indication of worsening lung compliance.

While the patient is supported with mechanical ventilation, airway obstruction should be aggressively treated with bronchodilators (**Chapter 4**). As airflow improves, the patient will tolerate higher V_T levels and longer inspiratory times.

C. Asymmetric Lung Disease

Asymmetric lung disease or injury that occurs after aspiration, contusion, or a localized pneumonia may cause abnormal distribution of ventilation and gas exchange during mechanical ventilation. Because the conditioned gas from the ventilator follows the path of least resistance along the bronchi, the V_T is distributed primarily to the less-affected (more-compliant) lung and may overexpand it. Overdistension of the less-affected lung and poor expansion of the diseased/injured lung worsen ventilation-perfusion relationships in both lungs, and hypoxemia and hypercapnia may occur, persist, or worsen. Standard settings and principles of ventilatory support should be initiated. However, if this is unsuccessful, expert consultation should be obtained to facilitate further efforts at patient management. Putting the less-involved lung in the gravitationally dependent (decubitus) position may be helpful in directing pulmonary blood flow to lung units receiving better ventilation. Other techniques, such as differential lung ventilation, and immediate expert consultation may be required.

D. Heart Disease

The major goal of ventilatory support in patients with myocardial ischemia is to decrease the work of breathing and ensure adequate oxygen delivery to the heart. Decreasing the work of breathing will reduce the consumption of oxygen by respiratory muscles, thus increasing oxygen availability to the heart. Patients with cardiogenic pulmonary edema who are mechanically ventilated find additional benefit from the decrease in preload as a result of increased intrathoracic pressure. Left ventricular afterload also decreases through application of positive juxtacardiac pressure during systole.

E. Neuromuscular Disease

Patients with peripheral neuromuscular disease typically have an intact respiratory drive and normal lungs. These patients may require a higher V_T level to avoid the sensation of dyspnea. Adjustments are made in other ventilatory parameters to ensure a normal arterial pH.

IX. MONITORING MECHANICAL VENTILATORY SUPPORT

Patients who receive mechanical ventilatory support require continuous monitoring to assess the beneficial and potential adverse effects of treatment (**Table 5-10**). Arterial blood gas measurements provide valuable information about the adequacy of oxygenation, ventilation, and acid-base balance. This information is essential during the initial phases of ventilatory support and during periods of patient instability. If available, a pulse oximeter (**Chapter 6**) and end-tidal capnometer (for measuring end-tidal CO_2) can be used to further monitor the patient's progress.

Table 5-10 Recommendations for Monitoring Mechanical Ventilatory Support

1. Obtain a chest radiograph after intubation and additional chest radiographs as indicated to evaluate any deterioration in status.
2. Obtain arterial blood gas measurements after initiation of mechanical ventilation and intermittently, based on patient status.
3. Measure vital signs frequently and observe the patient directly (including patient-ventilator interaction).
4. Measure inspiratory plateau pressure as clinically appropriate.
5. Use pulse oximetry to monitor oxygenation.
6. Use ventilator alarms to monitor key physiologic and ventilator parameters.

Ventilators are equipped with sophisticated alarms and monitors to assist with patient management and detection of adverse events. When initiating ventilatory support, the respiratory care practitioner usually establishes alarm parameters for low and high minute ventilation, high inspiratory pressures, and low exhaled volumes and pressures. Many ventilators allow for the measurement of auto-PEEP.

The low-pressure alarm is intended to alert the clinician to a leak in the circuit or to ventilator disconnection. A high-pressure alarm warns that the set maximum peak airway pressure has been exceeded; this alarm is usually set 10 cm H_2O above the patient's baseline peak airway pressure. If a patient receiving volume ventilation develops mucous plugging or a marked change in airway resistance or lung compliance, the peak pressure will rise acutely. If the peak pressure alarm sounds with volume ventilation, it implies that the patient is not receiving the set V_T, as inspiration ends when the pressure alarm limit is exceeded. Conversely, in pressure preset modes of ventilation, changes in airway resistance or lung compliance will trigger the low exhaled volume alarm. Some ventilators have substituted a low minute ventilation alarm in place of the low-pressure alarm to alert the clinician to leaks in the circuit or ventilator disconnection.

X. HYPOTENSION ASSOCIATED WITH INITIATION OF MECHANICAL VENTILATION

A. Tension Pneumothorax

When hypotension occurs immediately after initiation of mechanical ventilation, tension pneumothorax should be one of the first considerations. This diagnosis is based on a physical examination that finds decreased or absent breath sounds and tympany to percussion on the side of the pneumothorax. Tracheal deviation away from the side of the pneumothorax may be observed, although it is uncommon after placement of an endotracheal tube. Treatment includes emergent decompression by inserting a large-bore catheter or needle into the second or third intercostal space in the midclavicular line (**Appendix 8**). Treatment should not be delayed awaiting a chest radiograph. The insertion of a catheter or needle is both diagnostic and therapeutic: it improves blood pressure and reverses the findings of physical examination. The insertion of the catheter or needle must be followed by chest tube placement.

B. Conversion From Negative to Positive Intrathoracic Pressure

Normal intrathoracic pressure is slightly negative relative to the atmosphere. When positive pressure ventilation is initiated, intrathoracic pressure becomes positive. As intrathoracic pressure rises, right atrial pressure rises and the intravascular pressure gradient for return of blood from the large extrathoracic veins into the right heart decreases. As a result, blood return to the heart may be reduced. Left ventricular preload, stroke volume, cardiac output, and blood pressure then may decrease in sequence. Underlying intravascular volume depletion exacerbates the deleterious effects of the increased intrathoracic pressure on cardiac output and blood pressure. Treatment of this common complication includes volume resuscitation by means of rapidly infused fluid boluses to raise extrathoracic venous pressure and increase venous return to the right heart until the blood pressure increases. Oxygen saturation should be monitored to avoid overly aggressive fluid resuscitation. Use of ventilation techniques associated with high mean airway pressure may exacerbate the deleterious hemodynamic consequences of mechanical ventilation.

C. Auto-PEEP

Auto-PEEP occurs when the combination of ventilator settings and patient physiology results in an inadequate expiratory time. Excessive end-expiratory pressure may increase intrathoracic pressure and cause hypotension due to decreased venous return to the heart. Although auto-PEEP may occur in any patient, those with obstructive airway disease are particularly predisposed to this condition. Assessment and treatment of auto-PEEP are performed as previously described.

D. Acute Myocardial Ischemia/Infarction

Stress from the cause of acute respiratory failure, as well as the stress of intubation itself, may lead to increased myocardial oxygen demand and to acute myocardial ischemia, infarction, and subsequent hypotension. Patients at high risk should be evaluated with serial electrocardiograms and myocardial markers of injury.

Key Points

Mechanical Ventilation

- The primary goals of noninvasive and invasive positive pressure ventilation are to support ventilation and oxygenation, and to reduce work of breathing while ensuring patient comfort.
- NPPV is best utilized in the alert, cooperative patient whose respiratory condition is expected to improve in 48 to 72 hours.
- The advantages and disadvantages of the different modes of invasive mechanical ventilation must be considered when determining the optimal ventilatory support for the patient's clinical condition.
- Guidelines for initiating mechanical ventilation should be carefully followed, with adjustments made based on patient assessment and monitoring.
- The complex interactions of inspiratory pressures, I:E ratio, FIO_2, and PEEP must be appreciated to evaluate the potential benefits and harmful effects in each patient.
- The primary determinants of oxygenation are FIO_2 and mean airway pressure, whereas alveolar ventilation primarily affects CO_2 exchange.
- During mechanical ventilation, a patient must be closely monitored using the ventilator alarm systems, continuous pulse oximetry, attentive physical assessment, measurement of inspiratory plateau pressure (as clinically appropriate), and intermittent arterial blood gases and chest radiographs as needed.
- The inspiratory plateau pressure should be maintained below 30 cm H_2O.
- Hypotension occurring immediately after initiation of invasive mechanical ventilation should prompt evaluation for tension pneumothorax, decreased venous blood return due to intrathoracic pressure, auto-PEEP, or myocardial ischemia.

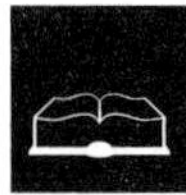

Suggested Readings

1. Acute Respiratory Distress Syndrome Network. Ventilation with lower tidal volumes as compared with traditional tidal volumes for acute lung injury and the acute respiratory distress syndrome. *N Engl J Med.* 2000;342:1301-1308.
2. Caples SM, Gay PC. Noninvasive positive pressure ventilation in the intensive care unit: A concise review. *Crit Care Med.* 2005;33:2651-2658.
3. Fink M, Abraham E, Vincent J, et al, eds. Controlled mechanical ventilation. In: *Textbook of Critical Care.* 5th ed. Philadelphia, PA: WB Saunders Co; 2005:chap 66.

4. Fink M, Abraham E, Vincent J, et al, eds. Patient-ventilator interaction. In: *Textbook of Critical Care.* 5th ed. Philadelphia, PA: WB Saunders Co; 2005:chap 67.

5. Hess DR, Kacmarek RM. *Essentials of Mechanical Ventilation.* 2nd ed. New York, NY: McGraw-Hill Companies; 2002.

6. Kallet RH, Jasmer RM, Pittet JF, et al. Clinical implementation of the ARDS network protocol is associated with reduced hospital mortality compared with historical controls. *Crit Care Med.* 2005;33:925-929.

7. Leisching T, Kwok H, Hill NS. Acute applications of noninvasive positive pressure ventilation. *Chest.* 2003;124:699-713.

8. MacIntyre N. Ventilatory management of ALI/ARDS. *Semin Respir Crit Care Med.* 2006;27:396-403.

9. MacIntyre N, Branson RD. *Mechanical Ventilation.* Philadelphia, PA: WB Saunders Co; 2000.

10. Marini JJ. Dynamic hyperinflation and auto-PEEP end-expiratory pressure: Lessons learned over 30 years. *Am J Respir Crit Care Med.* 2011;184:756-762.

11. Marini JJ, Gattinoni L. Ventilatory management of acute respiratory distress syndrome: A consensus of two. *Crit Care Med.* 2004;32:250-255.

12. Murray MJ, Cowen J, DeBlock H, et al. Clinical practice guidelines for sustained neuromuscular blockade in the adult critically ill patient. *Crit Care Med.* 2002;30:142-156.

13. Petrucci N, Iacovelli W. Ventilation with smaller tidal volumes: A quantitative systematic review of randomized controlled trials. *Anesth Analg.* 2004;99:193-200.

14. Tobin MJ. Advances in mechanical ventilation. *N Engl J Med.* 2001;344:1986-1996.

15. Tobin MJ. *Principles and Practice of Mechanical Ventilation.* Rev. ed. New York, NY: McGraw-Hill Companies; 2006.

Chapter 6

MONITORING OXYGEN BALANCE AND ACID-BASE STATUS

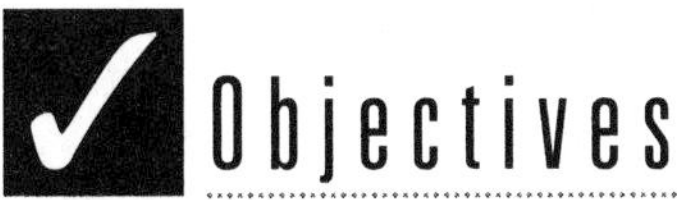

Objectives

- Outline the determinants of oxygen balance.
- Recognize disorders of oxygen delivery.
- Identify the principles and limitations of techniques for monitoring oxygen balance.
- Explain the use of acid-base status in monitoring the seriously ill patient.

Case Study

A previously healthy 40-year-old man presents to the emergency department with complaints of general malaise and lethargy after caring for his son with influenza. His vital signs at the triage desk are heart rate 145/min, blood pressure 118/82 mm Hg, respiratory rate 22/min, and oxygen saturation on pulse oximetry (Spo_2) 98% while breathing room air. As the evaluation is initiated, he is noted to be more tachypneic and anxious.

- What monitoring should be immediately implemented?
- What additional parameters should be assessed to determine if oxygen balance is adequate?

I. INTRODUCTION

Monitoring is never therapeutic, and information from monitoring tools must be integrated with patient assessment and clinical judgment to determine optimal care. In addition, the clinician must be aware of the risk-benefit ratio of a monitoring system. Monitoring may be as simple as measuring the pulse or temperature or as complex as invasive hemodynamic techniques with direct and calculated measurements. More invasive monitoring strategies that carry a higher risk should be considered if they provide sufficient new information to guide therapy. As an example, neuroendocrine responses to physiologic stress lead to early effects on heart rate, respiratory rate, vascular tone, and blood pressure. These combined signs may suggest the need for more intensive monitoring to appropriately evaluate and treat the patient. This chapter will emphasize basic monitoring techniques that can be accomplished in most care environments.

The goals of monitoring in seriously ill patients are to recognize physiologic abnormalities and to guide interventions to ensure adequate blood flow and oxygen utilization for maintenance of cellular and organ function. Tissue oxygenation cannot be directly measured or monitored, but estimates of the adequacy of oxygenation can be made based on knowledge of oxygen balance, which is determined by oxygen delivery and oxygen consumption. An understanding of these principles is required to appreciate the usefulness and limitations of various monitoring tools.

II. PRINCIPLES OF OXYGEN DELIVERY

Oxygen delivery is the amount of oxygen presented to the tissues, and it is the component of oxygen balance that can most often be altered by interventions in the seriously ill patient. Normally, the amount of oxygen delivered to the tissues is three to four times greater than the tissue needs. In critical illness, physiologic derangements that result in an absolute decrease in the oxygen delivered or an increase in tissue oxygen demand may compromise this margin of safety. In addition, sufficient oxygen delivery does not always guarantee adequate oxygen utilization at the tissue level. Delivery is dependent on cardiac output (blood flow) and the oxygen content of arterial blood. Invasive and/or more complex monitoring is required for exact measurement of cardiac output. However, an understanding of the variables that determine oxygen content in the blood and cardiac output, along with less invasive monitoring, may guide appropriate treatment.

A. Oxygen Content of Arterial Blood

Arterial oxygen content (Cao_2) is defined as the amount of oxygen bound to hemoglobin plus the amount of oxygen dissolved in arterial blood. The components of arterial oxygen content are related by the formula:

$$Cao_2\ (mL\ O_2/dL) = [\text{Hemoglobin}\ (g/dL) \times 1.34 \times Sao_2\ (\%)] + [0.0031 \times Pao_2\ (mm\ Hg)]$$

where Sao_2 is the arterial oxyhemoglobin saturation and Pao_2 is the partial pressure of oxygen in arterial blood. Each fully saturated gram of hemoglobin transports 1.34 to 1.39 mL of oxygen, depending on the affinity of hemoglobin for oxygen. Hemoglobin is the major contributor of oxygen for tissue demands and releases bound oxygen based on cellular uptake of dissolved oxygen as blood flows through the capillaries. The ability of hemoglobin to release more oxygen when supply is inadequate or cellular demand is increased is one of the main compensatory mechanisms to sustain cellular function. The oxyhemoglobin dissociation curve shows the relationship of hemoglobin saturation and partial pressures of oxygen (Po_2) (**Figure 6-1**). When the Po_2 drops to approximately 40 mm Hg (5.3 kPa) in the capillaries, the decrease in oxyhemoglobin saturation to 75% reflects the amount of oxygen released to the tissues. During physiologic stress, oxyhemoglobin saturation at the tissue level may decrease to <20%, reflecting the release of additional oxygen to tissues. Acidosis and fever will shift this curve to the right, resulting in a lower affinity of oxygen for hemoglobin and greater delivery of oxygen to the tissues.

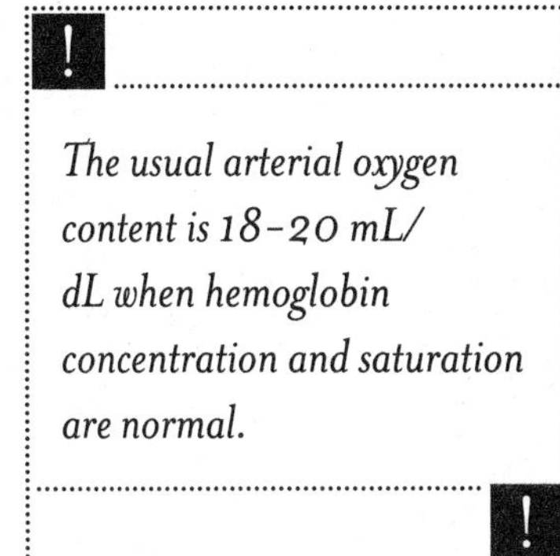

Figure 6-1. Oxyhemoglobin Dissociation Curve

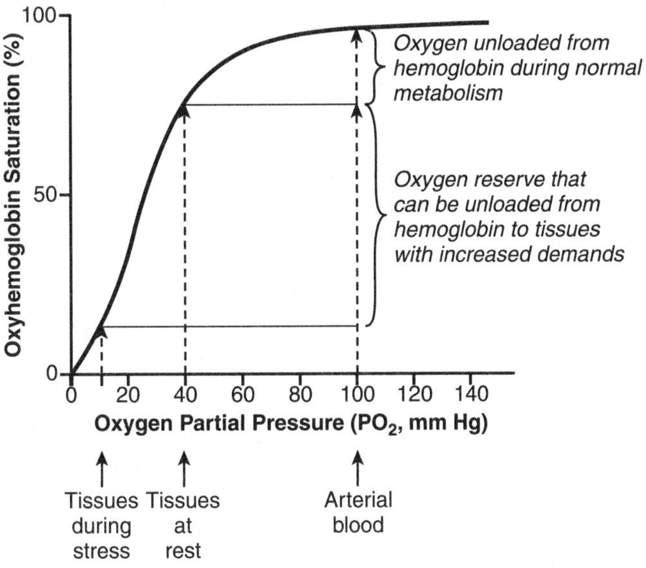

The oxyhemoglobin dissociation curve relates the partial pressure of oxygen (Po_2) to oxyhemoglobin saturation. Near-maximal saturation of hemoglobin occurs at a Po_2 of 60 mm Hg (8.0 kPa). Po_2 values above this point provide only a modest increase in oxyhemoglobin saturation. Note, however, that a rapid decrease in oxyhemoglobin saturation occurs when the Po_2 drops below 60 mm Hg (8.0 kPa).

Arterial oxygen content can be estimated by using the direct measurement of the hemoglobin concentration and arterial oxyhemoglobin saturation in intermittent blood samples, as dissolved oxygen ($0.0031 \times Pao_2$) contributes minimally to oxygen content. Although hemoglobin is not monitored continuously, oxyhemoglobin saturation measured by pulse oximetry (Spo_2) allows continuous assessment of this determinant of arterial oxygen content.

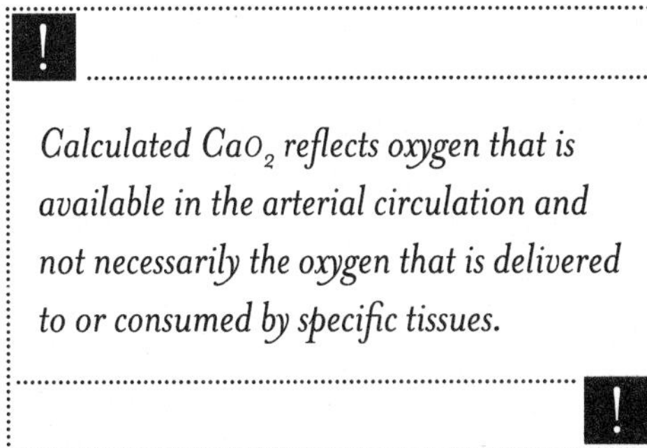

B. Cardiac Output

If the oxygen content of arterial blood is optimum, then an appropriate cardiac output is needed to ensure delivery of oxygen to the tissues. Cardiac output (in mL/min or L/min) is the product of heart rate and stroke volume (**Figure 6-2**). Stroke volume is the quantity of blood pumped out of the heart with each beat and is determined by the difference between the end-diastolic volume and end-systolic volume of the ventricle. Variables that determine stroke volume are preload, afterload, and contractile function. The first compensatory mechanism to increase oxygen delivery is an increase in heart rate. Patients who are unable to increase the heart rate (eg, beta blockade) will have a limited ability to compensate. Although the heart rate is easily measured and evaluated, an evaluation of stroke volume must be performed with echocardiography or invasive methods. The option of measuring cardiac output depends on the expertise and resources available. The clinician must be aware of the limitations of any chosen technique. If cardiac output is not directly measured, an indirect assessment of variables involved in determining cardiac output (**Table 6-1**) and knowledge of hemodynamic principles are useful.

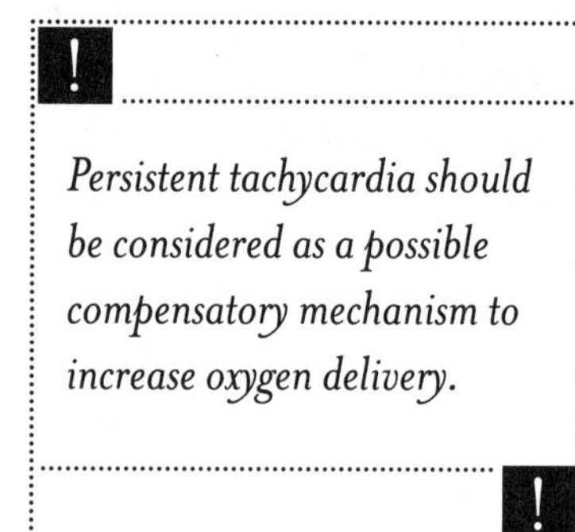

Figure 6-2. Cardiac Output As the Product of Heart Rate and Stroke Volume

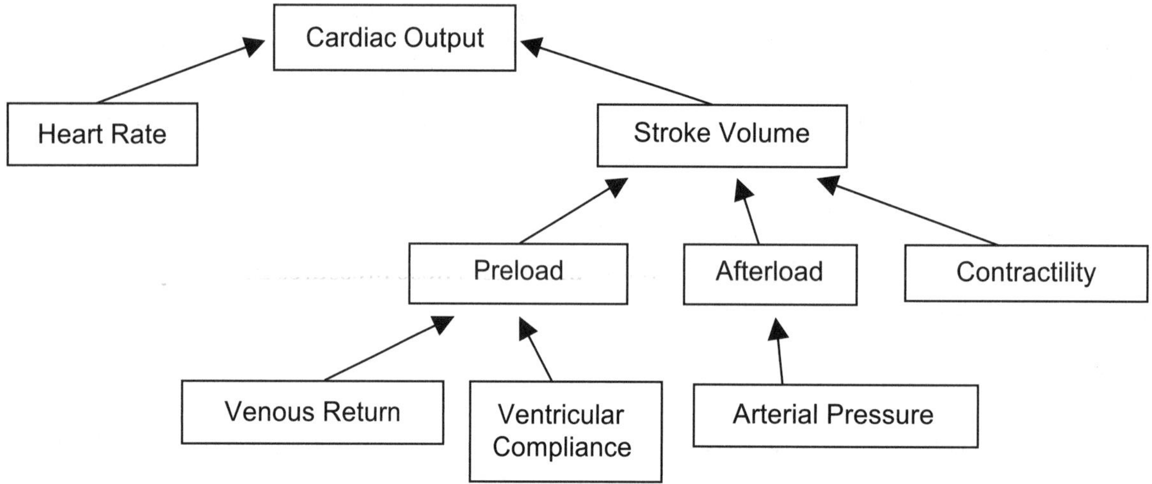

1. Contractility

Contractility is the ability of myocardial fibers to shorten during systole. It is highly dependent on preload and afterload and is difficult to measure as an independent variable. Additional factors that can affect contractility in the critically ill patient are endogenous sympathetic activation, acidosis, ischemia, inflammatory mediators, and vasoactive agents. An increase in contractility would result in a larger stroke volume. There are no readily available methods for monitoring the contractile state of the myocardium in the acutely ill patient.

Table 6-1 Clinical Assessment of Determinants of Cardiac Output

Variable	Method of Assessment
Heart rate and rhythm	Finger on pulse
	Pulse oximetry
	Electrocardiography
Preload	
Right heart	Neck vein distension, liver enlargement, dependent edema
	Central venous pressure
Left heart	Presence of dyspnea on exertion, orthopnea
	Pulmonary edema, rales on lung examination
	Pulmonary artery occlusion pressure
Afterload (left heart)	Mean arterial blood pressure
	Systemic vascular resistance
Contractility	Ejection fraction by echocardiography

2. Preload

Preload is a measure or estimate of the ventricular volume at the end of diastole (end-diastolic volume) and is determined by venous return and ventricular compliance. The distensibility (compliance) of the ventricle and the volume load (venous return) it can accept are the basis for the Frank-Starling curve. In general, a greater end-diastolic volume leads to increased stretch on the myocardium, resulting in a larger stroke volume (**Figure 6-3**). Because it is difficult to measure volume, preload is most often estimated from the ventricular end-diastolic pressure, which is transmitted and reflected in the atrial pressure. The atrial pressure is estimated by the measurement of pressure in a central vein or the pulmonary artery. Thus, right ventricular preload is estimated by measurement of the central venous pressure (CVP) and left ventricular preload by the measurement of pulmonary artery occlusion pressure. These pressures indirectly reflect the end-diastolic volume as well as the compliance of the ventricular wall.

Figure 6-3. Relationship Between Ventricular Preload and Stroke Volume

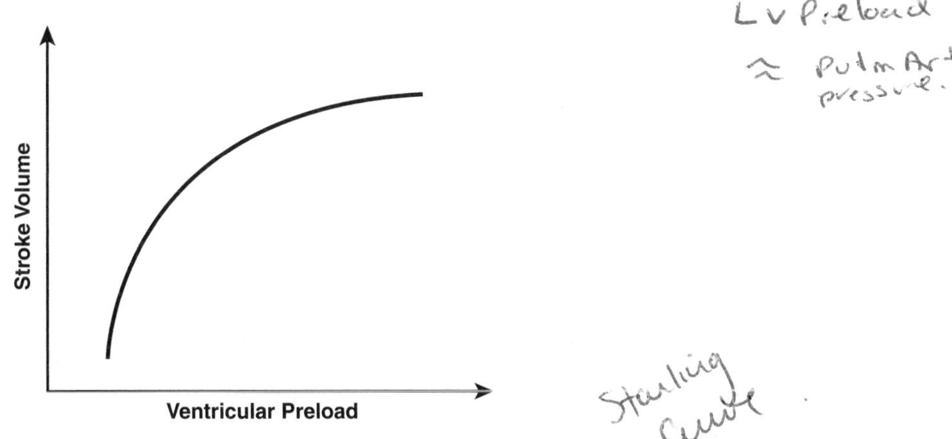

When end-diastolic volume of the ventricle (preload) increases, stroke volume usually increases proportionately.

The relationship between the measured pressure and volume in the ventricular chambers depends upon the compliance or distensibility of the ventricle. During myocardial ischemia, sepsis, valvular dysfunction, and even tachycardia, the ventricles may become less compliant and may not fully relax during diastole. This diastolic dysfunction reduces the ventricular volume at end diastole but may be associated with a higher filling pressure; therefore, the clinician may misinterpret pressure measurements to indicate adequate volume loading. Changes in intrathoracic pressures (eg, tension pneumothorax, positive pressure ventilation) may also affect the filling pressures.

3. Afterload

Afterload is the myocardial wall tension required to overcome the resistance, or pressure load, that opposes ejection of blood from the ventricle during systole. The higher the afterload, the more tension the ventricle must develop, the more work is performed, and the less efficient the contraction may become. Afterload is usually estimated from the systemic mean arterial pressure (left ventricle) and mean pulmonary artery pressure (right ventricle) and by calculations of aortic and pulmonary vascular resistance.

III. ASSESSMENT OF OXYGEN BALANCE

In addition to oxygen delivery, oxygen consumption by the tissues affects oxygen balance. However, less is known about the factors that determine oxygen utilization at the cellular and tissue levels, and no direct routine measures of oxygen consumption are available. Indirect calculated measurement of oxygen consumption requires invasive or complex techniques. These measures reflect global oxygen utilization and do not provide information on oxygen utilization by specific tissues or organs.

Measurements of global oxygen balance that may be useful in monitoring the seriously ill patient include central venous oxyhemoglobin saturation ($Scvo_2$) and lactate concentrations. $Scvo_2$ can be obtained continuously or intermittently from a catheter placed in the internal jugular or subclavian vein and correlates with the mixed venous oxyhemoglobin saturation (Svo_2) obtained from a pulmonary artery catheter. The Svo_2 measures the oxyhemoglobin saturation of blood from the superior vena cava and the inferior vena cava that has been mixed in the right ventricle. These measures of venous oxyhemoglobin saturation represent the amount of oxygen still bound to hemoglobin after traversing the tissue capillaries; the decrease from the Sao_2 estimates the amount of oxygen utilized (**Figure 6-4**). In normal individuals, the Svo_2 is >65% and the $Scvo_2$ is 2% to 3% lower. However, in patients with shock and/or hypoperfusion, the $Scvo_2$ may be 5% to 7% higher than the Svo_2 due to greater desaturation of venous blood from the gastrointestinal tract contributing to Svo_2. Low values of $Scvo_2$ suggest an imbalance in the oxygen supply and demand. This imbalance may be due to decreases in cardiac output, hemoglobin concentration, or Sao_2, or increases in tissue oxygen consumption. Patients may have more than one abnormality contributing to oxygen imbalance. A normal $Scvo_2$ may still be associated with tissue hypoxia in conditions such as severe sepsis and certain poisonings (eg, cyanide). Further evaluations of lactate concentration and organ function are needed to assess oxygen balance in the seriously ill patient when the $Scvo_2$ is normal.

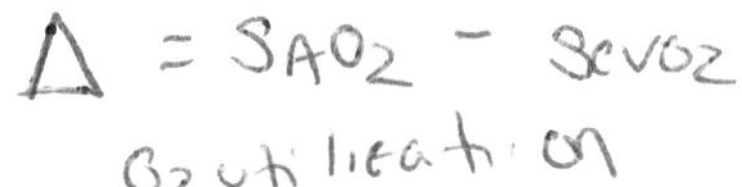

Figure 6-4. Determinants of Oxygen Balance

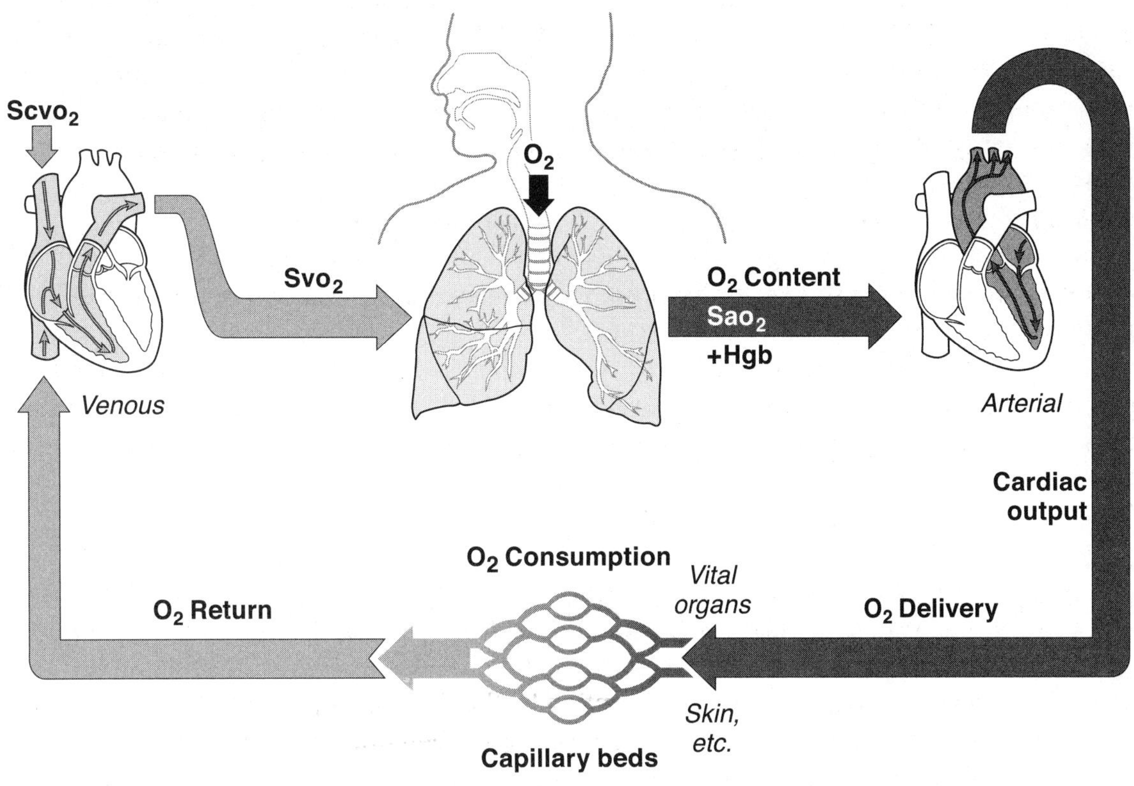

Abbreviations: Hgb, hemoglobin; Sao_2, arterial oxyhemoglobin saturation
Oxygen balance depends on the oxygen delivered to the tissues and the metabolic needs of those tissues. An estimate of the oxygen utilized by the tissues is provided by the central venous oxyhemoglobin value ($Scvo_2$) and mixed venous oxyhemoglobin saturation (Svo_2).

Lactate is another indicator of overall oxygen balance. It is produced during anaerobic metabolism when cellular hypoxia occurs. The elevation of blood lactate in shock and hypoperfusion may be due to inadequate oxygen supply to tissue but also may be affected by altered hepatic metabolism, use of vasoactive drugs, and other factors. Lactate concentrations do not have high sensitivity or specificity for inadequate tissue oxygenation, but elevated concentrations often are associated with tissue hypoperfusion. A decreasing lactate concentration may be a useful indicator of intervention success.

!

Elevated lactate concentrations correlate with worse prognosis in severely ill patients.

!

IV. MONITORING DETERMINANTS OF OXYGEN BALANCE

Precise monitoring of oxygen balance is not easily accomplished because techniques may not be available to assess some variables (contractility, tissue oxygen consumption) or special expertise and resources are required (pulmonary artery catheter, echocardiography). However, monitoring of variables such as oxyhemoglobin saturation, blood pressure, CVP, $Scvo_2$, and lactate concentration, combined with other clinical information, may provide guidance in evaluating the adequacy of oxygen balance in seriously ill patients.

> !
>
> *Trends in the values of measured variables are usually more helpful than single values.*
>
> !

A. Monitoring of Oxyhemoglobin Saturation

1. Principles

The pulse oximeter is a simple, noninvasive device that estimates arterial oxyhemoglobin saturation. The transmission of red and infrared light through the capillary bed creates several signals throughout the pulsatile cardiac cycle. These signals measure the absorption of the transmitted light by the tissue or venous and arterial blood. Calculations made from the processed signals provide estimates of the oxygen saturation of hemoglobin, expressed as a percentage. This is not the same as the Pao_2 in the blood, although Pao_2 is a primary determinant of the saturation of hemoglobin. Neither does it reflect adequacy of oxygen delivery. The value measured by the device is commonly called the Spo_2 to distinguish it as the oxyhemoglobin saturation measurement by a pulse oximeter rather than the Sao_2, which is determined directly from an arterial blood sample by co-oximetry.

2. Clinical Issues

Studies have shown that to ensure a Pao_2 of 60 mm Hg (8.0 kPa), an Spo_2 of 92% should be maintained in patients with light skin, whereas 94% saturation may be needed in patients with dark skin. Oximetry sensors can be applied to the finger, toe, earlobe, bridge of nose, mouth, or any skin surface from which a reliable pulsatile signal can be obtained. Factors that can affect signal detection or fidelity are listed in **Table 6-2**. Pulse oximeters display a digital heart rate derived from the pulsatile signal detected by the sensor. This rate should equal the patient's heart rate as measured by another method, so these two rates should be compared as the first step in the analysis of an Spo_2 measurement. Additional hemodynamic information may be obtained from the pulse oximeter waveform, which is related to the arterial blood pressure waveform. Variation in the pulse oximeter waveform with positive pressure ventilation may suggest hypovolemia and responsiveness to fluid administration (see next section).

Table 6-2 Factors That Affect Accuracy of Pulse Oximetry

Anatomic or Physiologic Factors
Dark skin
False nails
Nail polish
Hypothermia
Vasoconstriction
Hypotension
Poor regional perfusion
Hematocrit <15%
Hyperlipidemia
Carboxyhemoglobin
Tachycardias
External Factors
Lipid suspensions, propofol (falsely elevate the Spo_2)
Bright room lighting
Electrical interference
Poorly adherent probe
Excessive motion of the sensor

B. Blood Pressure Monitoring

Although blood pressure is not a direct determinant of oxygen balance, an appropriate driving pressure is necessary for oxygen delivery at the tissue level. Blood pressure is determined by the cardiac output and systemic vascular resistance according to the following relationship:

Blood Pressure = Cardiac Output × Systemic Vascular Resistance

Blood pressure may be monitored invasively or noninvasively.

1. Automated Noninvasive Devices

a. Principles

Automated blood pressure devices are frequently used to obtain intermittent blood pressure measurements. These devices use one of several methods to measure systolic and diastolic pressure, but the most common method is oscillometry. Systolic and diastolic pressures and the mean arterial pressure are directly measured via appearance, disappearance, and amplitude of oscillating waves. The arm is the preferred measurement site in adults, but alternative sites include the calf, forearm, or thigh, the latter being the least comfortable site for patients. The cuff should not be placed on an extremity that is being used for intravenous infusion or in an area susceptible to circulatory compromise. The appropriate cuff size is necessary for accurate measurements. A cuff that is too large will underestimate the true blood pressure, and a cuff that is too small yields artificially high measurements.

b. Clinical Issues

An adequate blood pressure measurement does not ensure adequate tissue perfusion. Automated blood pressure devices are less accurate in clinical situations commonly encountered with the critically ill patient, such as shock, vasoconstriction, mechanical ventilation, and arrhythmias. Shivering, muscle contraction, and movement of the extremity can lead to erroneous measurements. Device malfunction can distract the attention of the caregiver. Blood pressure monitoring via an arterial catheter is preferable to the use of an automated blood pressure device in hemodynamically unstable patients.

2. Arterial Cannulation

a. Principles

An indwelling arterial catheter allows for continuous measurement of blood pressure, pulse volume or pressure, and mean arterial pressure (**Figure 6-5**) by transduction of pressure via a specialized monitoring setup. It may also be used for continuous arterial blood gas measurement. The primary indications for insertion of an arterial cannula are the need for frequent arterial samples and continuous assessment of arterial blood pressure. Use of an arterial catheter should be considered for arterial blood sampling if more than four samples are required in 24 hours. The complication rate is lower for inserting a 20-gauge, 2-inch radial artery catheter than for performing four 22-gauge needlesticks in a single artery. Arterial pressure monitoring may also be used with special systems to evaluate cardiac output, stroke volume, and/or systolic pressure variation (as an estimate of volume responsiveness).

Figure 6-5. Appearance of Arterial Pressure Wave With Invasive Monitoring

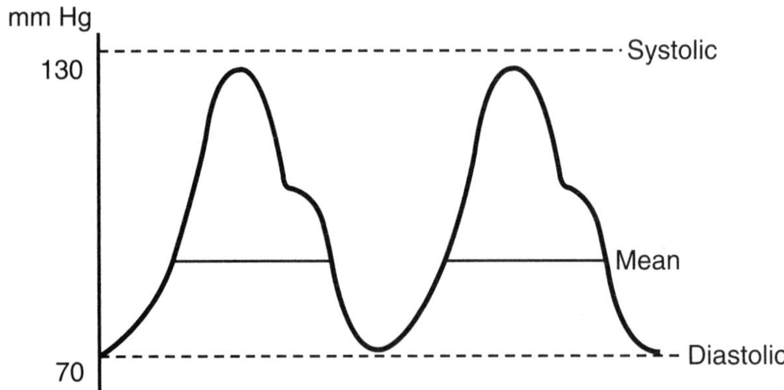

When invasive monitoring is used, the calculation of the mean arterial pressure is based on the area under the curve.

The most common insertion sites for arterial catheters are (in order of preference for adults) the radial, femoral, axillary, and dorsalis pedis arteries. Brachial artery cannulation is usually avoided if possible because it is an end artery and hand ischemia is a potential complication. Shorter catheters are used for radial and dorsalis pedis artery insertion and longer catheters for insertion in femoral and axillary sites. Preferred sites have alternative collateral circulations. The choice of site is based on the presence of palpable pulses, general hemodynamic state, and other anatomic or physiologic factors unique to each patient.

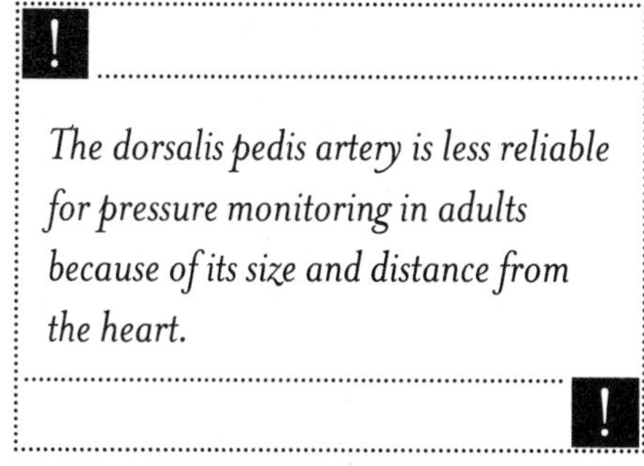

b. Clinical Issues

The arterial catheter is never used for infusion of any medications or fluids and must be monitored continuously. Concern about the accuracy of the intra-arterial pressure measurements should lead to a return-to-flow assessment with a manual blood pressure cuff. Measurements should be made with the catheter/transducer system at or near the level of the heart.

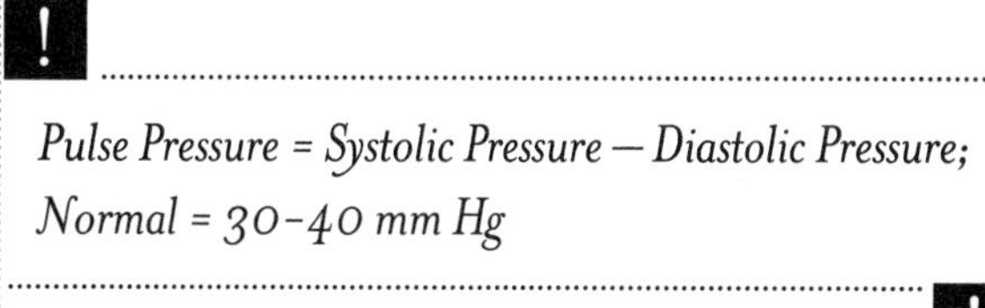

Several technical and anatomic factors may affect the accuracy of the pressures obtained with the catheter system. Distortion of the arterial waveform signal may occur due to vascular alterations, the hydraulic coupling system of the transducer, the calibration of the transducer, or the maintenance of the pressurized system tubing. Inspection of the result may show an overdamped and domed waveform or the high-spiking, "overshoot or ringing" pattern of the underdamped waveform. Both distortions have the greatest effect on the systolic and diastolic pressures, whereas the mean arterial pressure is less affected.

As with noninvasive monitoring, intra-arterial blood pressure monitoring may not be a sensitive indicator of hypoperfusion because of compensatory vasoconstriction. Additional clinical information regarding volume status can be obtained by inspection of the arterial blood pressure waveform in mechanically ventilated patients (**Figure 6-6**). Positive pressure during inspiration may decrease the stroke volume in patients with inadequate intravascular volume due to decreased venous return. The decrease in stroke volume leads to a decreased pressure that is visually represented as a systolic variation of blood pressure and a decrease in the pulse pressure. The pulse pressure is the difference between the systolic and diastolic arterial blood pressure measurements. Significant variation in the systolic pressure and pulse

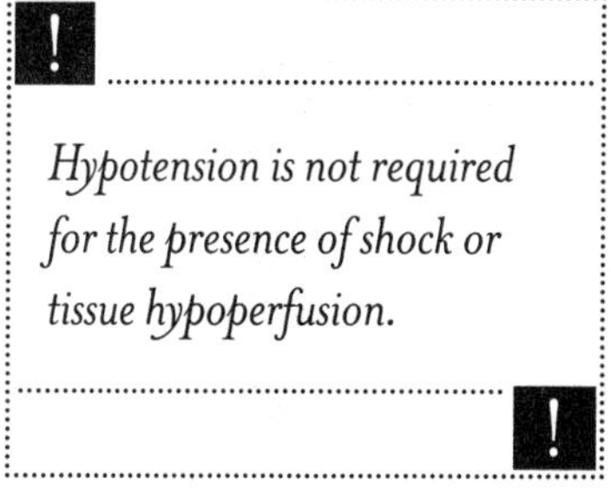

pressure (greater than 10% to 15%) may suggest the need for additional fluids to optimize cardiac output or the need to reduce intrathoracic pressures by decreasing tidal volume or positive end-expiratory pressure.

Figure 6-6. Variation of Blood Pressure in a Mechanically Ventilated Patient With Hypovolemia

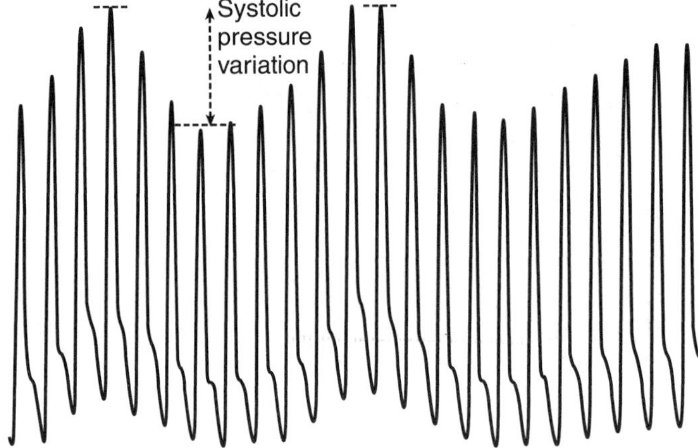

With positive pressure applied during inspiration, the decrease in systolic pressure is greater than the decrease in diastolic pressure.

Possible complications associated with arterial catheter insertion are listed in **Table 6-3**. These can be minimized by careful insertion technique, appropriate catheter size for the artery, proper site care, and a continuous flush system. The arterial waveform must be continuously monitored and displayed, with alarm settings to prevent inadvertent blood loss through a catheter that is accidentally opened to the atmosphere. The extremity with the arterial catheter should be inspected frequently for evidence of ischemia or infection. Any sign of ischemia distal to the catheter or infection at the site of insertion requires immediate removal of the catheter. Arterial catheters should be removed as soon as possible to minimize the risk of infection.

Table 6-3 Possible Complications of Arterial Catheters

Possible Complications of Arterial Catheters
Hematoma formation
Blood loss
Arterial thrombosis
Proximal or distal embolization
Arterial pseudoaneurysm
Infection
Accidental administration of fluids or medications

C. Monitoring Right Ventricular Filling Pressures and $Scvo_2$

A central venous catheter in the internal jugular or subclavian vein allows measurement of CVP and $Scvo_2$. Placement of a central venous catheter may be indicated for other reasons as well (**Table 6-4**). Confirmation of catheter placement in the internal jugular or subclavian vein by chest radiography is recommended to ensure accurate measurements of CVP and $Scvo_2$ and to detect complications of the procedure.

Table 6-4 Common Indications for Central Venous Cannulation

Common Indications for Central Venous Cannulation
Measurement of mean central venous pressure
Measurement of $Scvo_2$
Large-bore venous access
Difficult or long-term venous access
Administration of irritating drugs and/or parenteral nutrition
Hemodialysis
Placement of a temporary pacing wire
Placement of a pulmonary artery catheter

CVP, obtained from an appropriately positioned catheter, estimates the right ventricular filling pressure as a reflection of preload (end-diastolic volume). Normal values for CVP are 2 to 8 mm Hg, and measurements should be made at the end of expiration. Significant variation of the CVP waveform may occur during spontaneous breathing and mechanical ventilation, requiring visual assessment of the waveform to identify the end of expiration (**Figure 6-7**). In general, a low CVP indicates a low intravascular volume associated with a low preload. Normal or high CVP measurements must be evaluated cautiously, as they may not predict adequate or increased preload volume due to changes in intrathoracic pressures or ventricular compliance. Additional clinical assessment is required to estimate preload with normal or elevated CVP measurements. Right ventricular preload estimates do not necessarily correlate with left ventricular preload.

Figure 6-7. Typical Cyclic Pattern for CVP Waveform

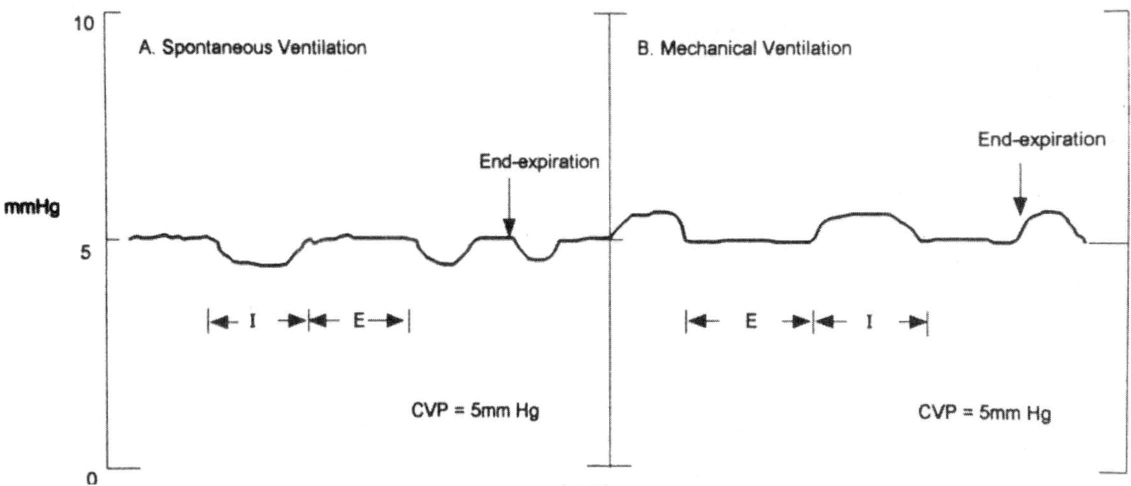

Typical cyclic pattern for central venous pressure (CVP) waveform showing inspiration (I) and expiration (E). **A**, Respiratory variation during spontaneous ventilation: CVP decreases during spontaneous inspiration as intrapleural pressure decreases. **B**, Respiratory variation during positive pressure mechanical ventilation: CVP increases during delivery of the mechanical breath as positive pressure is transmitted from the airway to the intrapleural space and great vessels. The vertical arrows denote the point of end-expiration during spontaneous and mechanical ventilation.

$Scvo_2$ can be monitored intermittently by withdrawal of blood for analysis or continuously with a catheter containing an oximeter to evaluate oxygen balance. Clinical protocols have used $Scvo_2$ measurements along with other parameters to determine adequacy of resuscitation. Normal $Scvo_2$ values are usually >65%.

D. Measuring Left Ventricular Filling Pressures

Left ventricular filling pressures are estimated from measurement of the pulmonary artery occlusion pressure. A pulmonary artery catheter (PAC) is necessary to obtain this information but requires expertise in insertion, data collection, and data interpretation. The clinician should consult with a critical care practitioner if invasive monitoring with a PAC is needed to obtain additional hemodynamic information.

E. Measuring Cardiac Output

Cardiac output plays a key role in determining oxygen delivery to the tissues. Measurement methods – such as thermodilution with a PAC, esophageal Doppler ultrasonography, and arterial waveform pulse contour analysis – require varying degrees of invasiveness as well as special expertise. In the absence of direct measurement of cardiac output, less specific indicators of tissue oxygenation, such as lactate concentration and $Scvo_2$, may guide specific interventions until critical care expertise is available.

V. ACID-BASE DISORDERS

Acid-base disorders are common in the critically ill patient, and assessment of acid-base status may indicate specific diagnoses and/or therapeutic interventions. The presence of a metabolic acidosis should suggest hypoperfusion and prompt further assessment of the adequacy of the oxygen balance. Appropriate evaluation of acid-base status requires accurate interpretation of simultaneous measurements of electrolytes, albumin, and arterial blood gases, as well as knowledge of compensatory physiologic responses.

A. Evaluation of Acid-Base Disorders

Analysis of acid-base disorders in seriously ill patients requires a systematic approach. Although several methods can be utilized (base excess, strong ion difference), the approach below relies on traditional analysis using formulas based on hydrogen ion and bicarbonate (HCO_3) concentrations.

1. Determine the overall acid-base condition by measuring pH. Is acidemia or alkalemia present?
2. If an abnormality is present, determine if the primary process is metabolic (change in $[HCO_3]$) or respiratory (change in $Paco_2$).
3. If a respiratory disturbance is present, determine if it is an acute or a chronic process.
4. If a metabolic disturbance is present, determine if respiratory compensation is adequate.
5. Always calculate the anion gap (AG).
6. If an AG metabolic acidosis is present, calculate the delta gap (Δgap) to determine if other metabolic disturbances are present.

B. Metabolic Acidosis

Metabolic acidosis results from an increase in endogenous acid production that overwhelms renal excretion (eg, ketoacidosis, lactic acidosis), exogenous acid input (eg, toxin ingestion), excessive loss of bicarbonate (eg, diarrhea), or decreased renal excretion of endogenous acids (eg, renal failure). Compensation is achieved primarily by increasing minute ventilation to eliminate CO_2. The adequacy of respiratory compensation can be estimated by the following formulas:

Appropriate $Paco_2 = 1.5 \times [HCO_3] + 8 \pm 2$; or $\Delta Paco_2 = 1.2 \times \Delta[HCO_3]$

The lower limit of respiratory compensation is $Paco_2$ of approximately 10 mm Hg (1.3 kPa).

Metabolic acidosis is further characterized by a normal or increased anion gap. Normally, unmeasured anions exceed unmeasured cations, and the difference results in the AG, which is estimated by the following formula:

$$AG = [Na] - ([Cl] + [HCO_3])$$

The normal AG value is approximately 10 ± 4 mmol/L but the normal range varies by laboratory. An increased AG indicates an increase in unmeasured anions and/or a decrease in unmeasured cations. An increased AG has limitations as the sole indicator of a metabolic acidosis. In patients with severe hypoalbuminemia, an AG acidosis can exist even when a normal AG is measured. In such patients, the expected AG may be as low as 4 to 5 mmol/L. For every albumin decrease of 1 g/dL, a decrease of 2.5 to 3 mmol in AG will occur. The corrected AG can be calculated using the following formula:

$$AG_{corrected} = AG_{observed} + 2.5 \times [\text{normal albumin-measured albumin (in g/dL)}]$$

Another exception can occur when an elevated AG does not reflect an underlying acidosis. In patients with significant alkalemia (usually pH >7.5), albumin is more negatively charged, which increases unmeasured anions.

In an uncomplicated AG metabolic acidosis, every AG increase of 1 mmol/L beyond the normal value should result in a concomitant decrease of 1 mmol/L in $[HCO_3]$. Deviation from this relationship suggests a mixed acid-base disorder. The difference between the change in the AG and the change in $[HCO_3]$ from the normal values is the Δgap, which can be expressed as follows:

$$\Delta gap = (\text{deviation of AG from normal}) - (\text{deviation of } [HCO_3] \text{ from normal})$$

The normal value for Δgap should be 0. However, variance in measurements can result in a Δgap of 0 ± 6. If the Δgap is positive, then a simultaneous metabolic alkalosis exists. If the decrease in $[HCO_3]$ is greater than the increase in AG, which results in a negative Δgap, then a concomitant normal AG acidosis (hyperchloremic) may exist. Small deviations of the Δgap may not indicate mixed acid-base disorders, and clinical information must always be considered.

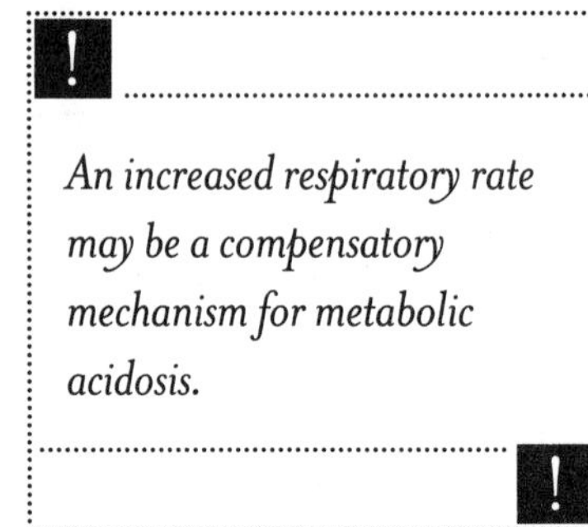

The most common causes of metabolic acidosis with an increased AG in seriously ill patients are lactic acidosis, renal failure, and diabetic ketoacidosis. Metabolic acidosis with a normal AG, often called *hyperchloremic acidosis*, may result from gastrointestinal or renal loss of HCO_3 or volume resuscitation with normal saline.

C. Metabolic Alkalosis

Metabolic alkaloses are usually characterized as chloride-depleted (hypovolemic) and chloride-expanded (hypervolemic). Hypokalemia is common to both types of metabolic alkalosis. Measurement of urine chloride is helpful in distinguishing the two categories, with urine chloride $<$20 mmol/L in chloride-depleted metabolic alkaloses and urine chloride $>$20 mmol/L in chloride-expanded metabolic alkaloses. Diuretic therapy is a common cause of hypovolemic metabolic alkalosis in hospitalized patients. Normal compensation for metabolic alkalosis is hypoventilation, which is limited by hypoxemia as $Paco_2$ increases in patients breathing spontaneously. $Paco_2$ may rise 6 to 7 mm Hg (0.8 to 0.9 kPa) for every increase of 10 mmol/L in $[HCO_3]$. Treatment includes volume replacement for chloride-depleted states and assessment of the renal-adrenal axis for chloride-expanded conditions. Potassium deficiencies should be corrected. Severe alkalemia is associated with high mortality and requires aggressive treatment.

D. Respiratory Acidosis

Respiratory acidosis is most commonly due to ineffective alveolar ventilation. If the respiratory acidosis is acute, the pH decreases by 0.08 units for each increase of 10 mm Hg (1.3 kPa) in $Paco_2$. A very small increase in plasma $[HCO_3]$ can be seen acutely because of titration of intracellular non-bicarbonate buffers. For each acute increase of 10 mm Hg (1.3 kPa) in $Paco_2$, the $[HCO_3]$ increases by 1 mmol/L to a maximum of 30 to 32 mmol/L. In chronic respiratory acidosis, the pH decreases 0.03 units and the $[HCO_3]$ increases 3.5 mmol/L for each increase of 10 mm Hg (1.3 kPa) in $Paco_2$. The limit of normal renal compensation in chronic respiratory acidosis is an $[HCO_3]$ of approximately 45 mmol/L. Higher values suggest an associated metabolic alkalosis. Treatment of respiratory acidosis involves the rapid identification of the etiology and implementation of corrective action. In some circumstances, intubation and mechanical ventilation may be necessary to support alveolar ventilation.

E. Respiratory Alkalosis

Respiratory alkalosis results from primary hyperventilation due to a variety of etiologies. Acute pulmonary processes or an acidosis should be considered in the seriously ill patient. Similar to changes noted in respiratory acidosis, pH increases 0.08 for every decrease of 10 mm Hg (1.3 kPa) in $Paco_2$ in acute respiratory alkalosis, and pH increases 0.03 for each decrease of 10 mm Hg (1.3 kPa) in $Paco_2$ in chronic respiratory alkalosis. The $[HCO_3]$ decreases 2 mmol/L in acute respiratory alkalosis and 5 mmol/L in chronic respiratory alkalosis for each decrease of 10 mm Hg (1.3 kPa) in $Paco_2$. Chronic respiratory alkalosis is unique among acid-base disorders in that pH may return to normal if the condition is prolonged. Therapy is directed to the underlying cause.

F. Complex Acid-Base Disorders

Simple acid-base disorders result from a single process such as metabolic alkalosis. In many critically ill patients, multiple acid-base disturbances exist concurrently and result in complex acid-base disorders. For example, septic shock often presents with respiratory alkalosis and metabolic acidosis. A systematic approach to acid-base analysis is needed to identify the ongoing disturbances and determine appropriate diagnoses and interventions. Formulas that are helpful in evaluating acid-base status are listed in **Table 6-5**.

Table 6-5 Acid-Base Formulas

Acid-Base Disorder	Equation
Respiratory Acidosis	
Acute	Decrease in pH = $0.08 \times \frac{(Paco_2 - 40)}{10}$
	Increase in $[HCO_3]$ = $\frac{\Delta Paco_2 \pm 3}{10}$
Chronic	Decrease in pH = $0.03 \times \frac{(Paco_2 - 40)}{10}$
	Increase in $[HCO_3]$ = $3.5 \times \frac{\Delta Paco_2}{10}$
Respiratory Alkalosis	
Acute	Increase in pH = $0.08 \times \frac{(40 - Paco_2)}{10}$
	Decrease in $[HCO_3]$ = $2 \times \frac{\Delta Paco_2}{10}$
Chronic	Increase in pH = $0.03 \times \frac{(40 - Paco_2)}{10}$
	Decrease in $[HCO_3]$ = $5 - 7 \times \frac{\Delta Paco_2}{10}$
Metabolic Acidosis	Anion Gap = $[Na] - ([Cl] + [HCO_3])$
	Expected $Paco_2 = 1.5 \times [HCO_3] + 8 \pm 2$ or expected $\Delta Pco_2 = 1.2 \times \Delta[HCO_3]$
	Δgap = (Measured Anion Gap – Normal Anion Gap) – $(24 - [HCO_3])$
Metabolic Alkalosis	Increase in $Paco_2 = 0.6 - 0.7 \times \Delta[HCO_3]$

Key Points

Monitoring Oxygen Balance and Acid-Base Status

- Oxygen delivery is dependent on cardiac output (blood flow) and the oxygen content of arterial blood.
- Hemoglobin is the major contributor of oxygen for tissue demands.
- Normal ventricular filling pressure measurements may not indicate adequate preload volume.
- Measurements of global oxygen balance that may be useful to monitor in the seriously ill patient include central venous oxyhemoglobin saturation ($Scvo_2$) and lactate concentrations.
- Low $Scvo_2$ values suggest an oxygen imbalance that may be due to decreases in cardiac output, hemoglobin concentrations, or arterial oxyhemoglobin saturation, or increases in tissue oxygen consumption.
- The pulse oximeter estimates arterial oxyhemoglobin saturation but does not reflect adequacy of oxygen delivery.
- Blood pressure monitoring via an arterial catheter is preferable to the use of an automated blood pressure device in unstable patients.
- Assessment of acid-base status may suggest specific diagnoses and/or therapeutic interventions.

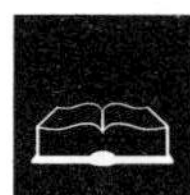

Suggested Readings

1. Gauthier PM, Szerlip HM. Metabolic acidosis in the intensive care unit. *Crit Care Clin.* 2002;18:289-308.
2. Huang YC. Monitoring oxygen delivery in the critically ill. *Chest.* 2005;128:554S-560S.
3. Kellum JA. Disorders of acid-base balance. *Crit Care Med.* 2007;35:2630-2636.
4. Magder S. Central venous pressure monitoring. *Curr Opin Crit Care.* 2006;12:219-227.
5. Marx G, Reinhart K. Venous oximetry. *Curr Opin Crit Care.* 2006;12:263-268.
6. McMorrow RC, Mythen MG. Pulse oximetry. *Curr Opin Crit Care.* 2006;12:269-271.
7. Michard F. Changes in arterial pressure during mechanical ventilation. *Anesthesiology.* 2005;103:419-428.

8. Nguyen HB, Rivers EP, Knoblich BP, et al. Early lactate clearance is associated with improved outcome in severe sepsis and septic shock. *Crit Care Med.* 2004;32:1637-1642.

9. Shelley KH. Photoplethysmography: Beyond the calculation of arterial oxygen saturation and heart rate. *Anesth Analg.* 2007;105:S31-S36.

10. Whittier WL, Rutecki GW. Primer on clinical acid-base problem solving. *Dis Mon.* 2004;50:122-162.

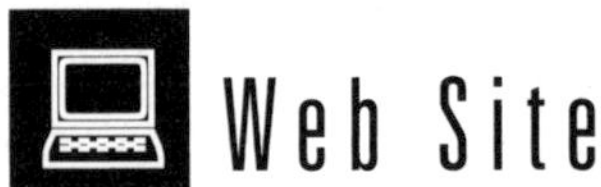

Web Site

1. Ortega R, Hansen CJ, Elterman K, et al. Pulse Oximetry. *N Engl J Med.* 2011;364:e33. http://www.nejm.org/multimedia/medical-videos. *Demonstration of use of pulse oximetry.*

Chapter 7

DIAGNOSIS AND MANAGEMENT OF SHOCK

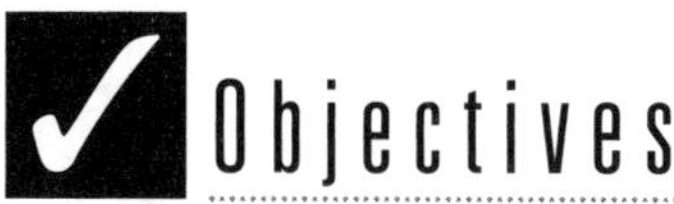

Objectives

- Identify the four main categories of shock.
- Discuss the goals of resuscitation in shock.
- Summarize the general principles of shock management.
- Describe the physiologic effects of vasoactive and inotropic agents.
- Discuss the differential diagnosis of oliguria.

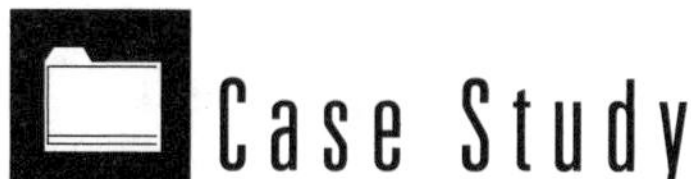

Case Study

A 25-year-old woman presents to the emergency department complaining of a cough productive of tenacious greenish yellow mucus. Vital signs are temperature 101.8°F (38.8°C), heart rate 129/min, respiratory rate 27/min, and blood pressure 112/68 mm Hg.

- What information is needed to determine if this patient has shock?
- What initial interventions are needed to stabilize the patient?

I. INTRODUCTION

Shock is a syndrome of impaired tissue oxygenation and perfusion due to a variety of etiologies. Prompt recognition of shock and early, effective intervention is needed to prevent irreversible injury, organ dysfunction, and death. Inadequate tissue oxygenation and perfusion may result from one or more of the following mechanisms:

- An absolute or relative decrease in systemic oxygen delivery (inadequate cardiac output, low blood oxygen content)
- Ineffective tissue perfusion (maldistribution of blood flow to tissues or inadequate perfusion pressure)
- Impaired utilization of delivered oxygen (cellular or mitochondrial dysfunction)

Shock results when the oxygen balance is disturbed and demand exceeds supply. Shock is not defined by hypotension, although hypotension is frequently associated with shock. In some patients with shock, the blood pressure initially may be normal even though it has significantly dropped from baseline, or it may be preserved due to compensatory sympathetic responses. Management of shock should be directed toward correcting the oxygen balance and hypoperfusion as the primary end points.

II. CLINICAL ALTERATIONS IN SHOCK

The presentation of patients with shock may be subtle (mild confusion, tachycardia) or easily identifiable (profound hypotension, anuria). Shock may be the initial manifestation of an underlying condition or it may develop as the condition progresses. A strong index of suspicion and vigilant clinical assessment are needed to identify the early signs and initiate appropriate treatment. The clinical manifestations of shock result from inadequate tissue oxygenation and perfusion, compensatory responses, and the specific etiology of shock. Hypoperfusion of end organs may result in hypotension, altered mental status, oliguria/anuria, and other organ dysfunction. In addition, hypoperfusion is associated with some degree of inflammatory response that may contribute to organ injury. Direct and indirect effects of hypoperfusion may be reflected in laboratory findings of abnormal oxygenation, blood urea nitrogen, creatinine, bilirubin, hepatic transaminases, and coagulation parameters. An anion gap metabolic acidosis is one of the most common findings of hypoperfusion. Acidosis is often associated with an elevated lactate concentration. Although neither sensitive nor specific for the diagnosis of shock, the lactate concentration is an indicator of hypoperfusion and a relevant monitoring tool for assessment of therapeutic interventions.

Compensatory mechanisms in shock involve complex neuroendocrine responses that attempt to increase tissue perfusion and oxygenation. In many forms of shock, sympathetic vasoconstriction redirects blood flow from low-oxygen-requiring organs (eg, skin) toward oxygen-dependent organs (eg, brain and heart). Compensatory vasoconstriction can maintain blood pressure early

> *The increased systemic vascular resistance present in cardiogenic, hemorrhagic, and obstructive shock is the body's attempt to maintain blood pressure (perfusion pressure).*

in shock and lead to an increase in the diastolic pressure and a narrowing of the pulse pressure. Intense vasoconstriction correlates with cold, clammy extremities and contributes to organ hypoperfusion. Hypothermia also may be a manifestation of severe vasoconstriction. Patients with distributive shock (see next section) often have vasodilation and warm extremities, but other signs of hypoperfusion are usually present. Tachycardia, mediated by the sympathetic response, reflects an attempt to increase cardiac output in shock. Tachypnea may be a compensatory response to metabolic acidosis, a response to lung injury, or a reaction to direct stimulation of the respiratory center.

Additional changes in shock alter oxygenation at the tissue level. As discussed in **Chapter 6**, hemoglobin releases more oxygen as it traverses the capillaries in order to meet tissue demands. A rightward shift of the oxyhemoglobin saturation curve due to acidosis or increased temperature facilitates release of hemoglobin-bound oxygen. The greater extraction of oxygen is reflected in lower venous oxyhemoglobin saturation (Svo_2) or central venous oxyhemoglobin saturation ($Scvo_2$) measurements in many forms of shock (**Chapter 6**). However, a normal value of Svo_2 does not imply that tissue oxygenation is adequate because some forms of shock (eg, septic shock) may lead to impaired tissue or cellular utilization of oxygen or result in maldistribution of blood flow.

III. CLASSIFICATION OF SHOCK

There are four main categories of shock based on cardiovascular characteristics: hypovolemic, distributive, cardiogenic, and obstructive (**Table 7-1**). A careful history and a physical examination often provide information that is helpful in determining the likely cause of shock. However, many patients will have components of more than one type (mixed shock). Septic shock is a form of distributive shock, but it may have a hypovolemic component before fluid resuscitation. Likewise, myocardial dysfunction may be present in septic shock and hypovolemic shock.

Table 7-1 Classifications of Shock

Hypovolemic	**Cardiogenic**
Hemorrhagic	Myopathic (ie, ischemic)
Nonhemorrhagic	Mechanical (ie, valvular)
	Arrhythmic
Distributive	**Obstructive**
Septic	Massive pulmonary embolism
Adrenal crisis	Tension pneumothorax
Neurogenic (spinal shock)	Cardiac tamponade
Anaphylactic	Constrictive pericarditis

Knowledge of the expected hemodynamic profiles associated with different types of shock is helpful in determining appropriate therapy, even when specific measurements are not available. **Table 7-2** presents the usual hemodynamic profiles for more common forms of shock, but variations occur depending on the patient's specific etiology, cardiac function, and resuscitation status.

Table 7-2 Hemodynamic Profiles of Shock

Type of Shock	Heart Rate	Cardiac Output	Ventricular Filling Pressures	Systemic Vascular Resistance	Pulse Pressure	$Svo_2/Scvo_2$
Cardiogenic	↑	↓	↑	↑	↓	↓
Hypovolemic	↑	↓	↓	↑	↓	↓
Distributive	↑	↑ or N[a]	↓	↓	↑	↑ or N[a]
Obstructive	↑	↓	↑ or N[b]	↑	↓	↓

Abbreviations: Svo_2, mixed venous oxyhemoglobin saturation; N, normal; $Scvo_2$, central venous oxyhemoglobin saturation

[a]May be decreased prior to or early in resuscitation.

[b]Left ventricular filling pressures may be normal or low in massive pulmonary embolism.

A. Hypovolemic Shock

Hypovolemic shock occurs when intravascular volume is depleted relative to the vascular capacity as a result of hemorrhage, gastrointestinal or urinary fluid losses, dehydration, or third-space fluid losses. Third-space fluid losses resulting from interstitial fluid redistribution may be prominent in burn injury, trauma, pancreatitis, and any severe form of shock. The hemodynamic findings in hypovolemic shock are decreased cardiac output, decreased right and left ventricular filling pressures (preload), and an increased afterload (systemic vascular resistance [SVR]) due to compensatory vasoconstriction. The Svo_2 or $Scvo_2$ is decreased as a result of decreased cardiac output with unchanged or increased tissue oxygen demands and potentially decreased hemoglobin concentration (hemorrhage). In addition to the usual clinical findings, patients with hypovolemic shock have flat, nondistended jugular veins.

B. Distributive Shock

Distributive shock is characterized by loss of peripheral vascular tone (vasodilation). However, these patients often have components of hypovolemic shock and cardiogenic shock. The most common form of distributive shock is septic shock, with neurogenic shock and anaphylactic shock being much less common. The hemodynamic profile usually includes a normal or increased cardiac output with a low SVR and low to normal ventricular filling pressures. A consistent finding is increased pulse pressure. A decreased cardiac output may result if intravascular volume is not optimized. $Scvo_2$ or Svo_2 may be normal or increased due to shunting of blood in the microvasculature or the inability of tissue to utilize oxygen. In contrast to other forms of shock, the vasodilation of fluid-resuscitated distributive shock results in warm extremities, decreased diastolic pressure, and increased pulse pressure. Neurogenic shock may be associated with bradycardia rather than tachycardia. Fever may be present in septic shock and adrenal crisis.

C. Cardiogenic Shock

In cardiogenic shock, forward blood flow is inadequate because of cardiac pump failure due to loss of functional myocardium (ischemia, cardiomyopathy), a mechanical or structural defect (valvular failure, septal defect), or arrhythmias. Most commonly, cardiogenic shock results from acute myocardial infarction or a subsequent complication. Cardiogenic shock is the most severe form of heart failure and is distinguished from less severe chronic heart failure by the presence of hypoperfusion, hypotension, and the need for different therapeutic interventions (**Chapter 10**). The typical hemodynamic characteristics are decreased cardiac output, elevated ventricular filling pressures, and increased afterload (SVR). When cardiac output is low, the Svo_2 or $Scvo_2$ declines due to increased extraction of oxygen from hemoglobin at the tissue level. Clinical manifestations associated with cardiogenic shock may include distended jugular veins, pulmonary edema, and S_3 gallop.

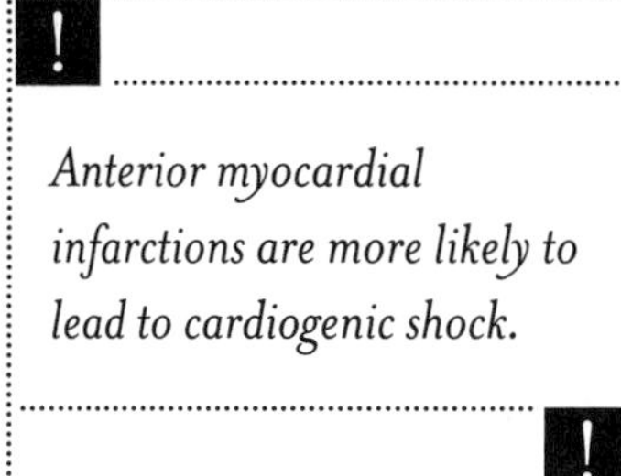
Anterior myocardial infarctions are more likely to lead to cardiogenic shock.

D. Obstructive Shock

The common features in obstructive shock are obstruction to flow due to impaired cardiac filling and excessive afterload. Cardiac tamponade and constrictive pericarditis impair diastolic filling of the right ventricle, while tension pneumothorax limits right ventricular filling by obstruction of venous return. Massive pulmonary emboli increase right ventricular afterload. The hemodynamic profile is characterized by decreased cardiac output, increased afterload, and variable left ventricular filling pressures, depending on the etiology. In cardiac tamponade, the pressures of the right heart chambers, the pulmonary artery, and the left heart chambers equilibrate in diastole. A drop of >10 mm Hg in systolic blood pressure during inspiration (pulsus paradoxus) is an important clinical finding in patients with suspected cardiac tamponade. Distended jugular veins may be seen, depending on the time course of development and intravascular volume status.

IV. GENERAL PRINCIPLES OF SHOCK MANAGEMENT

The overall goal of shock management is to improve oxygen delivery or utilization in order to prevent cellular and organ injury. Effective therapy requires treatment of the underlying etiology, restoration of adequate perfusion, monitoring, and comprehensive supportive care. Interventions to restore perfusion center on achieving an adequate blood pressure, increasing cardiac output, and/or optimizing the oxygen content of blood. Oxygen demand should also be decreased when possible. These goals are usually accomplished with a combination of interventions, as summarized in **Table 7-3**.

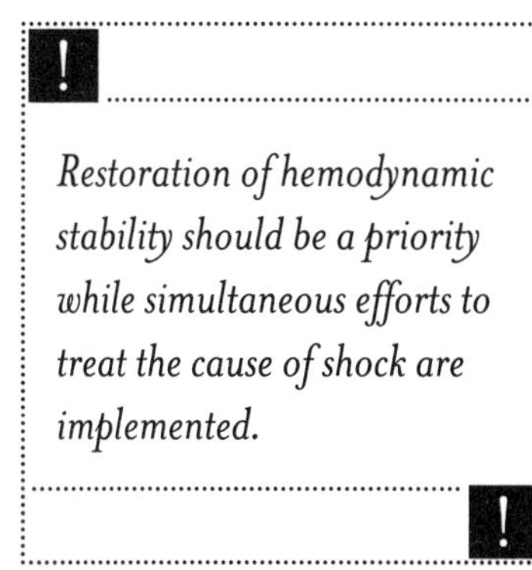
Restoration of hemodynamic stability should be a priority while simultaneous efforts to treat the cause of shock are implemented.

Table 7-3 Interventions for Managing Shock

Component	Intervention
Blood pressure	Fluids, vasopressor or vasodilator agents[a]
Cardiac Output	
Preload	Fluids, vasodilator agents[a]
Contractility	Inotropic agents
Afterload	Vasopressor or vasodilator agents[a]
Oxygen Content	
Hemoglobin	Blood transfusion
Hemoglobin saturation	Supplemental oxygen, mechanical ventilation
Oxygen demand	Mechanical ventilation, sedation, analgesia, antipyretics

[a]Vasodilator agents are used only when blood pressure is adequate (see text).

The first goal in treating hypotensive shock is to achieve a minimum blood pressure (driving pressure). This is needed to maintain blood flow to the heart and other organs while optimizing other components of oxygen delivery. A mean arterial pressure (MAP) ≥65 mm Hg is usually recommended as an initial goal. A higher MAP may be needed in patients with myocardial ischemia or chronic hypertension, but an increase in blood pressure is beneficial only if it translates into improved perfusion. Otherwise, higher blood pressures may increase myocardial oxygen demands. Following initial resuscitation, the MAP goal should be individualized based on further assessment of the adequacy of systemic and organ perfusion. A blood pressure goal is usually achieved with fluids and/or vasoactive agents (discussed later).

The next goal in the management of shock is to optimize oxygen delivery. As outlined in **Chapter 6**, this can be enhanced by increasing cardiac output, hemoglobin concentration, or oxyhemoglobin saturation. In the absence of specific measurement of cardiac output, an assessment of adequacy depends on the etiology of shock and the presence of hypoperfusion abnormalities (discussed later). Fluids and/or vasoactive agents are often needed to optimize cardiac output. The determinants of the oxygen content of blood (hemoglobin and oxyhemoglobin saturation) can be easily measured and optimized when indicated. Increasing hemoglobin concentration by transfusion may be one of the most efficient ways of improving oxygen delivery in some patients. For example, increasing the hemoglobin concentration from 7 g/dL to 9 g/dL increases oxygen delivery by almost 30%, even if cardiac output remains constant. The oxyhemoglobin saturation can be increased raising the Pa_{O_2} with oxygen supplementation and mechanical ventilation. However, once the Pa_{O_2} has been increased to a range of 60 to 70 mm Hg (8-9.3 kPa), little additional benefit is gained by increasing it further. An oxyhemoglobin saturation ≥95% is recommended in patients with shock.

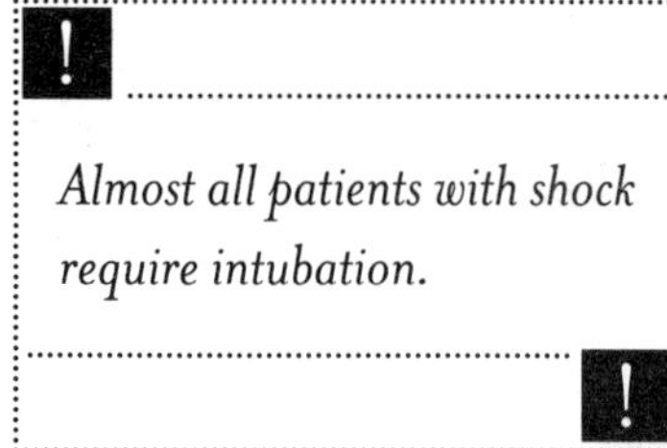

A. Monitoring

Patients with shock require monitoring to determine the appropriate interventions and to assess their response to interventions (**Chapter 6**). Continuous electrocardiographic monitoring is needed to assess changes in heart rate and rhythm. Blood pressure is best watched with an arterial catheter due to the inaccuracy of noninvasive devices in patients with shock. Pulse oximetry should be monitored routinely to ensure adequate oxyhemoglobin saturation. Central venous pressure (CVP) may be helpful in selected patients as an indicator of right ventricular preload. Measurement of $Scvo_2$ via a central venous catheter may be useful as an indicator of oxygen balance, but a normal $Scvo_2$ value does not rule out hypoperfusion. A urinary catheter should be inserted to monitor urine output as an indicator of renal perfusion, with a suggested goal of 0.5 to 1 mL/kg/h. Lactate concentrations should be measured initially and at appropriate intervals. A normal or decreasing lactate concentration suggests improved oxygen balance. Other laboratory data should be monitored with the goal of assessing progression or improvement of organ dysfunction.

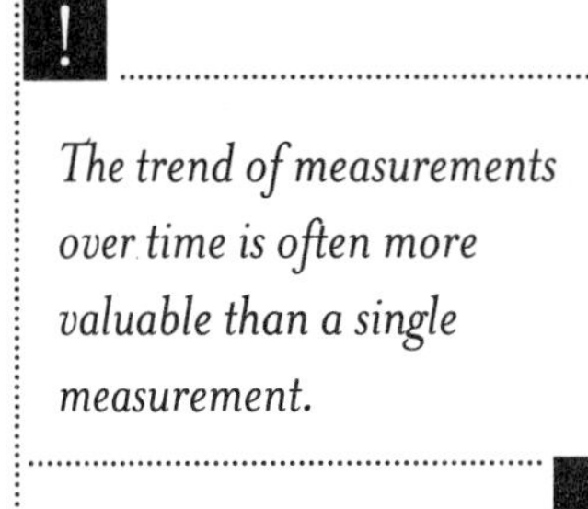

The trend of measurements over time is often more valuable than a single measurement.

B. Fluid Therapy

The initial therapy for most forms of shock is replacement of intravascular volume. Physical examination may provide valuable information about the intravascular volume status. Diffuse or dependent crackles, as well as distended neck veins, suggest high ventricular filling pressures, unless acute respiratory distress syndrome or diffuse pneumonia is present. Clear lung fields and flat neck veins suggest inadequate preload in the hypotensive patient. Although orthostatic changes in blood pressure and heart rate may be helpful in assessing the degree of volume depletion, patients with hypotension or severe tachycardia should not be subjected to such positional changes. The nature and degree of fluid deficit should be determined to identify the necessary type of fluid replacement. Pulse pressure variation noted on a pulse oximeter or arterial pressure waveform may be used to determine fluid responsiveness (**Chapter 6**).

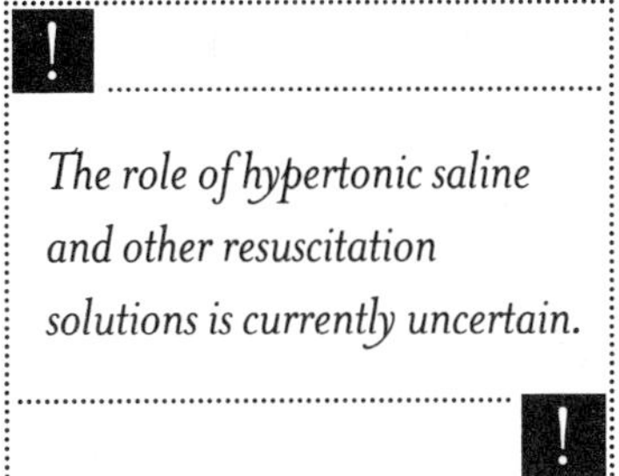

The role of hypertonic saline and other resuscitation solutions is currently uncertain.

Intravascular volume deficiency in the patient who is not anemic may be replenished with either crystalloid or colloid solutions. Crystalloids are less expensive than colloids and typically accomplish the same goals, although a higher total volume is needed due to their higher volume of distribution. Isotonic crystalloid solutions, such as lactated Ringer's solution or normal saline, should be used for volume resuscitation. Dextrose 5% in water offers little expansion of intravascular volume since it is quickly distributed throughout body fluid compartments and should not be used to treat hypovolemic shock. For the same reasons, 0.45% saline is not appropriate for volume expansion. Colloid solutions include hetastarch, albumin, and gelatins. Crystalloid in titrated boluses of 500 to 1000 mL (10-20 mL/kg) or colloid in titrated boluses of 250 to 500 mL may be given initially to most adult patients and repeated as necessary while appropriate parameters are closely monitored. Smaller bolus amounts are indicated for patients with suspected or known cardiogenic shock.

In addition to crystalloid or colloid solutions, packed red blood cells are indicated to increase oxygen-carrying capacity in the patient with significant bleeding or anemia. In many critically ill patients, a hemoglobin concentration of 7 to 9 g/dL may be adequate after stabilization, but a higher hemoglobin may be needed during acute resuscitation. Fresh frozen plasma should be used only for correction of a coagulopathy and not for volume replacement. Priorities in the administration of fluids are resuscitation and then replacement of ongoing losses. As the patient's clinical course continues, the solution that most closely approximates the patient's losses should be used with serum electrolytes guiding therapy.

The first target in fluid resuscitation is correction of hypovolemia. Often, correction of hypovolemia manifests clinically as resolution of tachycardia, hypotension, or oliguria. However, these end points may remain altered despite euvolemia in states such as septic (distributive), neurogenic, or obstructive shock. Vasoactive drug support is indicated in patients who continue to have a low blood pressure or impaired cardiac output after euvolemia has been established. The potential deleterious effects of overly aggressive fluid resuscitation include deterioration of oxygenation due to pulmonary edema, ileus or bowel edema, and compartment syndromes. Therefore, frequent auscultation of the chest for the presence of crackles, monitoring of Pao_2 or oxyhemoglobin saturation by pulse oximetry, and CVP monitoring should be performed during fluid resuscitation. Intra-abdominal pressure monitoring should be considered in patients requiring massive fluid resuscitation (**Chapter 13**). In the absence of invasive hemodynamic monitoring, volume therapy should be administered carefully in patients with persistent hypotension and/or hypoperfusion until no further change is noted in the blood pressure following a fluid bolus. This suggests that the patient has obtained a euvolemic state and administration of more fluid can lead to the deleterious effects noted. Further correction of hypotension or other perfusion abnormalities may require pharmacologic support with vasoactive drugs. This approach to volume therapy presents minimal risk in patients with adequate oxygenation.

C. Vasoactive Agents

Vasoactive agents for the acute management of shock include medications with vasopressor, inotropic, and vasodilator effects. A vasopressor is a medication that has α_1-adrenergic activity resulting in arteriole constriction, rise in systemic vascular resistance, and rise in arterial blood pressure. An inotrope is a medication that augments cardiac contractility through β_1-adrenergic effects. Many agents have more than one hemodynamic effect, and results may vary among individual patients and with dosage. The goals of resuscitation are usually more important than the specific agent chosen. **Table 7-4** summarizes each vasoactive drug and its mechanism of action. An intensivist should be consulted when the decision to use vasoactive medications is made.

> !
>
> *No one vasoactive agent or combination of agents has been demonstrated to be superior in managing shock.*
>
> !

Table 7-4 Vasoactive Agents

	DA-R (↑UOP)	B_1[a] (↑ HR)	B_2[b] (↓BP)	α_1[c] (↑ BP)
Dopamine 1-20 µg/kg/min	1-5 µg/kg/min	6-10 µg/kg/min		>10 µg/kg/min
Phenylephrine (Neo-Synephrine®) 1-300 µg/min				+++
Norepinephrine (Levophed®) 0.01-0.5 µg/kg/min		+		++++
Epinephrine 0.01-0.5 µg/kg/min		++++	+++	++++
Dobutamine (1-20 µg/kg/min)		+++	++	
Milrinone (0.125-0.5 µg/kg/min)		+++	+++	

Abbreviations: DA-R, dopamine receptor; UOP, urine output; HR, heart rate; BP, blood pressure
Potency scale is from 1+ to 4+
[a]B_1 = adrenergic receptor which increases cardiac contractility and/or heart rate
[b]B_2 = adrenergic receptor which mediates bronchodilation and also arteriole dilation
[c]α_1 = adrenergic receptor which mediates arteriole constriction and increase in peripheral vascular resistance

1. Norepinephrine

Norepinephrine is one of two vasoactive drugs of choice in the treatment of septic shock, with dopamine being the other. It is a potent α-adrenergic vasoconstrictor with greater potency than either dopamine or phenylephrine, and it also has β1-mediated inotropic and chronotropic effects. In adults, the infusion rate of norepinephrine starts at 0.05 µg/kg/min and is titrated to desired effects. As with other vasoconstrictors, cardiac output may decrease as afterload and blood pressure are increased. Norepinephrine usually increases renal blood flow in patients with adequate volume resuscitation. An increase in heart rate is uncommon with use of norepinephrine.

2. Dopamine

Dopamine is a frequently used vasoactive agent with dose-dependent inotropic and vasopressor effects. It is one of two vasoactive drugs of choice in the treatment of septic shock, with norepinephrine being the other agent. Although dose response varies greatly among patients, some generalizations about dose and anticipated effect may be helpful. At low rates of infusion (2-3 µg/kg/min), dopamine has modest inotropic and chronotropic effects. In this dose range, it acts on the dopaminergic receptors in the kidney and may increase urine output; however, its use for renal effects is not recommended because it does not prevent renal dysfunction or improve outcomes. At intermediate rates of infusion (6-10 µg/kg/min), dopamine has primarily inotropic effects. At higher infusion rates (≥10 µg/kg/min), dopamine has significant α-agonist effects that produce dose-related vasoconstriction. At infusion rates ≥20 µg/kg/min, dopamine usually offers no advantage over norepinephrine, which may have greater vasopressor effect. Potential adverse effects include arrhythmias and tachycardia.

3. Epinephrine

Epinephrine has both α-adrenergic and β-adrenergic effects, potent inotropic and chronotropic effects; at higher doses, it has vasopressor effects. Doses start at 0.05 µg/kg/min and can be titrated as desired. The epinephrine-induced increase in myocardial oxygen consumption may limit the use of this agent in adults, especially in the presence of coronary artery disease. Mesenteric ischemia is more common with epinephrine than with other vasopressors.

4. Phenylephrine

Phenylephrine is a pure α-adrenergic vasoconstrictor. In adults, the infusion rate starts at 25 µg/min and can be titrated to the desired blood pressure. Because its mechanism of action involves solely arterial constriction, it is most useful in states with arterial dilation without concomitant cardiac depression, such as neurogenic shock or hypotension caused by an epidural catheter.

5. Vasopressin

Vasopressin is a potent vasopressor that acts through V_1 receptors to produce vasoconstriction. As blood pressure is increased, cardiac output may decrease, similar to the effect of norepinephrine. The recommended dose in adults is 0.01 to 0.04 units/min. Higher doses may lead to ischemic events. Vasopressin may be considered for use in hypotensive shock refractory to other agents and fluid resuscitation, but it has not been found to improve mortality. Further study is needed to define the role of vasopressin in the management of shock.

6. Dobutamine

Dobutamine is a non-selective β-adrenergic agonist with inotropic effects. It is used in doses of 5 to 20 µg/kg/min and is usually associated with an increase in cardiac output, which is mediated mostly by an increase in stroke volume. Arterial blood pressure may remain unchanged, decrease, or increase slightly. Dobutamine must be introduced with care in the hypotensive patient; in the face of inadequate intravascular volume replacement, blood pressure can drop precipitously, and tachycardia may be problematic. This agent has variable chronotropic effects.

7. Milrinone

Milrinone is a phosphodiesterase inhibitor that inhibits the breakdown of cyclic adenosine monophosphate, the second messenger for catecholamines. Therefore, milrinone is a sympathomimetic agent with mostly β-adrenergic-like effects. It will increase cardiac output mostly by increasing stroke volume and will decrease afterload by causing arteriole dilation. It should be used with caution in hypovolemic patients because it can cause significant hypotension.

D. End Points of Resuscitation

No one end point can be used to assess resolution of shock and return to normal homeostasis. Furthermore, for any end point, the trend is more important than static value, and fluid and pharmacologic therapy should be titrated based on the trend for the particular end point rather than its absolute value.

Blood pressure, pulse, and urine output are the most commonly used end points in resuscitation of shock. All parameters can be easily measured but lack sensitivity and specificity for either detection of impending shock or its resolution. As such, they may be normal if the patient is in a state of compensated shock, and they may remain abnormal despite appropriate therapy (eg, low blood pressure and urine output despite reaching a euvolemic state). Similarly, urine output may not be a reliable end point in patients with pre-existing, advanced renal dysfunction.

Invasive monitoring may be helpful in guiding therapy. CVP and pulmonary capillary occlusion pressure measure preload, but normal values for these indices vary based on cardiac compliance and transpulmonary pressure. Therefore, although the trend in the filling pressure values may help guide fluid therapy, the absolute value can be misleading. Correlation of the ventricular or venous pressure with an echocardiogram allows one to discern the cardiac response to specific therapies and may be an ideal way of directing fluid resuscitation.

Biochemical tests also can be followed as markers of hypoperfusion and end points for resuscitation of shock. Two of the most commonly ordered tests include the base deficit, which is calculated from the arterial blood gas, and the serum lactate. The base deficit is a measure of base or acid that is required to normalize the arterial pH and is used as an index of the severity of acid (or base) accumulation. The base deficit will be negative in under-resuscitated shock and will approach zero as perfusion is reestablished. Similarly, lactate is produced under anaerobic cellular conditions associated with end-organ hypoperfusion and clears once homeostasis is reached. Of note, neither end point assesses the need for fluid versus pharmacologic support of the circulation.

V. MANAGEMENT OF SPECIFIC TYPES OF SHOCK

A. Hypovolemic Shock

The treatment goals for hypovolemic shock are restoration of intravascular volume and prevention of further volume loss. Therapy of hypovolemic shock should be targeted to reestablish normal blood pressure, pulse, and organ perfusion. For initial resuscitation, either colloid or crystalloid fluids are effective if given in sufficient volume. Subsequently, the fluid that is used should replace the fluid that has been lost. For example, blood products may be needed to replace blood loss (**Chapter 9**), and crystalloid should be used for vomiting and dehydration. For hypotension, the crystalloid of choice is normal saline or lactated Ringer's solution because of the osmolality needed to restore intravascular volume. In large volume resuscitation, however, normal saline infusion may produce hyperchloremic metabolic acidosis. Vasoactive medications should be considered only as a temporizing measure while fluid resuscitation is ongoing or when hypotension persists despite adequate volume resuscitation. CVP monitoring may help to guide fluid resuscitation in patients without significant heart or lung disease. Resuscitation of rapidly exsanguinating patients may be optimally performed by transfusing near-equivalent amounts of packed red blood cells, fresh frozen plasma, and platelets (**Chapter 9**).

B. Distributive Shock

The initial approach to the patient with septic shock is restoration and maintenance of adequate intravascular volume. Obtaining cultures and prompt institution of appropriate antibiotics are essential, as are other interventions to control the infection (removal of catheter, surgery, drainage, debridement). Early goal-directed therapy using CVP monitoring and measurement of $Scvo_2$ has been shown to reduce mortality in severe sepsis and septic shock (**Figure 7-1**).

Figure 7-1. Protocol for Resuscitation of Hypovolemic and Distributive Shock

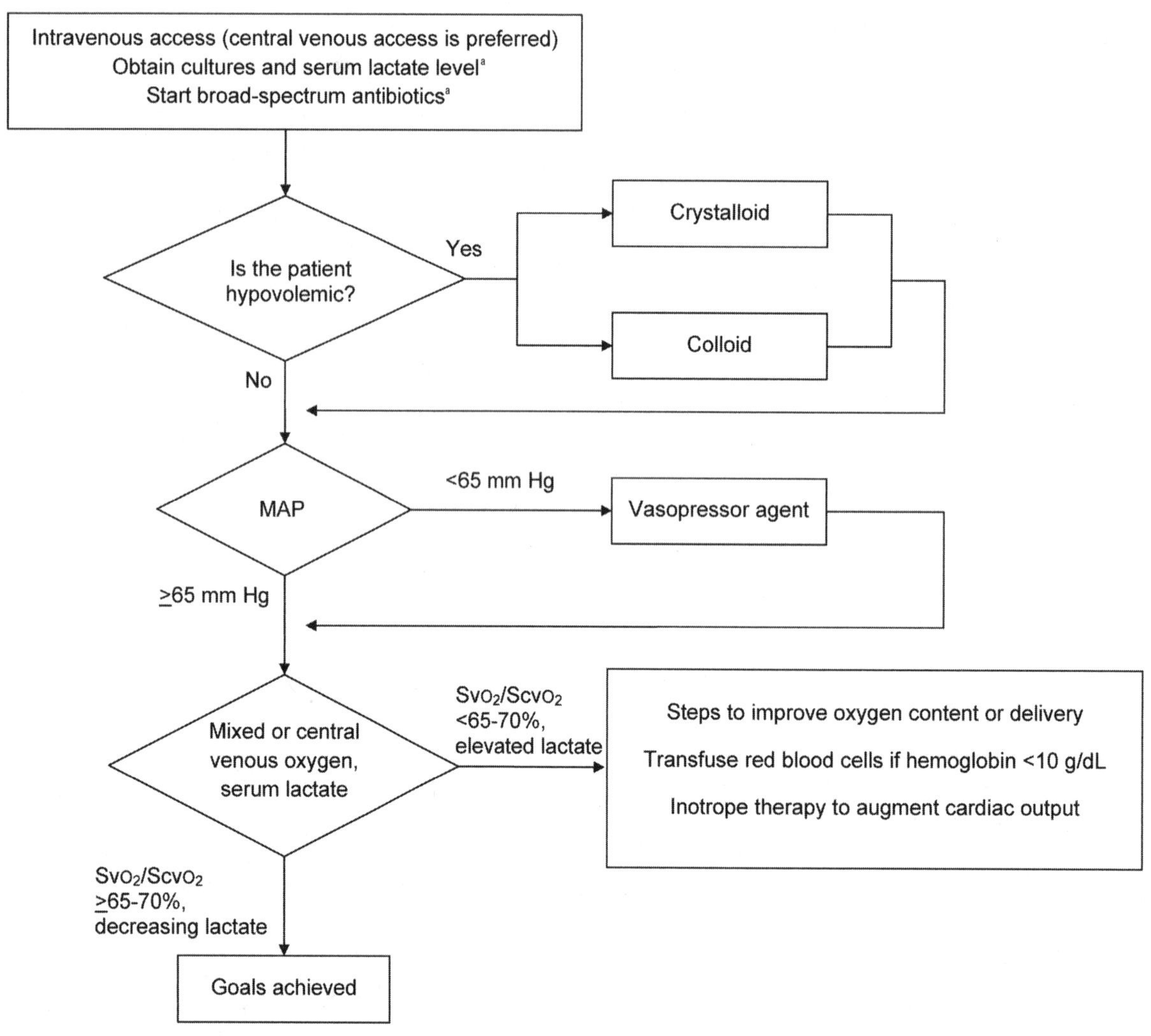

Abbreviations: MAP, mean arterial pressure; $Svo_2/Scvo_2$ = mixed or central venous oxygenation saturation
[a]Where infection is possible

Volume expansion can be initiated with isotonic crystalloid or colloid solutions. Vasodilation and diffuse capillary leaks are common in septic shock, and fluid requirements may be large. If the patient with septic shock remains hypotensive despite adequate fluid resuscitation, dopamine or norepinephrine is recommended as the initial vasoactive drug. Low-dose vasopressin or epinephrine can be considered for patients who fail to respond adequately to first-line vasoactive agents, but these agents have not been shown to improve survival. Dobutamine should be considered in patients with adequate blood pressure who have hypoperfusion and low cardiac output with adequate ventricular preload. Reversible myocardial dysfunction with ventricular dilation and decrease in ejection fraction frequently occurs in septic shock. An initial MAP <65 mm Hg may require initiation of vasoactive pharmacologic therapy until fluid resuscitation is optimized. Corticosteroids (hydrocortisone 200-300 mg in 24 hours administered as boluses or continuous infusion) should be considered in patients with septic shock when the blood pressure is poorly responsive to fluids and vasoactive medications. Anaphylactic shock is treated with volume resuscitation and subcutaneous epinephrine. In circumstances of very low blood pressure and poor peripheral perfusion, titrated intravenous epinephrine is indicated. Acute adrenal insufficiency is treated with volume therapy, intravenous corticosteroids, and vasoactive medications, if needed (**Chapter 12**). See **Chapter 9** for information about the management of neurogenic shock.

C. Cardiogenic Shock

The primary goal in treating cardiogenic shock is to improve myocardial function. Arrhythmias should be treated promptly. Reperfusion by percutaneous intervention is the treatment of choice in cardiogenic shock due to myocardial ischemia (**Chapter 10**). Diastolic dysfunction during myocardial ischemia may decrease ventricular compliance and elevate the left ventricular filling pressures, falsely indicating adequate preload. Therefore, a cautious trial of fluid administration may be warranted (250-mL bolus amounts). When blood pressure is decreased in cardiogenic shock, initial therapy with a single agent that has inotropic and vasopressor effects (eg, norepinephrine or dopamine) is indicated. Severely hypotensive patients (systolic arterial pressure <70 mm Hg) should be treated with norepinephrine to rapidly raise the systolic arterial pressure. The addition of an intravenous inotrope, such as milrinone or dobutamine (or dopexamine, which is available in some countries), may be considered to augment myocardial contractility after blood pressure stabilizes, with the goal of decreasing vasopressor therapy. If moderate hypotension is not responsive to initial therapy, consultation should be sought for steps such as intra-aortic balloon counterpulsation or left/right ventricular assist devices.

The elevated afterload (SVR) may also impair cardiac output if it is a primary hemodynamic alteration, as occurs in chronic congestive heart failure. Often in acute cardiogenic shock, the SVR is secondarily elevated to maintain vascular perfusion pressure. Treatment aimed primarily at reducing afterload with a vasodilator, such as nitroprusside, should be initiated very cautiously and only in patients with hypoperfusion accompanied by adequate blood pressure.

> **!** *Afterload and preload reduction should be avoided in cardiac failure when hypotension is present.*

When cardiac failure is characterized by low cardiac output, normal or elevated blood pressure, and hypoxemia due to high pulmonary capillary pressure, reduction of preload and afterload is helpful in improving hypoxemia. High pulmonary capillary pressure is diagnosed clinically. Preload reduction is accomplished with loop diuretics (furosemide or bumetanide) and venodilators (nitroglycerin and morphine), whereas afterload reduction is accomplished with arterial vasodilators (angiotensin-converting enzyme inhibitors or, occasionally, nitroprusside). If the blood pressure can be increased to normal levels with inotropes, then the cautious addition of afterload and preload reduction is feasible in the presence of low cardiac output or high pulmonary capillary pressure.

D. Obstructive Shock

In the patient with obstructive shock, relief of the obstruction is the treatment of choice. Additionally, maintenance of intravascular volume is vitally important. Fluid resuscitation may improve the patient's cardiac output and hypotension temporarily. Inotropes or vasopressors have a minimal role in the management of obstructive shock, and these agents provide only temporary improvement, if any. Pulmonary embolus is a common cause of obstructive shock. Treatment is centered on fluid resuscitation to maintain cardiac output and prompt anticoagulation to prevent clot propagation (**Chapter 13**). Thrombolytic therapy or thrombectomy is needed in rare cases of refractory cardiac collapse. If cardiac tamponade is present, pericardiocentesis may be lifesaving. Tension pneumothorax must be treated promptly by needle decompression and subsequent tube thoracostomy (**Appendix 8**).

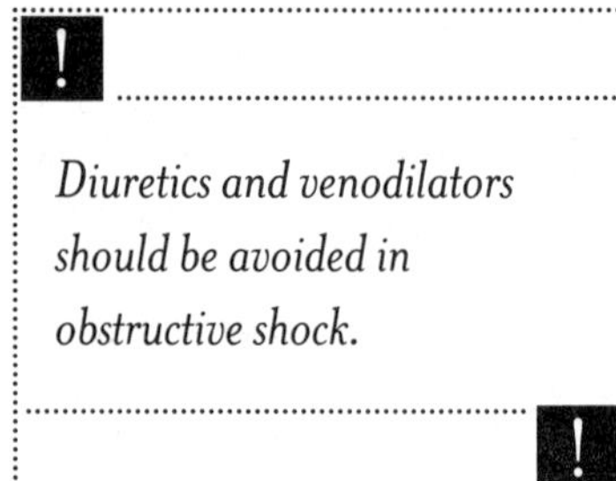

VI. OLIGURIA

Glomerular filtration rate (GFR) is a measure of fluid filtration through the glomerulus of the kidney into the renal tubule system. A significant decrease in GFR results in a rise in the serum creatinine and blood urea nitrogen, the most common measure of renal function, and a decrease in urine output. Oliguria, defined as urine output <0.5 mL/kg/h for >2 hours, is an important manifestation of hypoperfusion or decreased GFR. Oliguria also may be due to inherent renal injury or postrenal obstruction, in which case urine output cannot be used as a goal of adequate resuscitation. Causes of oliguria are categorized as prerenal, renal, and postrenal, as outlined in **Table 7-5**.

Table 7-5 Differential Diagnosis of Oliguria

Prerenal

- Decreased cardiac output (eg, volume depletion, cardiac failure, tamponade)
- Redistribution of blood flow (distributive shock) with peripheral vasodilation and/or shunting

Renal

- Glomerular disease (glomerulonephritis)
- Vascular disease (eg, vasculitis)
- Interstitial disease (eg, antibiotics)
- Renal tubular disease
- Ischemia
- Nephrotoxic drugs

Postrenal (Obstructive)

- Bilateral ureteral obstruction
- Urethral stricture
- Bladder outlet obstruction
- Urinary catheter obstruction

Assessment of volume status by physical examination is often difficult in the critically ill patient, and invasive hemodynamic monitoring may be of benefit. Additional laboratory tests can help differentiate prerenal causes of oliguria from acute kidney injury. Some laboratory tests of renal function are shown in **Table 7-6**. Results of these tests should be obtained before the administration of diuretics. **Figure 7-2** shows the RIFLE criteria (Risk, Injury, Failure, Loss of kidney function, End-stage kidney disease), a consensus-based definition of renal dysfunction that has been shown to correlate with probability for need for dialysis and mortality. The key point demonstrated by the RIFLE criteria is that seemingly small alterations in creatinine or urine output portend a high risk of subsequent renal failure and should not be discounted. Studies should be undertaken for the underlying cause of renal injury, and nephrotoxic agents should be discontinued while renal blood flow is optimized.

Table 7-6 Laboratory Tests to Distinguish Prerenal Conditions From Acute Tubular Necrosis

Laboratory Tests	Prerenal	Acute Tubular Necrosis
Blood urea nitrogen/creatinine ratio	>20	10–20
Urine specific gravity	>1.020	>1.010
Urine osmolality (mOsm/L)	>500	<350
Urinary sodium (mmol/L)	<20	>40
Fractional excretion of sodium (%)[a]	<1	>2

[a]Fractional excretion of sodium = ([urine sodium ÷ serum sodium] ÷ [urine creatinine serum creatinine]) × 100.

Figure 7-2. RIFLE Criteria Defining Acute Kidney Injury and Renal Failure[a]

Risk	Increased creatinine x 1.5 or GFR decrease >25%	UO <0.5 mL/kg/h x 6 h
Injury	Increased creatinine x 2 or GFR decrease >50%	UO <0.5 mL/kg/h x 12 h
Failure	Increased creatinine x 3 or GFR decrease 75% or creatinine ≥4 mg/dL or acute rise of ≥0.5 mg/dL creatinine	UO <0.3 mL/kg/h x 24 hr or anuria x 12 h
Loss	Persistent ARF = complete loss of renal function >4 weeks	
ESRD	End-stage renal disease	

Abbreviations: RIFLE, Risk, Injury, Failure, Loss of kidney function, End-stage renal disease; GFR, glomerular filtration rate; UO, urine output; ARF, acute renal failure; ESRD, end-stage renal disease
[a]Adapted with permission from BioMed Central Ltd. Copyright 2004. Bellomo, et al; licensee BioMed Central Ltd. http://www.ncbi.nlm.nih.gov/pmc/articles/PMC522841/?tool=pubmed.[2]

VII. MANAGEMENT OF ACUTE RENAL INSUFFICIENCY

Shock-induced hypoperfusion may lead to renal insufficiency or failure, as may other direct renal insults associated with critical illness. Reversible causes of acute renal insufficiency should always be excluded. A urinary catheter and renal ultrasound will exclude urinary obstruction in most patients. The urinary catheter is also a useful device to monitor urine output. Intravascular volume should be optimized with crystalloid and/or colloid solutions. If the patient remains oliguric after an adequate fluid challenge, a high dose of a loop diuretic (eg, furosemide 200 mg slow intravenous push) will often induce a nonoliguric state. Although the conversion to a nonoliguric state may not change outcome, fluid management is usually easier and dialysis may be avoided. No evidence supports the use of low-dose dopamine in oliguric patients. Once oliguric acute renal failure is confirmed, fluids should be restricted to the replacement of ongoing losses (including insensible losses). In disease states associated with ongoing loss of intravascular volume, fluid administration is necessary to maintain adequate left ventricular preload. These losses may be substantial, as in pancreatitis, severe sepsis, and large open wounds.

Because there is no specific treatment for most cases of acute renal failure, expectant and supportive care is maintained. Drug dosages need adjustment not only for GFR but also for the type of renal replacement therapy that is utilized. Nephrotoxic drugs should be avoided if possible. Problems with extracellular fluid overload, hyperkalemia, and hypermagnesemia should be anticipated and avoided if possible. Hyperkalemia usually can be managed medically until dialysis is available (**Chapter 12**). Bleeding may require red cell transfusion or desmopressin use. Nutritional supplements must be adjusted for renal function.

Renal replacement therapy is necessary when uremic symptoms develop or whenever extracellular volume excess, hyperkalemia, or metabolic acidosis is refractory to medical therapy. Various intermittent or continuous therapies are available to accomplish fluid removal (ultrafiltration) or solute removal (dialysis, hemofiltration, hemodiafiltration). Therapy selection depends on the circumstances of the individual patient and the resources available. Consultation with a nephrologist is advised to assist with determining the most appropriate treatment.

Key Points

Diagnosis and Management of Shock

- Shock is characterized by impaired tissue oxygenation and hypoperfusion.
- The four major categories of shock with characteristic hemodynamic patterns are hypovolemic, distributive, cardiogenic, and obstructive.
- The clinical manifestations of shock result from inadequate tissue oxygenation and perfusion, compensatory responses, and the syndrome's specific etiology.
- Interventions to restore perfusion center on achieving an adequate blood pressure, increasing cardiac output, optimizing the oxygen content of blood, and/or decreasing oxygen demand.
- The initial therapy for most forms of shock is replacement of intravascular volume with crystalloid or colloid solutions.
- The selection of a vasoactive agent to treat shock should be based on the hemodynamic effect desired for an individual patient and knowledge of the pharmacology of available agents.
- Reversible causes of acute oliguria should always be excluded, and intravascular volume should be optimized with crystalloid and/or colloid solutions.

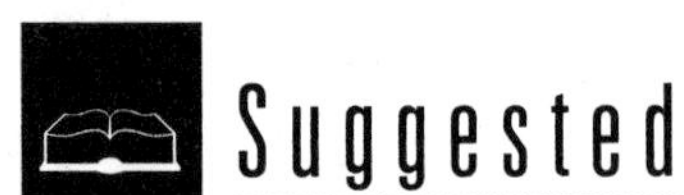

Suggested Readings

1. American Thoracic Society. Evidence-based colloid use in the critically ill: American Thoracic Society Consensus Statement. *Am J Respir Crit Care Med.* 2004;170:1247-1259.

2. Bellomo R, Ronco C, Kellum JA, et al. Acute renal failure – definition, outcome measures, animal models, fluid therapy and information technology needs: The Second International Consensus Conference of the Acute Dialysis Quality Initiative (ADQI) Group. *Crit Care.* 2004;8:R204-R212.

3. Dabrowski GP, Steinberg SM, Ferrara JJ, et al. A critical assessment of endpoints of shock resuscitation. *Surg Clin North Am.* 2000;80:825-844.

4. Dellinger RP, Levy MM, Carlet JM, et al. Surviving Sepsis Campaign: International guidelines for management of severe sepsis and septic shock: 2008. *Crit Care Med.* 2008;36:296-327.

5. Gutierrez G, Reines HD, Wulf-Gutierrez ME. Clinical review: Hemorrhagic shock. *Crit Care.* 2004;8:373-381.

6. Hébert PC, Wells G, Blajchman MA, et al. A multicenter, randomized, controlled clinical trial of transfusion requirements in critical care. Transfusion Requirements in Critical Care Investigators, Canadian Critical Care Trials Group. *N Engl J Med.* 1999;340:409-417.

7. Kellum JA, Bellomo R, Ronco C. Definition and classification of acute kidney injury. *Nephron Clin Pract.* 2008;109:c182-c187.

8. Müller M, Urbanek B, Havel C, et al. Vasopressors for shock [review]. *Cochrane Database Syst Rev.* 2004;(3):CD003709. doi:10.1002/14651858.CD003709.pub2.

9. Ricci Z, Cruz D, Ronco C. The RIFLE criteria and mortality in acute kidney injury: A systematic review. *Kidney Int.* 2008;73:538-546.

10. Rivers E, Nguyen B, Havstad S, et al. Early goal-directed therapy in the treatment of severe sepsis and septic shock. *N Engl J Med.* 2001;345:1368-1377.

11. Sprung CL, Annane D, Keh D, et al for the CORTICUS study group. Hydrocortisone therapy for patients with septic shock. *N Engl J Med.* 2008;358:111-124.

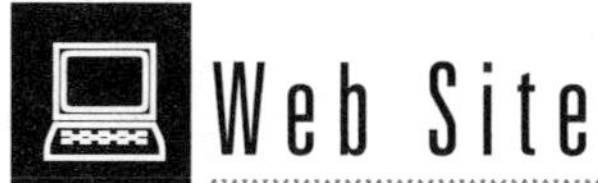

Web Site

Surviving Sepsis Campaign: www.survivingsepsis.org. *This Web site contains guidelines for the management of severe sepsis and septic shock, information on the Surviving Sepsis Campaign, and sepsis-related information and resources for healthcare professionals, patients, and the general public.*

Chapter 8

NEUROLOGIC SUPPORT

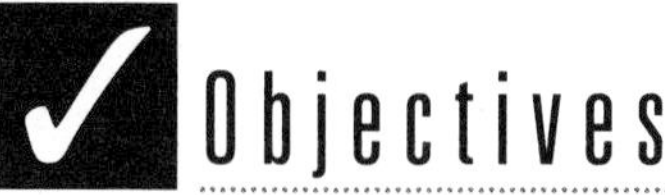

Objectives

- Review the principles of primary and secondary brain insult and the common mechanisms of neuronal injury.
- Apply the concepts of intracranial hypertension and brain oxygen delivery and consumption to the management of the brain-injured patient.
- Review the clinical and diagnostic assessment of a brain-injured patient.
- List general treatments that are common in brain injury.
- Review specific management principles and options for selected pathophysiologic conditions.

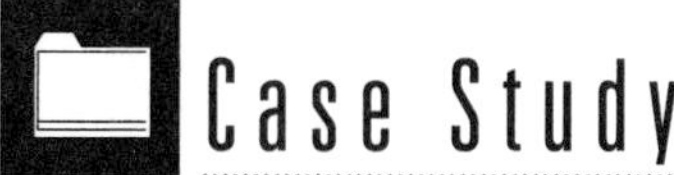

Case Study

A 16-year-old boy, riding his bicycle without a helmet, struck the post of a traffic sign and was thrown to the ground. According to bystanders, he was unconscious for approximately 30 to 45 seconds, then got up and began to walk around the scene. When paramedics arrived, his vital signs were: heart rate 110/min, respiratory rate 20/min, and blood pressure 124/62 mm Hg. He was oriented to name, place, and time but was slow to respond; his pupils were equal and reactive, and he showed no focal neurologic deficits. He was transported to the emergency department and, after a brief, unchanged neurological examination, an emergent computed tomography scan of his head without contrast was completed. Approximately 30 minutes later, the patient became less responsive, did not follow commands, and was moving his left arm significantly less than his right arm.

- What type of primary brain injury is likely to be present?
- What are the immediate concerns?
- What interventions and monitoring should be instituted in addition to the CT scan?

I. INTRODUCTION

Primary injuries to the brain include ischemic events, trauma, hemorrhage, and anoxia, which may occur either in isolation or in combination. Mechanisms for these and other primary injuries are shown in **Table 8-1**.

Table 8-1 Common Mechanisms of Primary Brain Injuries

- Trauma: concussion, contusion, shear injury, penetrating injury, and diffuse axonal injury
- Ischemia: global (eg, cardiac arrest with anoxia) or regional (eg, vasospasm, compression of blood vessels, stroke)
- Inflammation: meningitis, encephalitis
- Compression: tumor, cerebral edema, hematoma (eg, epidural, subdural, or intraparenchymal)
- Metabolism: encephalopathies (eg, hepatic, electrolyte disorders, drugs, toxins)

Often, little can be done to reverse the immediate and frequently devastating effects of the primary cerebral insult that produces neuronal injury or death. In some circumstances, the immediate effects of an injury may be reversed by prompt surgical intervention. Analogous to the injury seen in myocardial infarction, many types of brain insults produce a region of maximum injury associated with a surrounding area of tissue, or penumbra, that may survive and potentially recover if further damage can be prevented. Common mechanisms of secondary injury are shown in **Table 8-2**. Note that some also occur as primary injuries, as indicated in **Table 8-1**. The mechanisms of secondary brain injury may evolve over time from other primary insults. For example, edema after head trauma commonly develops and produces secondary brain compression, vasospasm after subarachnoid hemorrhage may cause regional ischemia and stroke, or secondary hemorrhagic conversion after an ischemic stroke may induce compression and further ischemia.

Table 8-2 Common Mechanisms of Secondary Brain Injuries

- Hypoperfusion: global (ie, secondary to high intracranial pressure, systemic arterial hypotension, or severe anemia) or regional (eg, secondary to high intracranial pressure, local edema, or vasospasm)
- Hypoxia: systemic hypoxemia, regional hypoperfusion, or high tissue consumption (ie, seizures, hyperthermia)
- Electrolyte or acid-base changes from systemic or regional ischemia
- Reperfusion injury with free radical formation

II. BRAIN INJURY MANAGEMENT PRINCIPLES

The focus of treatment for a neurologically compromised patient is the same as that for patients with other illnesses and injuries, that is, to ensure adequate oxygen delivery to meet the needs of both the damaged and the undamaged brain tissue. *The primary goal is prevention of secondary injury.* The initial care team must take early and aggressive action to ensure that secondary brain injury is prevented, minimized, or reversed with careful monitoring and treatment, particularly prevention and early treatment of hypoxia and hypotension. Optimizing oxygen delivery to the brain requires attention to oxygenation, hemoglobin concentration, cardiac output, and blood pressure. Prevention and early treatment of fever, seizures, pain, agitation, and anxiety can minimize oxygen demands.

A. Intracranial Hypertension

Intracranial pressure reflects the balance of volume-control mechanisms within the noncompliant cranial compartment. Because the brain is enclosed within the rigid skull and relatively inflexible dura, with tissues and water that are incompressible, control of the different intracranial components is essential to maintain brain homeostasis, regulate intracranial pressure, and preserve cerebral perfusion. The critical compartment relationship depends on the space occupied by each component. An increase in one component (eg, brain) must be accompanied by a decrease in another component (eg, blood). When the compensatory mechanisms are overwhelmed, intracranial pressure (ICP) increases and injury may ensue. In addition to the impaired cerebral perfusion, which may be a consequence of globally increased ICP, small pressure gradients within the skull may cause herniation of the brain around dural reflections (the falx and the tentorium), and shift of the midline structures. These movements within the skull may compromise function (eg, cause stupor or coma by disrupting the actions of the brainstem reticular formation) or lead to vascular compression and stroke.

An intensivist or a neurosurgeon should be consulted if intracranial hypertension is suspected. The patient may need a catheter inserted into a lateral ventricle for monitoring and drainage of cerebrospinal fluid, or into the brain parenchyma for monitoring (**Table 8-3**). Intracranial pressure, temperature, and/or brain oxygen can then be closely monitored. Measurements of cerebral oxygenation require special equipment and expertise that are not available in most facilities. When direct measures are not available, the initial care team must treat based on the principles of oxygen supply and demand.

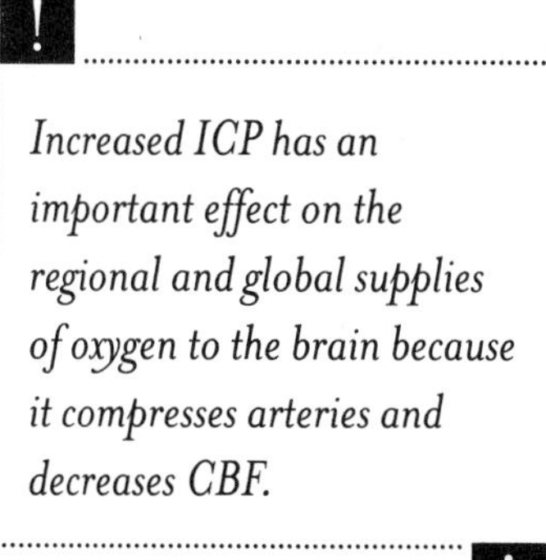

Table 8-3 Conditions Potentially Requiring Invasive Intracranial Pressure Monitoring

- Traumatic brain injury (see **Table 8-6**)
- Acute subarachnoid hemorrhage with hydrocephalus, coma, or clinical deterioration
- Intracranial hemorrhage with intraventricular blood
- Large ischemic stroke
- Fulminant hepatic failure
- Global brain ischemia/anoxia with increasing edema

B. Hypoperfusion

Cerebral autoregulation reflects the normal arteriolar dilation or constriction that controls regional cerebral blood flow (CBF) and links oxygen demand to its delivery; thus, global CBF normally remains constant over a defined range of mean arterial pressures (MAP). Loss of autoregulation occurs in many pathologic conditions and may lead to regional or global vasodilation and edema formation, which can further increase ICP. Increases in blood volume also profoundly affect the pressure inside the noncompliant cranial vault.

CBF is usually evaluated by the cerebral perfusion pressure (CPP), which is the MAP (the driving pressure) minus the ICP (the pressure impeding blood flow):

CPP = MAP – ICP

Normal CPP is between 60 and 100 mm Hg. If ICP increases without a change in MAP, CPP decreases and CBF will also decrease if autoregulation has failed. The decrease in CBF increases the risk of brain ischemia. Clinicians should pay particular attention to changes in mental status, as these may indicate inadequate perfusion (among many possibilities).

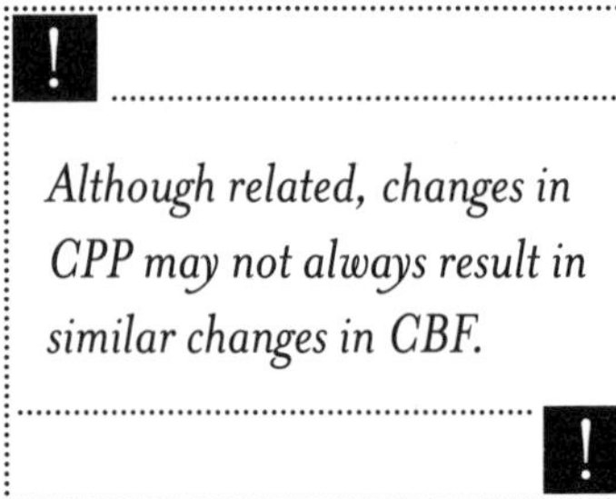

C. Recommendations for Therapy

To minimize damage to the brain, therapies are primarily designed to minimize oxygen demand and increase CBF and oxygen delivery. **Table 8-4** summarizes commonly accepted principles and therapeutic guidelines for treating a variety of brain insults and avoiding secondary brain injury. Note the focus on factors that minimize oxygen consumption and maximize oxygen delivery.

Table 8-4 General Principles of Managing Brain Injury

Prevent Abnormal Oxygen Demands

1. Avoid fever. Fever increases metabolic demand, resulting in neuronal injury and elevating intracranial pressure.
2. Avoid seizures. Prophylactic anticonvulsant administration is indicated after moderate or severe traumatic brain injury to prevent seizures in the first week, but the available evidence does not support longer use in head trauma or use in other neurologic injuries.
3. Avoid anxiety, agitation, or pain. Neuronal oxygen consumption may be decreased by an antianxiety agent, sedation, and analgesia.
4. Avoid shivering.
5. Minimize stimulation, particularly for the first 72 hours.

Promote Oxygen Delivery

1. Ensure systemic oxygen transport with adequate oxygenation, hemoglobin concentration, and cardiac output.
2. Ensure optimal blood pressure. Many primary insults are associated with hypertension that may be a physiologic compensation or may be injurious. Elevated blood pressure may be undesirable in patients with unsecured aneurysms and recent intracranial hemorrhage. *However, excessive lowering of blood pressure may result in secondary ischemia.*
3. Avoid prophylactic or routine hyperventilation because an increase in extracellular brain pH constricts responsive vessels and may reduce cerebral blood flow to ischemic zones. Brief hyperventilation while instituting other methods to lower elevated intracranial pressure may be lifesaving in the patient with evidence of herniation.
4. Ensure euvolemia because hypovolemia may result in systemic hypotension and hypoperfusion of brain tissue.
5. Rapid-sequence intubation should be used for patients with increased intracranial pressure. Consider administration of intravenous lidocaine (1.5 mg/kg) or intravenous thiopental (5 mg/kg) to blunt the rise in intracranial pressure associated with intubation.
6. Institute nimodipine immediately in patients with subarachnoid hemorrhage.

III. ASSESSMENT

After appropriate management of airway, breathing, and hemodynamic concerns, the priority in neurologic assessment is to distinguish among ischemic, structural, metabolic, and infectious injuries. Suspected ischemic stroke requires an immediate decision regarding thrombolytic therapy, and emergent neurologic consultation should be obtained. The presence of an expanding mass lesion accompanied by significant brain shift may indicate the need for immediate surgical evaluation and possible intervention. The most common causes of such an event include epidural, subdural, and intracerebral hematomas. Intracranial hematomas should be suspected in the settings of head trauma, recent neurosurgery, anticoagulant therapy, alcohol abuse, coagulopathies, and chronic or acute hypertension. The diagnostic procedure of choice, computed tomography (CT) scan of the brain, characterizes the extent of structural injury. Medical treatment may be a temporizing option until more definitive therapy is available and implemented.

> **!** *Early identification of patients with ischemic stroke or potential surgical lesions provides the best opportunity to minimize secondary brain injury.* **!**

Serial examinations are necessary to detect the possible sequelae of many brain insults. Any change in the examination is a sensitive indicator of deterioration and should prompt an immediate and thorough reevaluation. For example, decreased consciousness without lateralizing findings may be due to elevated ICP, hydrocephalus, fever, toxic ingestants, or worsening of an encephalopathy, among others.

> !
>
> *When physical examination or CT scan suggests significant brain compression, medical therapy to reduce ICP should be instituted immediately while awaiting definitive treatment.*
>
> !

The Glasgow Coma Scale score is widely used in the initial and serial assessment of patients with head trauma, and it may be useful in evaluating patients with other brain insults. **Table 8-5** lists its components.

Table 8-5 Components of Glasgow Coma Scale Score

Clinical Parameters	Adults	Points
Eye opening	Spontaneous	4
	Response to speech	3
	Response to pain	2
	No response	1
Verbal response	Oriented and appropriate	5
	Disoriented and confused	4
	Inappropriate words	3
	Incomprehensible sounds	2
	No response	1
Best motor response	Obeys commands	6
	Localizes pain	5
	Withdraws from pain	4
	Flexor response	3
	Extensor response	2
	No response	1

Total Glasgow Coma Scale score = eye + verbal + motor scores; best possible score = 15 and worst possible score = 3.

Serial examinations, including evaluation of brainstem and cranial nerve function, should be performed. Pupillary asymmetry may be an important sign of horizontal shift of the brain, which commonly precedes downward herniation in patients with supratentorial masses. Disconjugate eye movements, a change in respiratory pattern, or deterioration in motor response may suggest an increase in intracranial mass effect and should be investigated immediately.

> !
>
> *Cushing reflex with hypertension, bradycardia, and altered respiration may be an indication of brain herniation.*
>
> !

When clinical findings suggest herniation, emergent administration of mannitol or hypertonic saline should be initiated to lower ICP, and emergent neurosurgical assistance should be obtained. A brief period of hyperventilation may be considered. Whether repetition of an imaging study or immediate surgical therapy is required depends upon the nature, location, and progression of the pathologic process.

Neurosurgical consultation is advised for any patient who: (1) is at risk for developing an expanding intracranial mass lesion; (2) has an open or depressed skull fracture or acute ventricular obstruction; (3) demonstrates blood in the fourth ventricle, cerebellar bleeding, or subarachnoid hemorrhage; or (4) has cerebrospinal fluid leakage. Nontraumatic disease processes, such as spontaneous intracerebral hematoma, large brain tumors, or brain abscesses, require urgent neurosurgical consultation if clinical findings or an imaging study indicate significant mass effect (midline deviation, ventricular obliteration, brainstem or basal cistern compression).

Urgent neurosurgical consultation should be obtained for hemorrhages and infarcts in the posterior fossa regardless of the level of consciousness. Although such patients may have few findings on initial clinical examination, progressive swelling around the lesion may necessitate emergent surgical decompression. Typically, any cerebellar mass >3 cm in diameter with hydrocephalus or brainstem compression requires evacuation.

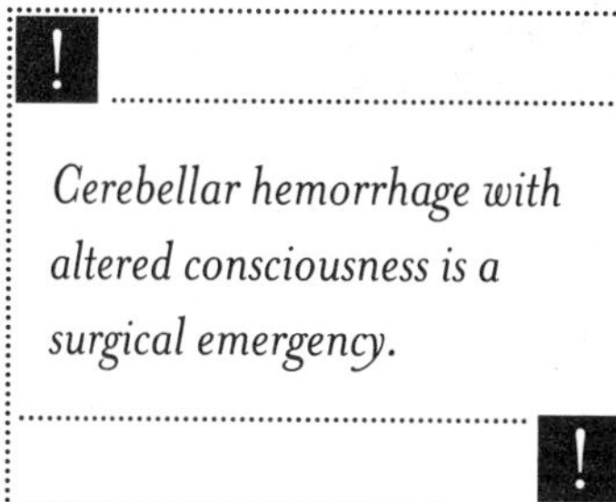

IV. SPECIFIC DIAGNOSES AND CONSIDERATIONS

A. Traumatic Brain Injury

Approximately 25% of patients who experience blunt head trauma require urgent evacuation of a subdural hematoma (**Figure 8-1A**) or an epidural hematoma (**Figure 8-1B**) to relieve compression of the brain. Consider neurosurgical consultation early. Because 20% of patients with severe traumatic brain injury will have concomitant cervical spinal cord injuries, immobilization of the cervical spine until it can be appropriately assessed is very important.

Figure 8-1A. Subdural Hematoma

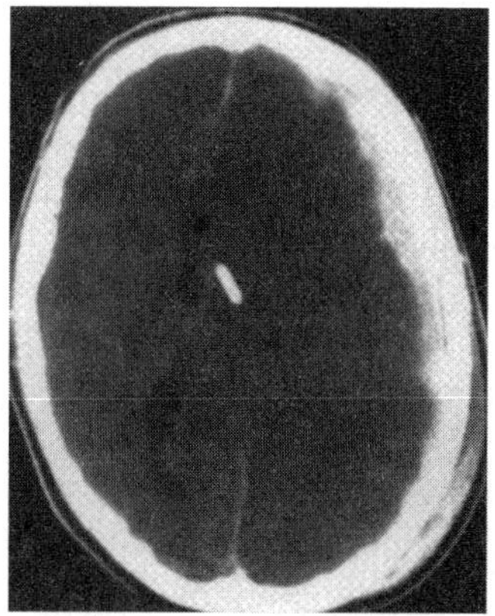

Figure 8-1B. Epidural Hematoma

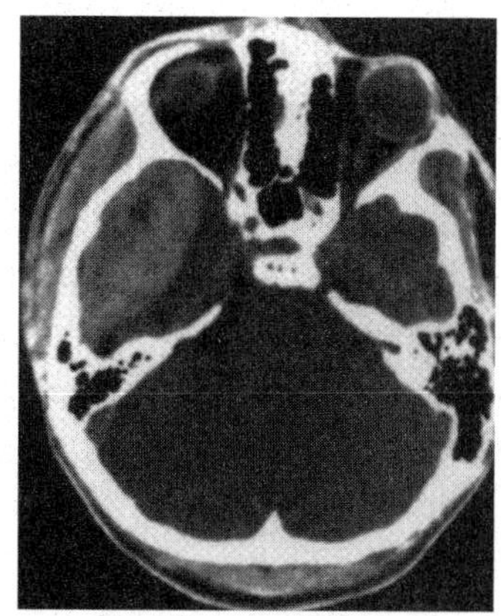

Penetrating and nonpenetrating head injuries are often associated with the formation of cerebral edema, brain contusions, or hemorrhage within the parenchyma. Because the skull cannot expand to accommodate increased intracranial volume and the compensatory space in the subarachnoid space of the spinal canal is very limited, the ICP commonly becomes elevated. Monitoring and treatment of increased ICP are considered important in such patients.

Guidelines for the management of severe traumatic brain injury have been developed by the Brain Trauma Foundation on the basis of established evidence. These principles are included in the recommendations in **Table 8-6**.

Table 8-6 General Principles for Treatment of Traumatic Brain Injury

- Ensure the ABCs of resuscitation.
- Avoid hypotension and maintain systolic blood pressure >90 mm Hg. Although it may be valuable to maintain mean arterial pressure higher than the systolic pressure, the actual target value is unknown.
- Avoid hypoxemia (Pa_{O_2} <60 mm Hg [8.0 kPa] or Sp_{O_2} <90%) while adequate oxygenation is maintained.
- Maintain alignment between head and trunk to avoid jugular compression.
- Keep the head of the bed at 30° to 45° elevation unless the patient is hypotensive. Elevation of the head promotes venous drainage and cerebrospinal fluid displacement to the spinal compartment. Adjust any devices that may constrict the neck, including cervical collars.
- Maintain the Pa_{CO_2} at 35 to 40 mm Hg (4.7-5.3 kPa). Prophylactic hyperventilation is not recommended. Hyperventilation is recommended as a temporizing measure for reduction of elevated intracranial pressure. Cerebral blood flow is often reduced in the first 24 hours after head trauma, and hyperventilation should be avoided in this period to prevent further reductions.
- Use normal saline as the primary maintenance fluid. Do not use hypotonic fluids.
- Actively treat fever to maintain body temperature at normal levels.
- Control harmful agitation with sedation if necessary. Use medications with a relatively short half-life to facilitate reliable and ongoing neurologic assessments.
- Maintain the usual electrolyte homeostasis and treat hyperglycemia/hypoglycemia.
- Assess and treat coagulation defects.
- Provide nutrition to attain full caloric replacement as tolerated.
- Do not use anticonvulsants prophylactically to prevent post-traumatic epilepsy. Although prophylactic anticonvulsants prevent early seizures, they do not improve risk of mortality. If seizures occur, they should be aggressively treated.
- Give mannitol (0.25-1 g/kg intravenous push) for signs of herniation or for neurologic deterioration not attributable to other factors. There are no specific recommendations for use of hypertonic saline, and expert consultation should be obtained if this type of hyperosmolar therapy is considered.
- Avoid steroid use. These are contraindicated in patients with head trauma.
- Initiate appropriate intracranial pressure monitoring:
    - For a patient with a Glasgow Coma Scale score of 3-8 after resuscitation or a score of 9-12 with an abnormal computed tomography scan
    - For a patient who has normal computed tomography scan results but at least 2 of the following factors:
        1. Age >40 years
        2. Systolic blood pressure <90 mm Hg
        3. Unilateral or bilateral motor posturing (decerebrate/decorticate)
- Maintain the lowest perfusion pressure compatible with adequate cerebral blood flow. The target cerebral perfusion pressure is in the range of 50 to 70 mm Hg, although patients with intact autoregulation may tolerate higher values. The ideal is the pressure that provides adequate cerebral perfusion and oxygenation while intracranial pressure is maintained <20 mm Hg.

B. Intracerebral Hemorrhage

Patients with intracerebral hemorrhage frequently have a history of hypertension. Blood pressure control is controversial in these cases. Elevated blood pressure may contribute to rebleeding and edema formation but may also preserve regional CPP. If the elevated blood pressure is causing considerable systemic effects, such as cardiac stress, modest reductions may be safe. The target blood pressure should take into account the patient's age, baseline blood pressure, presumed cause of hemorrhage, and intracranial pressure (if known). If elevated ICP is suspected, expert consultation is advised for assistance with blood pressure management. Preferred agents include labetalol and nicardipine. Use of vasodilators remains controversial, but drugs that cause substantial intracranial vasodilation (eg, nitroprusside, nitroglycerin) should be avoided.

Expansion of the hematoma occurs commonly, especially in patients taking anticoagulants or who have liver disease or low platelet counts. Some neurosurgeons may consider removal of the hematoma, especially in a young, clinically deteriorating patient with a large lobar hemorrhage or when the hemorrhage is associated with a surgically treatable lesion, such as an aneurysm, arteriovenous malformation, or cavernous angioma. Deep basal ganglionic hemorrhages do not yet have a commonly accepted surgical therapy.

C. Subarachnoid Hemorrhage

Characteristics from the patient history ("worst headache of their life") and CT findings usually confirm the diagnosis of subarachnoid hemorrhage. Classification systems (eg, the Hunt and Hess scale) have been used to categorize findings and suggest prognosis but do not alter the care provided by the primary team, as outlined in **Table 8-7**. Early aneurysm repeat rupture is frequently fatal, so initial therapy is aimed at decreasing its risk. Guidelines are available from the American Heart Association/American Stroke Association (AHA/ASA). Prompt consultation with a center experienced in the care of these patients is essential. Almost all patients, regardless of severity, should be stabilized and evaluated for rapid transfer to such center for management.

Table 8-7 Treatment of Subarachnoid Hemorrhage

- Ensure the ABCs of resuscitation.
- Control blood pressure early, before definitive surgical therapy. Rebleeding is the major early complication until the aneurysm is clipped or coiled. A variety of intravenous antihypertensive agents have been useful. Labetalol and nicardipine have been selectively advocated. Nitroprusside should be avoided because of its tendency to induce cerebral vasodilation. Consider the effects of nimodipine on blood pressure when using other antihypertensive agents.
- Initiate oral nimodipine 60 mg every 4 hours. (An intravenous preparation is available in some countries.) Hypotension should be avoided.
- Maintain euvolemia. Some advocate gentle intravascular volume expansion. Significant cardiac injury can occur as a result of high circulating catecholamine levels; thus, careful attention to arrhythmias and cardiac function is necessary.
- Avoid hyponatremia, which is commonly encountered. Normal saline should be used as the primary intravenous fluid. Hyponatremia usually reflects cerebral salt wasting rather than the SIADH release; cerebral salt wasting should not be treated with the volume restriction utilized for SIADH. Both groups of patients will have inappropriately high urine osmolality, so this marker cannot be used to indicate SIADH. If salt administration is indicated for cerebral salt wasting, small amounts of hypertonic saline may be necessary. Hyponatremia should be corrected slowly, as central pontine myelinolysis can occur from rapid and aggressive sodium correction.
- Perform rapid evaluation of the aneurysm location for surgical clipping or coiling, which requires urgent neurosurgical and/or neurointerventional radiology consultation.
- Manage patients in centers with the capacity for aneurysm clipping and coiling, and for vasospasm treatment.

Abbreviation: SIADH, syndrome of inappropriate antidiuretic hormone

D. Ischemic Stroke

Ischemic stroke usually occurs due to the thromboembolic obstruction of arteries. Administration of intravenous recombinant tissue plasminogen activator during the first 3 to 4.5 hours following the known onset of ischemic stroke substantially improves outcome in one-third of patients.

Onset of symptoms, or the last time the patient was known to be at baseline, is the time used to determine whether a patient is a candidate for thrombolytic therapy. After an initial CT scan rules out the presence of hemorrhage, intravenous recombinant tissue plasminogen activator should be administered in a dosage of 0.9 mg/kg (10% as a bolus over 1 minute and 90% in a 1-hour infusion). Personnel who are not familiar with the use of recombinant tissue plasminogen activator for the acute treatment of nonhemorrhagic stroke should seek immediate neurologic consultation before administering therapy. Guidelines are available from the AHA/ASA.

> **!** *Determination of when the initial stroke symptoms appeared is critical.* **!**

Supportive care includes management of hypertension. Although elevated blood pressure is often present early, a decrease in pressure usually occurs in the first hours after stroke without specific medical treatment. No evidence defines a level of blood pressure that requires emergent intervention. The AHA/ASA have compiled consensus recommendations for patients who are candidates for thrombolytic therapy (**Table 8-8**). Emergency administration of antihypertensive agents is not indicated in other patients unless the diastolic blood pressure is >120 mm Hg, systolic blood pressure is >220 mm Hg, or there is evidence of end-organ injury (eg, pulmonary edema). If treatment is indicated, the blood pressure should be lowered cautiously with a reasonable goal of lowering the pressure approximately 15% in the first 24 hours after stroke onset.

Table 8-8 Blood Pressure Management in Patients Eligible for Recombinant Tissue Plasminogen Activator Treatment[a]

Blood Pressure	Treatment
Pretreatment	
SBP >185 or DBP	Labetalol 10-20 mg IV bolus (1-2 doses)
>110 mm Hg	Nicardipine infusion 5 mg/h titrated to goal BP
	(maximum 15 mg/h); reduce infusion to 3 mg/h when goal BP attained
Post-treatment	
SBP >230 mm Hg or	Labetalol 10-20 mg IV bolus; may repeat every 10-20 min to maximum 300 mg
DBP 121-140 mm Hg	Labetalol 10 mg IV bolus followed by infusion at 2-8 mg/min
	Nicardipine 5 mg/h IV infusion and titrate (maximum 15 mg/h)
SBP 180-230 mm Hg or	Labetalol 10 mg IV bolus; may repeat every 10-20 min to maximum 300 mg
DBP 105-120 mm Hg	Labetalol 10 mg IV bolus followed by infusion at 2-8 mg/min

Abbreviations: SBP, systolic blood pressure; DBP, diastolic blood pressure; BP, blood pressure.
[a]Adapted with permission from Wolters Kluwer Health. Adams HP, del Zoppo G, Alberts MJ, et al. Guidelines for the early management of adults with ischemic stroke. *Stroke.* 2007;38:1655-1711.[2]

Urgent anticoagulation with unfractionated or low-molecular-weight heparin is not indicated in acute stroke. Prophylactic heparin should be administered to immobilized patients to prevent venous thromboembolism, but the ideal time to start this therapy is not known. Aspirin administration within 24 to 48 hours of stroke onset is recommended for most patients after hemorrhage is excluded, but clopidogrel administration is not recommended. Significant edema formation, typically within the first 72 hours, or extensive hemorrhage within the ischemic zone may indicate emergent hemicraniectomy.

E. Anoxic Injury

Relative anoxia may be a part of other injuries and may be due to airway loss, systemic hypoxemia, hypoperfusion, and other causes. Anoxia may also be the primary brain insult, as occurs during cardiac arrest. Neuronal damage may occur as a direct result of the primary insult of hypoxemia or hypoperfusion

The initial team should maintain the usual standards of optimal oxygen delivery. Despite extensive studies of many agents and therapy options, none has proven selectively beneficial, nor has the poor prognosis from anoxic brain injury improved over time. Systemic cooling to approximately 91.4°F (33°C) for 12 to 24 hours improves neurologic outcome in comatose patients after out-of-hospital ventricular tachycardia/ventricular fibrillation arrests. Patients resuscitated after other forms of arrest (asystole, pulseless electrical activity), or who arrest in the hospital, may also be considered for cooling. At present, the inability to follow simple commands constitutes an acceptable threshold to consider cooling. Guidelines are available from the AHA and the International Liaison Committee on Resuscitation.

F. Metabolic Abnormalities, Infectious Emergencies, and Seizures

In adult patients with depressed consciousness after initial resuscitation, the use of 50% dextrose (50 mL intravenously) and thiamine (100 mg intravenously) should be considered for the treatment of potential hypoglycemia and the prevention of Wernicke encephalopathy if an immediate determination of the blood glucose concentration is not available. Intravenous naloxone should be administered if narcotic intoxication is a possibility. Other metabolic abnormalities, such as electrolyte disorders (ie, acute hyponatremia, hypercalcemia), liver failure, or uremia may also cause coma. Because headache or altered state of consciousness accompanied by fever, nuchal rigidity, and leukocytosis suggests meningitis or encephalitis, the cerebrospinal fluid should be submitted for physical, chemical, and bacteriologic (culture and Gram stain) studies. If clinical examination suggests a mass lesion or elevated ICP, a CT scan should be performed before lumbar puncture. If the scan reveals evidence of mass effect or generalized cerebral edema, a lumbar puncture may precipitate a herniation syndrome and should be postponed. When infection is part of the differential diagnosis, appropriate antibacterial and antiviral treatment should be initiated before performing the imaging study because early therapy for bacterial meningitis or encephalitis may be lifesaving. Blood cultures should be obtained before antibiotic therapy unless this would delay treatment. Antibiotics should also be given if lumbar puncture is delayed for any other reason. Treatment recommendations for adults are outlined in **Chapter 11** and those for children are in **Chapter 16**.

!

In the absence of papilledema or focal neurologic signs, a lumbar puncture may be performed without a prior CT scan for evaluation of meningitis.

!

Seizure activity after an acute brain injury increases cerebral oxygen requirements and typically elevates the ICP. Appropriate therapy should be administered to terminate seizure activity as soon as possible. The intravenous administration of anticonvulsants, many of which have a potent sedative effect, may depress respiratory function and requires appropriate supportive therapy. In addition, hypotension may occur, requiring additional intravenous fluids and/or vasopressors to preserve MAP and CPP.

Intravenous benzodiazepines are administered at the onset of prolonged or repeated seizure activity. Status epilepticus requires emergent neurologic consultation, and lorazepam 0.1 mg/kg should be administered. Anticonvulsants used in refractory status epilepticus include propofol (3 mg/kg loading dose, then infusion of 1-5 mg/kg/h) or midazolam (0.2 mg/kg loading dose, then infusion of 1-20 µg/kg/min) with electroencephalography and other ICU monitoring.

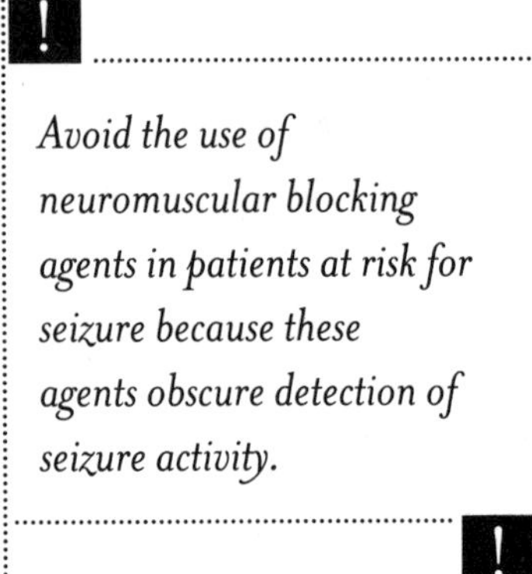

!

Avoid the use of neuromuscular blocking agents in patients at risk for seizure because these agents obscure detection of seizure activity.

!

G. Spinal Cord Injury

Cervical spine injury in awake patients is usually apparent from neck pain and weakness. If awareness is impaired, suspect cervical spinal cord injury in patients with respiratory weakness, extremity weakness without facial weakness, hypotension with bradycardia, and difficulty maintaining normothermia. Patients with lesions below C4 may breathe adequately on presentation but could progress to abrupt respiratory failure and thus must never be left unmonitored.

Thoracolumbar spine injury spares the upper extremities but involves leg weakness; depending on the level, the patients may have hypotension with tachycardia or unusual swings in blood pressure.

Initial management includes immobilization (cervical collar, backboard) while obtaining emergent neurosurgical consultation. Use of methylprednisolone is controversial and should be discussed with the consultant. To be most effective, methylprednisolone should be started within 3 hours, so it should not be delayed if it is to be employed.

Plain radiographs and CT scans of the spine can be obtained without removing immobilizing devices.

H. Other Neurologic Causes of Acute Respiratory Failure

Patients with conditions causing global weakness, such as myasthenia gravis and the Guillain-Barré syndrome, may have problems maintaining upper airway patency and clearing secretions in addition to respiratory muscle weakness. In such patients, endotracheal intubation may be needed for airway protection before being mandated by the falling tidal volume. Measurement of vital capacity and negative inspiratory pressure is important. Patients with <20 mL/kg vital capacity should be moved to an ICU and will likely need intubation soon. One should intubate based on tachypnea and discomfort without waiting for an elevation of $Pa{CO_2}$. Hypoxia due to atelectasis in patients with adequate airway protection may be treated with continuous positive airway pressure. Consultation with a neurologist should be obtained when the diagnosis is suspected, as treatment with intravenous immunoglobulin or plasma exchange may slow or halt disease progression and speed recovery.

Autonomic dysfunction is common in the Guillain-Barré syndrome, and may lead to large and rapid swings in blood pressure and heart rate requiring intravenous therapy.

I. Brain Death Criteria and Organ Donation

Despite the best efforts of medical and surgical teams, massive injury, cerebral infarction, or hemorrhage may result in a loss of all cerebral and brainstem functions. Evaluation of brain death and the guidelines for organ donation are variable, depending on the country, state, and facility.

Criteria for brain death vary from state to state and from country to country. For more information about brain death and organ donation, see **Appendix 9**.

Key Points

Neurologic Support

- Brain injury occurs as a consequence of a primary insult and secondary injury. The prevention of secondary brain injury is a critical goal for the initial care team.
- The most significant mechanisms for secondary injury in brain-injured patients are hypotension and hypoxia.
- Optimizing oxygen delivery while controlling oxygen consumption is a general treatment principle for all types of brain injury.
- Important principles/guidelines for initial treatment apply to all types of primary brain injury and help prevent harmful secondary sequelae.
- Blood pressure management is dependent on the initial brain injury. However, excessive lowering of blood pressure in any acute brain injury may induce secondary ischemia.
- Avoid prophylactic or routine hyperventilation in patients with brain injuries. Mannitol should be given and hyperventilation initiated for signs of herniation or if neurologic deterioration occurs that is not attributable to other factors.
- Ensure euvolemia using normal saline as the primary maintenance fluid. Avoid all hypotonic fluids; 5% dextrose in water is equivalent to free water when the glucose is metabolized and should be avoided.
- Seizure activity after acute brain injury should be terminated with an intravenous dose of a benzodiazepine, followed by an intravenous loading dose of phenytoin or fosphenytoin.

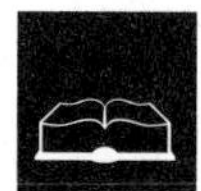

Suggested Readings

1. Adams HP Jr., del Zoppo G, Alberts MJ, et al. Guidelines for the early management of adults with ischemic stroke. *Stroke.* 2007;38:1655-1711.

2. Anderson CS. Medical management of acute intracerebral hemorrhage. *Curr Opin Crit Care.* 2009;15:93-98.

3. Bederson JB, Connolly ES Jr., Batjer HH, et al. Guidelines for the management of aneurismal subarchnoid hemorrhage: A statement for healthcare professionals from a special writing group of the stroke council, American Heart Association. *Stroke.* 2009;40:994-1025.

4. Brain Trauma Foundation, American Association of Neurological Surgeons, Congress of Neurological Surgeons, AANS/CNS Joint Section on Neurotrauma and Critical Care. Guidelines for the management of severe traumatic brain injury. 3rd ed. *J Neurotrauma.* 2007; 24(suppl 1):S1-S106.

5. Brisman JL, Song JK, Newell DW. Cerebral aneurysms. *N Engl J Med.* 2006;355:928-939.

6. Chiles BW, Cooper PR. Acute spinal injury. *N Engl J Med.* 1996;334:514-520.

7. Guidelines for the Management of Acute Cervical Spine and Spine Cord Injuries. *Neurosurgery.* 2002;50(suppl 3).

8. Kamel H, Navi BB, Nakagawa K, et al. Hypertonic saline versus mannitol for the treatment of elevated intracranial pressure: A meta-analysis of randomized clinical trials. *Crit Care Med.* 2011;39:554-559.

9. Legriel S, Azoulay E, Resche-Rigon M, et al. Functional outcome after convulsive status epilepticus. *Crit Care Med.* 2010;38:2295-2303.

10. Marik PE, Varon J. The management of status epilepticus. *Chest.* 2004;126:582-591.

11. McDonald JW, Sadowsky C. Spinal-cord injury. *Lancet.* 2002;359:417-425.

12. Morgenstern LB, Hemphill JC 3rd, Anderson C, et al. Guidelines for the management of spontaneous intracerebral hemorrhage: A guideline for healthcare professionals from the American Heart Association/American Stroke Association. *Stroke.* 2010; 41:2108-2129.

13. Naidech AM. Intracranial hemorrhage. *Am J Respir Crit Care Med.* 2011;184:998-1106.

14. Prasad K, Al-Roomi K, Krishnan PR, et al. Anticonvulsant therapy for status epilepticus (review). *Cochrane Database Syst Rev.* 2005;(4):CD003723.

15. Royal College of Physicians. National Clinical Guidelines for Stroke, 3rd ed. Prepared by the Intercollegiate Stroke Working Party. London, Royal College of Physicians, 2008.

16. Suarez JI, Tarr RW, Selman WR. Aneurysmal subarachnoid hemorrhage. *N Engl J Med.* 2006;354:387-396.

17. Vale FL, Burns J, Jackson AB, et al. Combined medical and surgical treatment after acute spinal cord injury: Results of a prospective pilot study to assess the merits of aggressive medical resuscitation and blood pressure management. *J Neurosurg.* 1997;87:239-246.

Web Sites

1. Brain Trauma Foundation. http://www.braintrauma.org. *In addition to guidelines for management of traumatic brain injury, this site offers Internet-based continuing education programs, including recorded presentations, live Web-based lectures, and interactive learning modules based on the latest scientific evidence. It also offers professional and academic resources for those interested in learning more about traumatic brain injury and quality improvement in healthcare.*

2. Brain Attack Coalition. http://www.stroke-site.org. *This Web site contains such practical information as guidelines for the diagnosis of strokes, order sets and checklists from a variety of institutions, and pathways — step-by-step approaches to the management of stroke. It also provides information and resources for stroke patients, families, and caregivers.*

Chapter 9

Basic Trauma and Burn Support

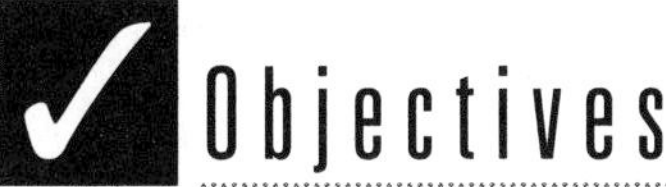

Objectives

- Prioritize and initiate a timely assessment of the traumatized patient.
- Initiate treatment of life-threatening traumatic injury.
- Utilize radiography in identifying significant traumatic injury.
- Identify and respond to significant changes in the patient's status after traumatic injury.
- Initiate early burn management.
- Review indications for initiating surgical consultation and/or transferring the patient to a higher level of care.

Case Study

A middle-aged man has been brought to the emergency department after his car collided with a large truck. He was not wearing a seat belt and was ejected. He is making incoherent sounds and is unable to clear his oral secretions. He has an open femur fracture with hemorrhage as well as bleeding from a scalp laceration. Contusions are present over the left chest wall and upper quadrant of the abdomen. Vital signs include a blood pressure of 90/60 mm Hg, pulse rate of 125/min, and respiratory rate of 35/min.

The patient is lethargic but moves all extremities voluntarily. His skin is cool and clammy.

- What does the primary survey indicate?
- What are the most urgent initial interventions?

I. INTRODUCTION

It is not the intention of the FCCS program to replace the Advanced Trauma Life Support (ATLS) course provided by the American College of Surgeons. The material presented here is intended to highlight evaluation and treatment issues for the provider confronted with a deteriorating patient in the setting of injury. Care providers who regularly encounter patients with traumatic injuries are encouraged to enroll in an ATLS course or obtain other similar training.

A. Death Following Injury

Death due to injury occurs in one of three periods. The first period is within seconds to minutes of injury. During this early period, deaths generally result from severe brain or high spinal cord injury, loss of the airway, or rupture of the heart, aorta, or other large blood vessels. Few of these patients can be salvaged because of the severity of injury, and prevention is the only way to reduce such trauma-related deaths. The second period occurs within minutes to hours following injury. These deaths are usually due to subdural and epidural hematomas, hemopneumothorax, solid organ rupture (spleen or liver), pelvic fractures, or other injuries associated with blood loss. The "golden hour" after trauma is characterized by the need for rapid assessment and resolution of these injuries. The third period occurs days to weeks after the initial injury and is most often due to sepsis with associated multiple organ failure.

Three principles guide the approach to injury. The most important is that the greatest threat to life must be treated first. For example, the inability to breathe kills more quickly than bleeding. The second premise is that it is not necessary to establish a definitive diagnosis before beginning lifesaving treatment. The third is that a detailed history is not essential to begin care in the setting of acute injury.

II. TRAUMA MANAGEMENT

Early management of the seriously injured patient requires simultaneous evaluation and treatment. The first goal is to ensure adequate oxygen delivery to vital organs by following an established sequence of priorities that allows identification and treatment of injuries causing immediate threats to life (primary assessment). Patient management should begin with the rapid primary evaluation with simultaneous resuscitation of vital functions, followed by a more detailed secondary assessment (head-to-toe examination), and finally, the initiation of definitive care. This process begins with the ABCDE of trauma care, which guides the identification of life-threatening conditions through the initial assessment sequence of airway, breathing, circulation, disability, and exposure (**Table 9-1**).

A surgeon skilled in trauma management should be consulted early in the course of all serious trauma cases. When a surgeon is not immediately available or when the patient is awaiting transfer, ongoing evaluation (tertiary assessment) and intervention should continue.

Table 9-1 Initial Assessment of Trauma

Airway: maintenance with cervical spine precautions
Breathing: ventilation and oxygenation
Circulation: hemorrhage control
Disability: brief neurologic examination
Exposure/environment: clothing removed, avoiding hypothermia

A. Primary Assessment: Initial Evaluation and Resuscitation

1. Airway and Breathing

If the patient is able to communicate verbally, the airway is unlikely to be in immediate jeopardy; however, repeated assessment of airway patency is essential. Patients with severe head injury (Glasgow Coma Scale [GCS] score of 8 or less) usually require placement of a definitive, protective airway. Nonpurposeful motor responses support the need for immediate airway management.

> **!** *Airway patency should be reassured frequently, particularly in patients with head injury, shock, and facial fractures.*

The airway should first be assessed for patency. Assessment for signs of airway obstruction includes inspection for foreign bodies and facial, mandibular, or tracheal/laryngeal fractures that may result in airway obstruction. Patients can develop signs of airway obstruction after benign initial presentation in the emergency department. Profuse bleeding from oropharyngeal injury may warrant a definitive airway placement.

After blunt trauma, airway control should proceed on the assumption that an unstable fracture or ligamentous injury of the cervical spine (C-spine) exists. Airway patency must be established, supplemental oxygen provided, and adequacy of ventilation ensured, as discussed in **Chapter 2**. If active airway intervention is needed before radiologic evaluation for possible C-spine fracture, the technique chosen for airway control (intubation, adjunctive device, or surgical airway) should take into account the expertise of available personnel, type of equipment available, patient factors, and injuries. If the patient is apneic or deteriorating rapidly, effective bag-mask ventilation can be lifesaving. Standard orotracheal intubation should be attempted with the use of in-line manual stabilization of the head and neck. Proper in-line stabilization may be accomplished from the front or the side of the patient. One care provider supports the occiput and mandible with both hands to maintain neck alignment without applying traction or distraction. With secure stabilization, the anterior portion of the cervical collar may be removed to allow airway interventions. In-line stabilization is continued until the cervical collar is replaced and the endotracheal tube or other airway device is secured. If an airway cannot otherwise be secured, a laryngeal mask airway, esophageal-tracheal double lumen airway device, or surgical cricothyrotomy is indicated.

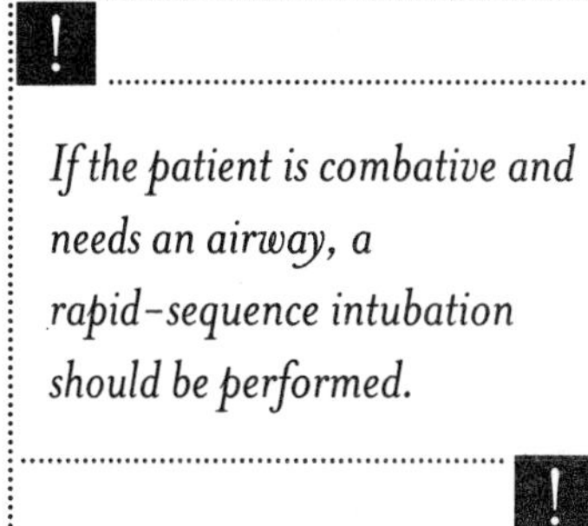

a. Key Issues in Airway Control

Facial fractures are not an immediate priority unless heavy bleeding or uncontrollable secretions are present. Similarly, facial fractures usually do not require that the patient be intubated. Mandibular fractures, however, are more likely to be associated with soft-tissue injury that may compromise the airway. Care should be taken to avoid nasotracheal intubation in patients with suspected midface and basal skull fractures.

Neurologic examination alone does not exclude a C-spine injury. The following considerations apply to patients at risk for C-spine injury:

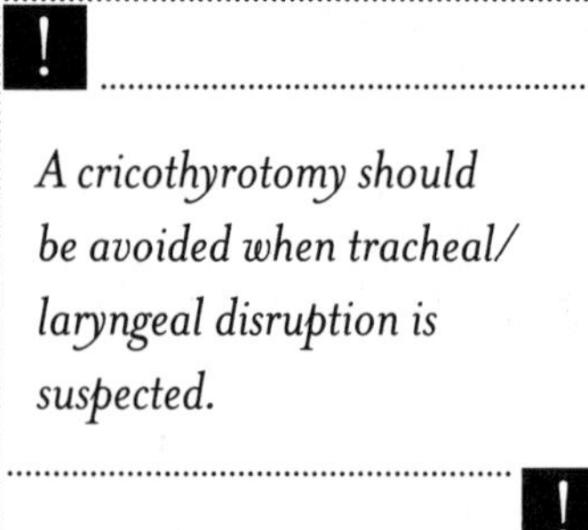

- Patients who are alert, awake, and have no changes in neurologic status or neck pain may be considered to have a stable C-spine and need no radiologic studies. Beware of injuries which could distract the patient with C-spine injury.
- Early computed tomographic (CT) scans may facilitate evaluation of the C-spine in any head-injured or intubated patient. Adding CT evaluation of the C-spine to the initial CT scan of the head is an appropriate strategy after injury.
- All other patients should have at least a lateral view of the C-spine that includes the base of the occiput to the upper border of the first thoracic vertebra.
- Presence of paraplegia or quadriplegia is presumptive evidence of spinal instability.
- Patients with neurologic deficits potentially due to a C-spine injury require neurosurgical consultation.
- Exclusion of bony injury does not eliminate the possibility of ligamentous disruption. Magnetic resonance imaging can facilitate clearance of ligamentous injury if the examination is not reliable.

Additional details regarding imaging in potential C-spine injury are given later in the section, "Radiologic Evaluation."

b. Key Injuries

Pneumothorax is frequently associated with rib fractures and usually requires tube thoracostomy (**Appendix 8**). Any patient who has a pneumothorax on plain chest films and is receiving general anesthesia should have a chest tube in place. Tension pneumothorax is evaluated and treated as discussed in **Chapter 5**. Open pneumothorax is generally associated with soft-tissue loss requiring dressing closure and chest-tube placement. Massive hemothorax is suggested by physical examination and chest radiograph. Rapid loss of 1,000 to 2,000 mL of blood or ongoing blood loss of >200 mL/h is an indication for thoracotomy.

Rib fractures are often missed on a chest radiograph; however, a fracture may be suspected and documented when tenderness over the fracture is identified during physical examination. Pain control may be required to ensure adequate spontaneous ventilation. Flail chest resulting from segmental rib fractures is manifested by paradoxical movement of the involved portion of the chest wall (ie, inward movement of the segment during inhalation). Frequently, flail chest is associated with contusion of the underlying lung, pain, and hypoxemia.

2. Circulation

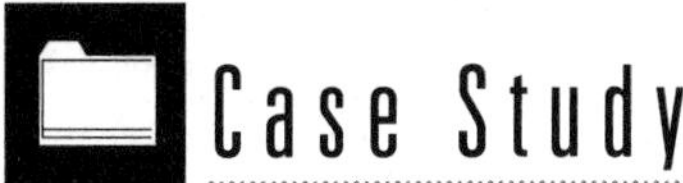

Case Study

A young man arrives in the emergency department with an epigastric stab wound, but the character of the weapon is unknown. Presenting systolic blood pressure is 90 mm Hg and the patient is tachycardiac. His systolic blood pressure improves (>100 mm Hg) with administration of intravenous fluids but deteriorates when bolus fluids are stopped. Extremities are cool and the patient is anxious.

- Is this patient in shock?
- What is the primary concern?
- What therapy is recommended?

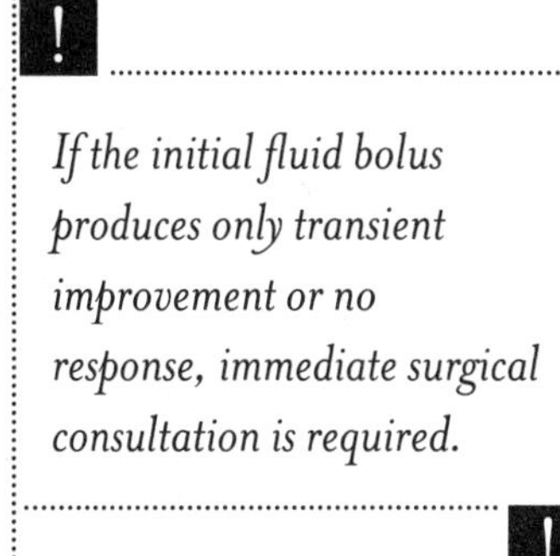

The leading cause of shock in a trauma patient is hemorrhage. Initial empiric treatment in adults consists of isotonic crystalloid infusion (2 L of warmed lactated Ringer's or normal saline solution) via two large-bore intravenous catheters and control of external hemorrhage by means of manual compression. Targets for empiric fluid therapy are normalization of blood pressure, reversal of tachycardia, and maintenance of adequate organ perfusion (**Chapter 7**). Patients with no traumatic brain injury, but extensive hemorrhage that may require operative intervention, are better managed by resuscitation to a systolic blood pressure of 90 to 100 mm Hg. This supports control of vessels that may have thrombosed and are not presently bleeding, but that may re-bleed if the blood pressure is normalized. When hypoperfusion and vascular compensation limit peripheral access, cannulation of a central vein (ideally with a 7F, 8.5F, or 9F introducer) is an alternative, as is saphenous vein cutdown or intraosseous access. Concomitant diagnostic studies for the source of bleeding can include chest radiographs (hemothorax), pelvic radiograph (pelvic fracture, open book, or vertical pelvic shear injury), focused assessment sonography in trauma (FAST), or diagnostic peritoneal lavage (DPL) (intraperitoneal hemorrhage). If the patient is hemodynamically stable, a CT scan of the abdomen and pelvis may be performed to better delineate the injuries unless a definitive indication to operate is present. A hemodynamically unstable patient should not be moved for CT scanning. Immediate control of external hemorrhage should proceed simultaneously with rapid resuscitation. In trauma to an extremity, direct pressure is recommended. Blind clamping at bleeding vessels is discouraged to avoid potential injury to adjacent structures.

As **Table 9-2** shows, a patient's systolic blood pressure, heart rate, respiratory rate, and mental status can be used to assess blood loss. The American College of Surgeons also validates a decrease in pulse pressure as a sign of occult hypoperfusion. Circulating blood volume corresponds to 7% of normal body weight (70 mL/kg) in an adult and 8% to 9% (80- 90 mL/kg) of normal body weight in children. Blood loss up to 1,200 mL may occur in a normotensive adult (70 kg) with minimal tachycardia. Class II hemorrhage is uncomplicated shock, but crystalloid resuscitation is required. Class III hemorrhage requires crystalloid resuscitation and often blood replacement. Class IV hemorrhage can be considered preterminal and requires aggressive measures to restore intravascular volume and red blood cell mass and to control bleeding. Treatment should be directed by the initial response to therapy rather than by a classification scheme. Patients will respond to fluid resuscitation in one of three ways. One group of patients will regain normal vital signs with small volumes of fluid. A second group of patients will initially respond to the fluid resuscitation, but then demonstrate signs of hemodynamic deterioration with time or a decrease in the fluid resuscitation; they will require additional fluids and focused evaluation of the etiology and treatment of the injuries. The third group of patients will not show signs of physiologic improvement despite volume resuscitation; these patients often need immediate operative intervention.

Table 9-2 Hemorrhage Classification[a]

	CLASS			
Variable	**I**	**II**	**III**	**IV**
Systolic blood pressure (mm Hg)	Normal	Normal	Decreased	Decreased
Pulse (beats/min)	<100	>100	>120	>140
Respiratory rate (breaths/min)	14-20	20-30	30-40	>35
Mental status	Anxious	Agitated	Confused	Lethargic
Blood loss (mL)	<750	750-1500	1500-2000	>2000
Blood loss (%)	<15	15-30	30-40	>40
Resuscitation fluid	Oral or crystalloid	Crystalloid	Crystalloid and blood	Blood and crystalloids

[a]Adapted with permission from the American College of Surgeons.[2] American College of Surgeons Committee on Trauma. *Advanced Trauma Life Support for Doctors (ATLS): Student Course Manual.* 8th ed. Chicago, IL: American College of Surgeons; 2008.

Isotonic crystalloid resuscitation, usually with 2 to 3 L of lactated Ringer's solution or 0.9% (normal) saline (>50 mL/kg), should be followed by the administration of packed red blood cells (PRBCs). Fully crossmatched blood is rarely available for emergency trauma resuscitation. Uncrossmatched type-specific blood can be safely administered and is available in most hospitals within 15 to 20 minutes after a request is received. If type-specific blood is not available and the patient is unstable,

> **!**
>
> *Citrate in PRBCs may chelate calcium, promoting a coagulation defect in patients receiving massive transfusion. Ionized calcium levels should be monitored and calcium administered as needed.*

O-negative PRBCs should be used. When these are not available, O-positive PRBCs may be used. The patient may become sensitized to the Rh factor, but this is significant only in female patients of childbearing age (who must be treated with Rh_0 (D) immune globulin injection to prevent antibody formation).

Transfusion of other blood products, such as fresh frozen plasma, platelets, or cryoprecipitate, is usually not part of the initial resuscitation but may be urgently required if bleeding persists and/or a coagulopathy develops. In patients with ongoing significant bleeding, serial coagulation profiles (ie, prothrombin time, partial thromboplastin time, hemoglobin, hematocrit, and platelet count) should be obtained. Platelet counts $<50{,}000/mm^3$ are usually treated with platelet transfusion in the setting of ongoing hemorrhage. Likewise, abnormalities of prothrombin time and partial thromboplastin time in the bleeding patient should be treated with fresh frozen plasma (10-20 mL/kg initially). Bleeding not due to coagulopathy should be addressed directly, usually in the operating room. Administration of large amounts of crystalloid solutions, a common cause of reduced coagulation factors and dilutional thrombocytopenia, requires platelet transfusion and fresh frozen plasma. Clinical manifestations of clotting dysfunction should be treated empirically with platelets and fresh frozen plasma when laboratory evaluation of these parameters is not available.

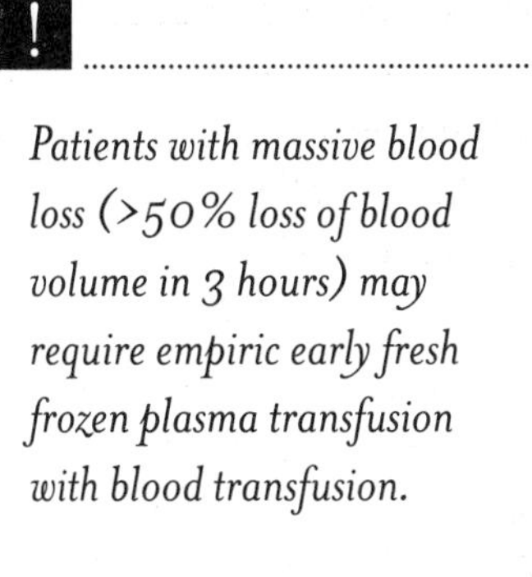
Patients with massive blood loss (>50% loss of blood volume in 3 hours) may require empiric early fresh frozen plasma transfusion with blood transfusion.

3. Disability/Exposure

Rapid neurologic evaluation is performed in the emergency department and includes determination of level of consciousness, pupillary size and reaction, lateralizing signs, and level of spinal cord injury. The GCS score is a quick, simple method for determining the level of consciousness and is predictive of outcome (particularly the best motor response). A decrease in the level of consciousness may reflect decreased cerebral perfusion or may be due to direct brain injury. Hypoglycemia, ethanol, narcotics, and other drugs may also be involved. An altered level of consciousness indicates the need for immediate reevaluation of oxygenation, ventilation, and tissue perfusion. Changes in consciousness should be assumed to be due to intracerebral conditions until proven otherwise. If a patient is to be sedated and intubated, initial attempts to determine the presence of any localizing spinal cord or cranial cord injury should be made, if the patient's condition permits.

Throughout the initial resuscitation period, efforts should be made to control and prevent hypothermia. Patients are often hypothermic after environmental exposure, and the body temperature may fall even more after administration of room temperature resuscitation fluids and cold blood, removal of clothing for examination purposes, loss of normal temperature-regulating reflexes in shock, or use of some medications. Hypothermia contributes to coagulation abnormalities, cardiovascular collapse, and poor outcome, and so should be avoided and treated. Warm intravenous fluids, heated respiratory gases in mechanical ventilation, warm rooms, insulating covers, and heating lamps can be used.

4. Monitoring

Improvements in parameters such as heart rate, blood pressure, pulse pressure, ventilatory rate, acid-base status, body temperature, and urinary output are the best guides to adequacy of resuscitation. Evaluation begins during the initial survey and should be repeated periodically. Pulse oximetry is a valuable adjunct for monitoring hemoglobin saturation with oxygen in injured patients, but it is not useful for evaluating the adequacy of ventilation. Blood pressure, as the sole marker of resuscitation, may be a poor measure of actual tissue perfusion. Additional metabolic markers, such as serum lactate, base deficit, and pH, will assist in the determination of the adequacy of resuscitation. Perfusion of extremities may be evaluated by examining capillary refill and hematoma formation, as well as the presence of the peripheral pulses.

A urinary catheter should be inserted as soon as is practical to monitor urine output as a gauge of renal perfusion, although it is contraindicated in male patients when urethral injury is suspected (eg, blood at the urethral meatus, scrotal hematoma, or abnormal prostate on rectal exam).

5. Hemorrhagic Shock

As resuscitation proceeds, it is crucial to identify potential causes of hypotension. A search for occult blood loss should be undertaken after any external hemorrhage is controlled. The most frequent sites for such blood loss are the chest, abdomen, pelvis, and the soft tissues adjacent to long bone fractures.

a. Hemothorax

A chest radiograph (ideally with the patient in upright or reverse Trendelenburg position if hemodynamically stable) is a reliable screen for intrathoracic bleeding. Ultrasonography of the chest also may reliably detect hemothorax or pericardial fluid. Hemothorax should be drained promptly by tube thoracostomy, with a subsequent radiograph to verify the location of the chest tube, blood evacuation, and lung expansion. As noted earlier, rapid loss of 1,000 mL of blood upon chest tube insertion or continued losses of >200 mL/h for 4 hours may necessitate thoracotomy. If available, autotransfusion devices should be attached to any chest tube drainage canister placed for massive hemothorax.

b. Intra-abdominal Hemorrhage

Abdominal examination is often misleading in the detection of acute bleeding, especially in patients with lower chest trauma, rib fractures, spinal cord injury, intoxication, or altered level of consciousness. Any patient who has sustained significant blunt torso injury from a direct blow or deceleration, or a penetrating torso injury must be considered to have an abdominal visceral or vascular injury. Focused ultrasound for trauma and DPL are the most expedient and reliable methods of identifying significant intraperitoneal hemorrhage, although the FAST exam has largely replaced the use of DPL in most institutions. When readily available and used by trained individuals, FAST has the sensitivity, specificity, and accuracy of DPL in detecting hemoperitoneum, an injury that requires immediate surgical evaluation to determine the need for an operative intervention. In stable cases, abdominal CT scan may be appropriate to identify the source of bleeding. Abdominal hemorrhage frequently comes from splenic or liver laceration, other visceral injury, or retroperitoneal hematoma. Patients with unstable or abnormal vital signs are usually not candidates for CT scanning and require surgery to control bleeding.

c. Pelvic Hemorrhage

Assessment of bony stability by means of physical examination and plain radiographs of the pelvis is crucial for early identification of major pelvic fractures. Patients with pelvic fractures (open book or vertical shear) are at high risk for major bleeding, which is usually venous. Initial management includes vigorous blood volume replacement and, possibly, mechanical tamponade with a bedsheet wrapped tightly around the pelvis or other strategies to produce circumferential compression. External skeletal fixation may be helpful if the fracture anatomy is appropriate, and an orthopedic surgeon should be consulted early in the course of treatment. In patients with arterial bleeding associated with pelvic injury, CT scanning will reveal a blush of contrast loss. Pelvic angiography for embolization should be considered in the persistently hypotensive patient due to an increased likelihood for arterial bleeding. Angiography may be required in approximately 10% of patients with pelvic fractures.

d. Long Bone Fractures

Patients with long bong fractures will likely have associated hemorrhage in the surrounding injured tissue. Humerus and femur fractures may result in 1 to 3 units of blood loss. This can be problematic in the patient with multiple long bone fractures. Repeated physical examination for soft tissue swelling and changes in the diameter of the extremity will assist in the management of these patients.

e. External Hemorrhage

External hemorrhage can be very dramatic, as with a lacerated artery where direct pressure will decrease blood loss. Other cases, such as scalp lacerations, may go unrecognized as a possible source of significant blood loss. Rapid application of direct pressure, temporizing suture repair, or application of a tourniquet to a bleeding extremity may be lifesaving. One technique employs a blood pressure cuff inflated to a pressure higher than the patient's systolic blood pressure. Tourniquet use should be followed by surgical consultation as the tourniquet places the extremity in jeopardy of ischemic injury.

6. Nonhemorrhagic Shock

The differential diagnosis of nonhemorrhagic shock in the trauma patient includes obstructive shock (tension pneumothorax, cardiac tamponade), blunt cardiac injury, air embolism, and neurogenic shock with acute spinal cord injury. Head injury is a rare cause of hypotension, but when it occurs, it is usually a preterminal event.

a. Tension Pneumothorax

Tension pneumothorax causes hemodynamic compromise and pulmonary dysfunction due to acute compression of the lung parenchyma and a shift of the mediastinum away from the hemithorax with the increased pressure. Do not wait for a chest radiograph to make this diagnosis. Breath sounds will be diminished, lung expansion will be asynchronous, and patients may develop respiratory distress, acute desaturation, bradycardia, and occasionally, distended neck veins. Classic venous distension may be absent in the setting of pneumothorax complicated by hypovolemia. All but gross changes in breath sounds may be difficult to detect in the resuscitation room. Tracheal shift is a late sign and may not be a presenting finding. In adults, needle thoracostomy is performed via the midclavicular line in the second intercostal space; this is a lifesaving intervention that is followed by placement of a chest tube.

! *If tension pneumothorax is suspected in an intubated patient, disconnect the patient from the ventilator and manually ventilate to evaluate for increasing resistance.* !

b. Cardiac Tamponade

The classic signs of cardiac tamponade — hypotension, distant heart sounds, jugular venous distension, and pulsus paradoxus — may be obscured due to noise and hypovolemia (decreasing jugular distention). Ultrasound (FAST) is a sensitive test for fluid in the pericardial sac. Pericardiocentesis via a surgical pericardial window should be considered for the patient with refractory shock, persistent central venous hypertension, and a high-risk penetrating wound (between the nipples, above the costal margin, below the clavicles). When surgical expertise is not available, a needle/catheter pericardiocentesis may be performed as a temporizing measure. Occasionally, major blunt chest trauma ruptures the cardiac surface. Most cases involve atrial tears and can be repaired if diagnosed early.

c. Blunt Cardiac Injury

The diagnosis of blunt cardiac injury should be suspected in a patient involved in a high-speed, frontal impact accident who has unexplained hypotension or arrhythmia or, less commonly, cardiogenic shock. Changes in the electrocardiograms (ECGs) are usually nonspecific and can include premature ventricular contractions, bundle branch block, atrial fibrillation, unexplained sinus tachycardia, and ST-segment changes. If blunt cardiac injury is a possibility, a screening ECG should be obtained in the emergency department. Abnormalities other than tachycardia warrant 24 hours of monitoring for arrhythmias. Hemodynamically stable individuals with no ECG abnormalities need no further cardiac evaluation or

! *The right ventricle is most frequently involved in blunt cardiac injury, and volume challenge is the initial therapy for hypotension in the absence of pulmonary edema.* !

observation. Echocardiography may be indicated in hypotensive patients to evaluate cardiac function. Use of cardiac troponins in diagnosing blunt cardiac injury is sometimes helpful. Treatment includes correction of acidosis, hypoxia, and electrolyte abnormalities; judicious administration of fluid; and pharmacologic treatment of life-threatening arrhythmias.

Inotropes may be indicated to support hemodynamic function. It is important to ensure that refractory hypotension is not due to ongoing blood loss. Patients may present with acute myocardial infarction secondary to cardiac injury, or an acute myocardial infarction may have led to trauma (ie, fall, motor vehicle crash).

d. Neurogenic Shock

Neurogenic shock occurs when a cervical or high thoracic spinal cord injury (above T6 level) causes sympathectomy. It is characterized by hypotension, frequently associated with relative or absolute bradycardia. Flaccid paralysis, loss of extremity reflexes, and priapism may be associated neurologic findings. Treatment for hypotension includes volume resuscitation and vasopressors (phenylephrine, norepinephrine, or dopamine) if volume loading does not reverse the hypotension. Atropine is indicated in the presence of bradycardia associated with hemodynamic instability.

B. Secondary Assessment: Diagnosis and Treatment of Other Injuries

Most patients with acute injuries can be resuscitated to a hemodynamically stable state. The primary survey should immediately identify acute life-threatening injuries. The next goal is to complete a secondary assessment to identify and treat other injuries. This assessment is crucial to allow proper triage to the operating room, radiology suite, or ICU.

1. History

Essential components of a patient's history include details of the mechanism of injury, previous medical illness, current medications, allergies, and tetanus immunization.

2. Physical Examination

The patient should be examined from head to toe. The skull is carefully inspected to identify occult injuries. Signs of basilar skull fracture include hematotympanum, rhinorrhea, or otorrhea; Battle sign (ecchymosis of the skin over the mastoid); and raccoon eyes. Facial bones, mandible, and neck are palpated for tenderness and crepitus. The GCS score and limited neurologic examination from the initial assessment are used to evaluate for head trauma (**Chapter 8**). Extraocular eye movements are checked to exclude muscle or nerve entrapment. The neck is inspected for distended neck veins, the position of the trachea, or subcutaneous emphysema. Neck pain or tenderness over the cervical spine warrants additional radiographs ("Radiologic Evaluation" section), CT, or magnetic resonance imaging. The chest is auscultated and palpated for tenderness and crepitus. The patient is log-rolled so that the thoracic and lumbar spine can be palpated for tenderness and other injuries can be detected. In penetrating trauma, exclude occult entrance or exit wounds in the axillary, cervical, or inguinal regions. The abdomen is likewise inspected, auscultated, and palpated. The pelvic bones are assessed for stability with lateral compression, anterior-posterior compression, and a gentle rocking motion; lack of pain with these motions in an awake patient without competing pain issues is usually sufficient to rule out significant pelvic bone fractures. The rectum is evaluated for tone and the presence or absence of blood and to ensure that the prostate gland is not displaced or difficult to palpate. The presence of perineal/scrotal hematoma and blood at the urethral meatus implies urogenital injury, which is a risk for urinary catheter insertion. The extremities are inspected, palpated, and evaluated for range of motion and neurovascular integrity.

3. Laboratory Studies

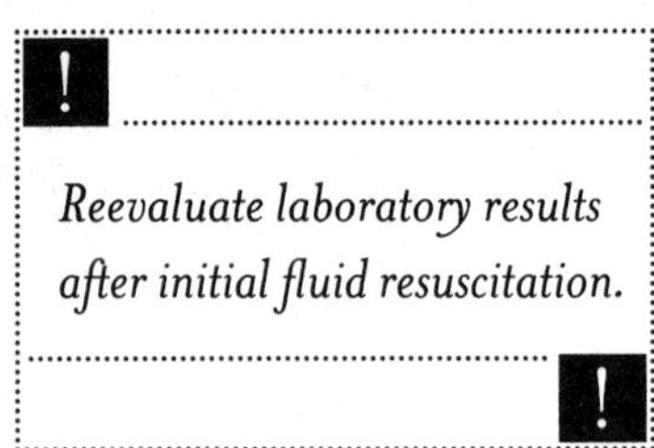

Minimal testing includes complete blood count, electrolytes, blood glucose, blood alcohol level, and toxicology screening. In any patient with evidence of hypovolemia, blood-group typing and a coagulation profile should be performed. In selected patients, blood may be drawn and held until tests are deemed necessary. Arterial blood gas measurements should be analyzed in selected patients to confirm adequate ventilation and perfusion (presence of acidosis). An elevated serum amylase level may be an indicator of pancreatic or bowel injury in the patient with blunt abdominal trauma. Creatinine phosphokinase should be checked if rhabdomyolysis is suspected. The hematocrit may not reflect the patient's acute volume status. Equilibration by transcapillary fluid shifts takes hours to be reflected as a decrease in hematocrit. In general, a fall of 3% in the hematocrit is equivalent to 1 unit of blood loss.

4. Radiologic Evaluation

a. General

In the evaluation of blunt multiple-system trauma, a lateral C-spine radiograph to the level of T1, a supine chest radiograph, and supine view of the pelvis are obtained as the primary survey is performed. This allows for interpretation of completed radiographs as the secondary survey begins. Plain films of the pelvis are crucial for early identification of major fractures.

b. Head

CT scanning is essential for initial evaluation of a head-injured patient or in any patient with a decreased or altered level of consciousness. Many centers will also obtain a CT scan of the cervical spine when the head scan is obtained.

c. Spine

The initial lateral C-spine radiograph is valuable in identifying major fractures that would affect decision making and support a diagnosis of catastrophic cervical spinal cord injury. A good quality lateral C-spine radiograph delineates many unstable fractures. The most common problems with lateral C-spine images are inadequate visualization of C7 to T1 and poor definition of the occiput. Most centers will now obtain a CT evaluation of any areas that cannot be cleared or that show a possibility of injury. In the patient with increased risk of C-spine injury, cervical immobilization is crucial until these studies are reviewed and correlated with a reliable physical examination for evidence of tenderness. Magnetic resonance imaging is helpful for disc, spinal cord, and ligament injuries. If a C-spine fracture is found, radiographic screening of the spine is indicated because ~10% of these patients will have a second, noncontiguous vertebral column fracture. Anteroposterior and lateral thoracic and lumbar radiographs should be obtained if these areas are tender to palpation, if ecchymosis or palpable irregularities are present, if the physical examination is not reliable, or if the mechanism of injury is suggestive. CT scans of chest and abdomen often can be reformatted to provide information on spine injury without the need for additional plain radiographs.

d. Chest

Once the spine is cleared for fractures, an upright (or reverse Trendelenburg) chest radiograph is indicated to better define or identify pneumothorax, hemothorax, mediastinal widening or irregularity (concern for aortic transection), or fractures and to confirm the position of various tubes. Chest radiographs are inadequate to rule out aortic injury when a significant lateral impact or deceleration injury exists. Suspect this lethal injury where the mediastinum is widened on chest radiographs and an appropriate mechanism is involved. CT angiography with newer helical scanners provides an alternative method to screen for aortic injury and define other thoracic injuries. Aortic angiography has largely been replaced by CT angiography to detect aortic injury.

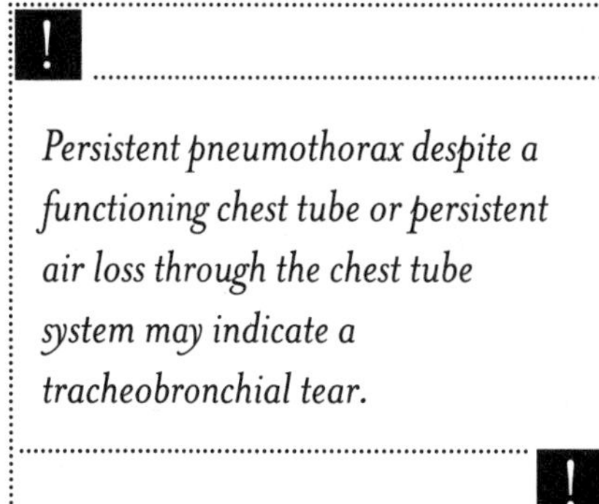
Persistent pneumothorax despite a functioning chest tube or persistent air loss through the chest tube system may indicate a tracheobronchial tear.

e. Abdomen

Plain abdominal radiographs are not usually helpful. In the hemodynamically stable patient, a CT scan of the abdomen and pelvis and the FAST examination are the mainstays of abdominal evaluation in a trauma patient. FAST can be followed up with a CT scan of the abdomen if free peritoneal fluid is identified. DPL may still be used in certain circumstances, but has generally been replaced by the CT scan of the abdomen and pelvis and the FAST. DPL may be used with penetrating abdominal trauma to determine the presence of bleeding.

f. Genitourinary Tract

Hematuria may be evaluated with a CT scan or other contrast studies. It provides anatomic detail about abdominal and retroperitoneal structures and any direct injury to the kidney(s). If physical examination suggests that a urethral injury is present, a urethrogram should be obtained before urinary catheterization. A cystogram may be indicated if bladder injury is suspected. Intravenous pyelograms are not commonly performed.

g. Skeletal Fractures

Films of the extremities (anterior posterior and lateral views) should be obtained on the basis of physical examination or patient complaint. Films should include the joint above and below the site of injury.

5. Other Issues

A nasogastric tube serves to decompress the stomach and may reduce the risk of pulmonary aspiration; however, it should be placed orally in patients with midfacial fractures or possible basilar skull fractures. Blood in the gastric aspirate may be the only sign of an otherwise occult injury to the stomach or duodenum, and further investigation may be indicated. Tetanus prophylaxis is routine (**Appendix 10**). Systemic antibiotics should usually be withheld until a specific indication is determined, but they are employed in three situations: (1) patients undergoing intracranial pressure monitoring or tube thoracostomy frequently receive gram-positive coverage when the device is inserted; (2) patients with penetrating abdominal trauma may be given coverage for gram-negative aerobic and anaerobic organisms for the first 24 hours after injury; and (3) patients with open fractures are given gram-positive coverage for 24 hours as orthopedic evaluation is arranged.

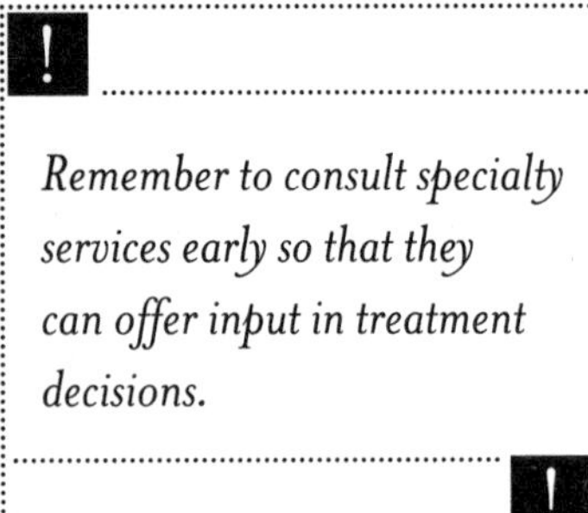

Female patients of childbearing age should be questioned about the possibility of pregnancy or be checked with a β-human chorionic gonadotropin test before extensive radiographic evaluation is performed. Anyone in her second or third trimester should be positioned with a wedge under her back to elevate the right side, avoiding compression of the vena cava. This is done only after examination of the spine and pelvis does not reveal any pain or tenderness, which may indicate a fracture. Remember that the optimal care of the mother yields optimal care for the fetus.

C. Tertiary Assessment: Ongoing Evaluation

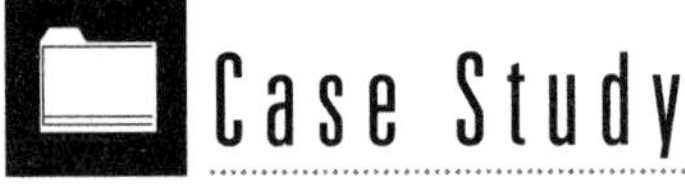

Case Study

A middle-aged man sustained multiple liver lacerations in a motor vehicle crash. He also had mesenteric lacerations and bowel resection was performed. The ends of the bowel were stapled, and the abdomen was filled with packs to control venous bleeding from the liver. He continues to require fluid resuscitation and administration of blood products due to coagulopathy. Several hours after admission to the ICU, increased airway pressures and falling urine output are noted.

- What are possible causes of increased airway pressures?
- Why has the urine output fallen?

After life- and limb-threatening injuries have been addressed and metabolic derangements have been corrected, periodic systematic assessment is done to identify occult injuries not evident at presentation.

1. Head Injury

Evaluation of the head-injured patient is an ongoing process requiring early neurosurgical consultation. Serial assessment of the GCS scores, pupil size and response, and presence or absence of lateralizing neurologic signs is crucial. Any changes in examination results are noted and acted upon as they are discovered.

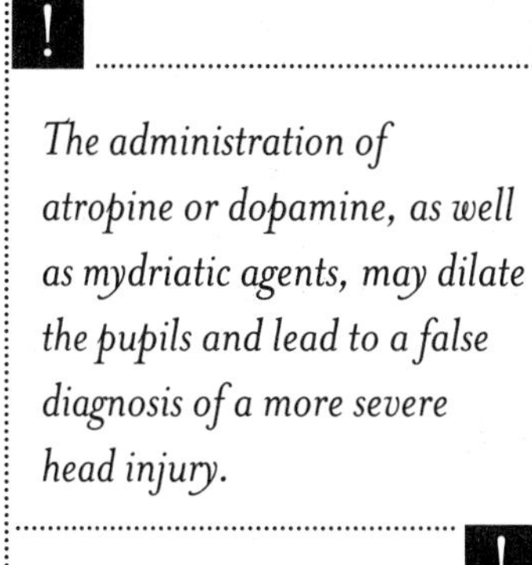

Serial CT scans of the head may offer clinically useful information, but the key to patient management is detection of changes in physical examination. Continued resuscitation is imperative to avoid secondary brain injury, which typically occurs when a patient becomes hypoxic or hypotensive during acute care. These secondary insults increase the likelihood of poor outcome (**Chapter 8**).

2. Pulmonary Injury

Trauma patients often have a full stomach at the time of injury and experience aspiration. The acidic gastric contents may cause a chemical pneumonitis initially and predispose patients to an infective pneumonitis or acute respiratory distress syndrome later. Antibiotics are not indicated in initial management. Bronchoscopy may be needed for removal of large particulate matter.

Delayed onset of pneumothorax or hemothorax may follow chest trauma. Additionally, pulmonary contusions and resulting acute respiratory distress syndrome may not become obvious until later (12-48 hours). Continued assessment includes physical examination, oximetry and/or arterial blood gas measurements, chest radiographs, and ventilatory mechanics.

3. Cardiac Injury

Continuous ECG monitoring and frequent measurements of blood pressure are mandatory in the emergency department and intensive care unit. Continuous arterial blood pressure monitoring may be indicated, as discussed in **Chapter 6**. Electrolyte disturbances may lead to cardiac contractile dysfunction or arrhythmias in the aggressively resuscitated trauma patient. Common electrolyte disturbances include hyperchloremia, hypokalemia and hyperkalemia, hypomagnesemia, and hypocalcemia.

4. Abdominal Injury

Substance abuse or neurologic injury may not allow reliable initial abdominal examination. Perforation of a hollow viscus in blunt trauma is sometimes difficult to diagnose. Free air under the diaphragm on an upright chest radiograph, over the liver on a left lateral decubitus radiograph, or on an abdominal CT indicates the need for operative exploration. CT scanning also provides information about the retroperitoneum. In the head-injured patient who is undergoing a head CT scan and has a nonoperative neurologic injury, abdominal scanning should be considered, as physical examination may be unreliable.

A frequently missed condition is the abdominal compartment syndrome. This condition occurs when there is an increase in intra-abdominal pressure due to intraperitoneal or retroperitoneal hemorrhage, ascitic fluid accumulation, edema secondary to massive fluid resuscitation, or intraoperative surgical closure of the abdomen under tension. Increased intra-abdominal pressure decreases cardiac output and compresses the vascular bed and kidneys. The diaphragm is displaced upward by increased intra-abdominal pressure, which results in decreased thoracic volume and compliance. Decreased volume within the pleural cavity predisposes to atelectasis, and ventilated patients with intra-abdominal hypertension require increased airway pressure to deliver a fixed tidal volume. Vascular compression can decrease blood flow to the liver and kidneys with resultant dysfunction. Finally, intra-abdominal hypertension significantly increases intracranial pressure (**Chapter 13**).

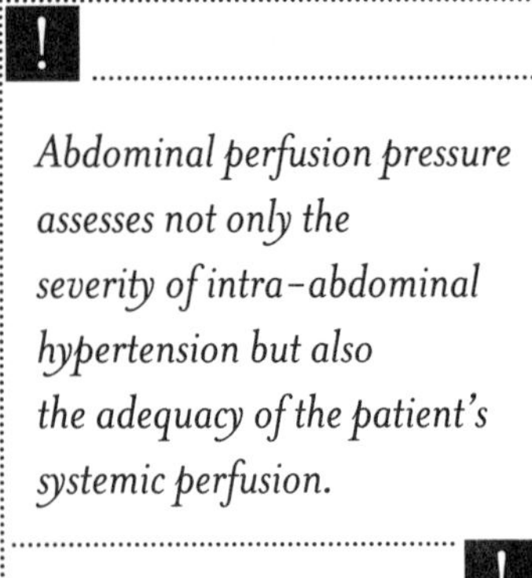

5. Musculoskeletal Injury

The neurologic and vascular evaluation of the extremities is an ongoing process. A swollen and tense extremity should be watched closely for the development of a compartment syndrome, particularly in patients with decreased responsiveness. In alert patients, serial physical examination is the best monitor. Classical signs include pain, pallor, pulselessness, paresthesia, and/or paralysis. Loss of pulse is a very late finding. The most helpful early signs are complaints of pain out of proportion to physical findings and severe pain on passive stretch of the involved muscle groups. In the unconscious patient or when the examination is unreliable, compartment pressure may be monitored using a needle with a standard gauge. Pressures >30 mm Hg warrant consideration of fasciotomy.

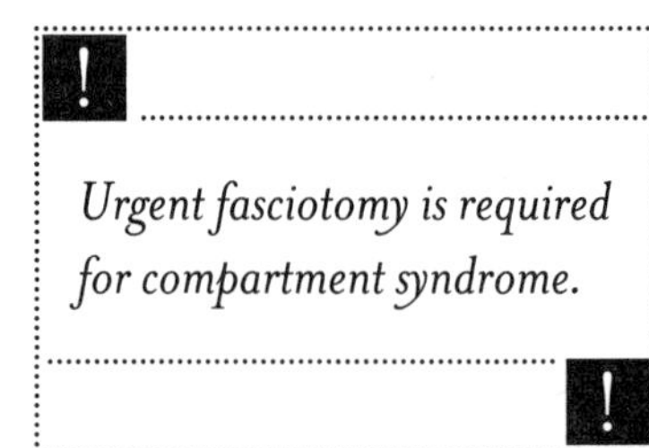

Musculoskeletal examination should be repeated, either as patients recover from other injuries or as their mental status clears, to identify new pain or tenderness. Plain radiographs should then be obtained to identify occult fractures. Commonly missed orthopedic injuries include fractures of the scapula, thoracic and lumbar spine, pelvis, ankle, and wrist.

Crush syndrome should be considered when patients have been trapped, injury to large muscle mass is involved, prolonged compression has occurred with protracted immobilization, or vascular compromise is present (such as tourniquet use or compartment syndrome). Crush syndrome develops when damaged myocytes lyse, releasing myoglobin, potassium, phosphorus, and calcium. Manifestations of this syndrome include cardiac dysrhythmias, renal failure, metabolic acidosis, and hypovolemia. Preemptive hydration before reperfusion of crushed muscle mass usually is accomplished before arrival at the hospital. Revascularization of ischemic extremities, fasciotomy for compartment syndrome, or release of tourniquets can mimic this situation. Before reperfusion, normal saline should be administered (1- to 2-L bolus or 10-15 mL/kg/h). Careful monitoring for cardiac signs of hyperkalemia should be instituted. After reperfusion, aggressive hydration to maintain urine output above 3 to 4 mL/kg/h helps prevent heme pigment-associated renal injury. Adjuvants such as bicarbonate and mannitol may be used.

6. Other Considerations

Resuscitation is an ongoing process. Traditional end points such as normalization of blood pressure, heart rate, and urine output may not always reflect complete correction of the shock state. The attainment of normal vital signs can occur even in the setting of tissue hypoperfusion resulting in a compensated state of shock. Lactate concentration and resolution of metabolic acidosis may provide more definitive end points for adequacy of resuscitation. Since the time to normalization of these parameters is predictive of survival, additional resuscitation in the form of volume replacement, red cell transfusion, or support with vasoactive agents may be indicated within the first 24 hours postinjury despite normal or near-normal vital signs. Persistence of a metabolic acidosis or elevated lactate concentration may be an early indicator of complications, including ongoing hemorrhage or abdominal compartment syndrome.

Damage control surgery (initially limited to control of bleeding and decontamination of hollow organ ruptures with spillage) may be needed in the first 24 to 48 hours, before definitive surgery is performed. Many trauma patients benefit from delayed definitive surgery, particularly the repair of fractures, during this period of ongoing stabilization. Decisions to proceed with surgery should be made after appropriate consultation with the primary surgical service, a critical care physician, and other consultants as indicated.

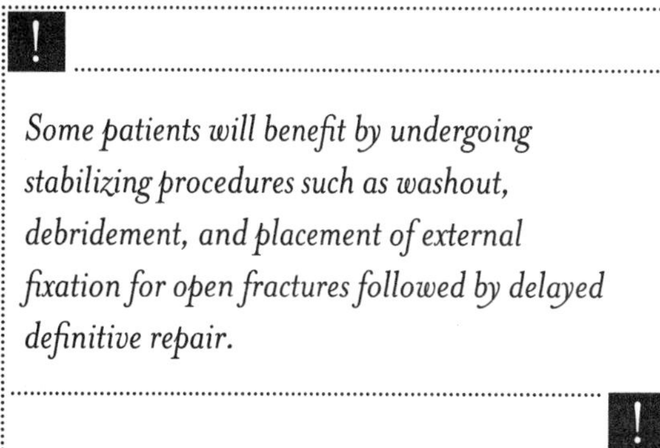

Some patients will benefit by undergoing stabilizing procedures such as washout, debridement, and placement of external fixation for open fractures followed by delayed definitive repair.

In the immediate resuscitation period, periodic reassessments are important. Once a patient is stabilized, all intravenous access sites should be reassessed. Because full sterile precautions to prevent line-related infections may not be feasible during emergency vascular access, many lines will need to be replaced. If central venous access is no longer indicated, it may be discontinued.

III. BURN INJURY: INITIAL EVALUATION AND STABILIZATION

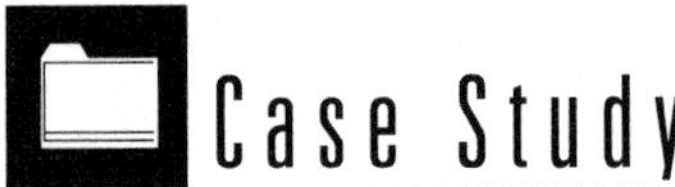

Case Study

A young man is brought in after a gasoline can exploded as he was burning brush. The patient sustained a full-thickness burn injury to both forearms and showed signs of flash-burn injury to his face. He is in no respiratory distress and has received no fluids since his injury. Although he has no abdominal burns, he complains of abdominal pain. Family members recall that the patient was thrown into a tree stump by the explosion. You are asked to follow up with the patient during his initial wound care in the burn unit.

- What are the initial evaluation priorities?
- What is the greatest risk to this patient?

A. General

Burn injuries represent a significant cause of morbidity and mortality. Deaths from burn injury occur with greatest frequency as a result of residential fires with smoke inhalation. Like other forms of injury, burns tend to be frequent in the young and the elderly. Scalds are the most common form of childhood injury, whereas electrical and chemical injuries affect adults in the workplace. Factors that affect burn mortality include size of cutaneous injury, patient age, and presence or absence of inhalation injury. Burn injuries should not distract providers from seeking other potential traumatic injuries. The initial evaluation and treatment of a serious burn injury follows the same pathway as trauma, including the primary and secondary surveys.

B. Airway/Breathing

The initial evaluation of the airway is directed, in part, by the history of the injury. Patients who are at the greatest risk of smoke inhalation injury typically have a history of being in a closed space with flame and smoke. With increased exposure time, the likelihood of smoke inhalation injury increases. Smoke inhalation can be described by three mechanisms of injury. These include particulate injury, toxic byproducts of combustion injury, and direct thermal injury. Particulates found in the soot and smoke of the fire are responsible for a reactive airway injury that may result in bronchospasm. Toxic exposure may have direct cytotoxic effect on alveolar tissue or affect energy generating pathways, or bind hemoglobin and reduce the availability of oxygen for intracellular use. Direct thermal injury can result in oral, nasal, and upper respiratory injury with airway swelling.

Inhalation injury is generally diagnosed by a combination of clinical signs and symptoms confirmed by bronchoscopy. Clinical findings include facial burns, parched oral mucosa, nasal singeing, soot in the oral and nasal passages, and symptoms of reactive airway exacerbation. Bronchoscopic findings include mucosal edema, ulceration, sloughing, and mucous plugging. Chest radiographs are frequently normal at admission, and hypoxemia often is not appreciated.

Three stages of inhalation injury have been identified:

1. Acute hypoxia with asphyxia typically occurs at the scene of the fire.
2. Upper airway and pulmonary edema may evolve during the first hours to days after injury.
3. Infectious complications that stem from exposure to heat and chemical irritants may appear later (eg, pneumonia).

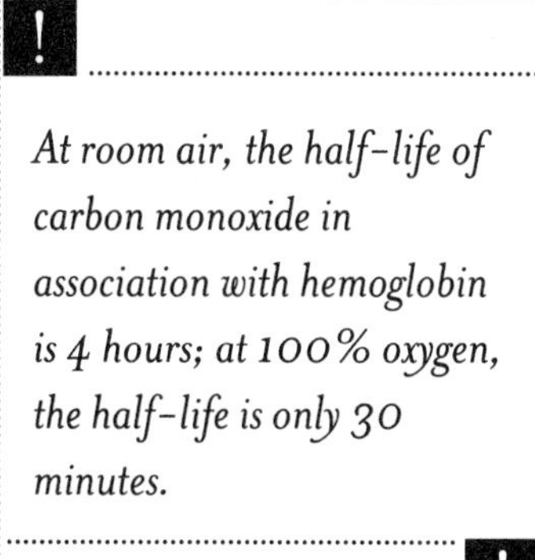

At room air, the half-life of carbon monoxide in association with hemoglobin is 4 hours; at 100% oxygen, the half-life is only 30 minutes.

Treatment of inhalation injury is largely supportive. If exposure to carbon monoxide is suspected, 100% oxygen should be provided. Early intubation is advocated, especially if the patient will be transferred, because pulmonary and laryngeal injury may quickly evolve even though the initial airway assessment is satisfactory. Caution should be exercised in the use of succinylcholine due to the possibility of clinically significant hyperkalemia. Intravascular resuscitation should not be delayed or withheld because inhalation injury increases resuscitation fluid requirements. Humidification of inhaled gases helps in secretion control and reduces desiccation injury to the airway.

C. Circulation

Patients sustaining small burns (<20% total body surface area [TBSA]) typically will have normal vital signs. Those with larger burns (>20% TBSA) may develop burn shock. This is due to a diffuse capillary leak syndrome resulting from the release of cytokines, interleukins, and vasoactive amines and causing third spacing of fluid. The combined loss of fluid from the burned surface area and the interstitial edema may result in the loss of circulating volume. Systemic hypotension may ensue. Resuscitation following the Parkland formula (discussed later) should be followed as it permits large volumes of fluid to be administered over an extended period. Large-bore peripheral intravenous catheters should be placed (through the burn, if necessary). The preferred resuscitation fluid is lactated Ringer's solution.

D. Assessment of Injury

The approach to the initial assessment is the same as in trauma. An initial primary survey (ABCDE) is performed, followed by a head-to-toe examination. All the clothes need to be removed to determine burn size, and the patient must be covered with blankets because heat is lost quickly. Depending upon the history, the patient may have other injuries and should be assessed for trauma in accordance with the guidelines outlined.

1. Depth of Burns

There are three burn depths:

1. First-degree (superficial): erythematous, painful
2. Second-degree (partial thickness): red, swollen, blistered, weeping, very painful
3. Third-degree (full thickness): white, leathery, painless

Third-degree or full-thickness injuries involve all layers of the epidermis and dermis and require surgical reconstruction. Burns that involve deep structures, such as tendon, muscle, and bone, have been called fourth-degree burns.

2. Burn Area (Rule of Nines)

The rule of nines is commonly used to estimate the TBSA that has been burned (**Figure 9-1**). The head and upper extremities each represent 9% of the TBSA. The anterior and posterior trunk and the lower extremities each represent 18%, and the perineum represents 1% of the TBSA. Alternatively, the patient's hand, which equals roughly 1% of TBSA, may be used to estimate the size of a small or irregular burn.

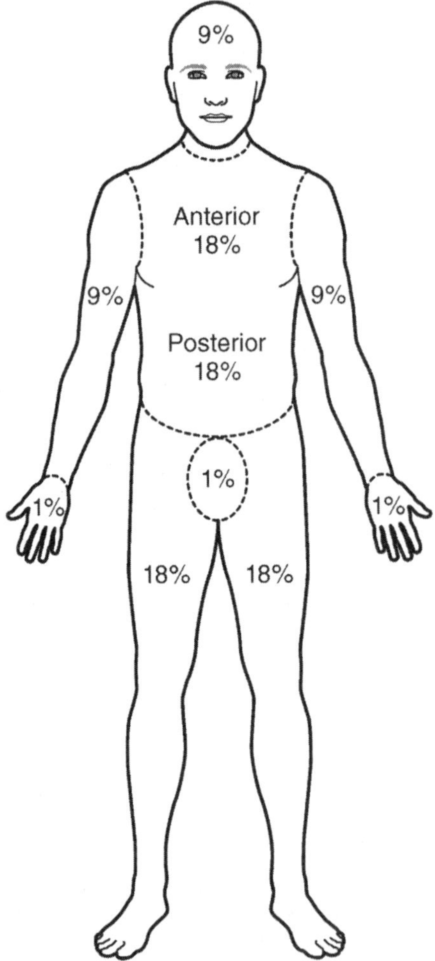

Figure 9-1. Rule of Nines

E. Resuscitation

Burn shock presents with profound hypovolemia, which has both interstitial and intracellular components. Increased capillary permeability is one of the key components of the burn shock response. In small burns, maximal edema is seen in 8 to 12 hours after injury, larger burns at 12 to 24 hours. Plasma volume loss coincides with edema formation and increased extracellular fluid. Edema is affected by fluid administration during resuscitation. Fluid and electrolytes should be replaced as dictated by organ perfusion indicators and electrolyte imbalance. Because fluid and electrolyte losses in burns are primarily insensible, fluid lost cannot be quantified adequately. Venous access should be obtained and a urinary catheter placed. The American Burn Association recommends the consensus formula of 2 to 4 mL/kg/% TBSA burned. Beginning at the low end of this range may reduce edema and extravascular complications such as abdominal compartment syndrome. The TBSA is calculated only for second- or third-degree burns. Resuscitation is carried out with Ringer's lactate solution. Half of the crystalloid resuscitation should be administered in the first 8 hours, the remaining over the next 16 hours. Surrogate markers of adequate resuscitation include normalization of blood pressure, heart rate, and urine output. Appropriate urine output in adults is 0.5 to 1 mL/kg/h and 1 to 1.5 mL/kg/h in children. An arterial blood gas measurement to monitor the pH and base deficit and serum lactate levels are also good markers of adequate resuscitation.

A circumferential burn to an extremity may develop significant edema that the underlying tissue cannot accommodate due to the constrictive nature of the burn wound. Impaired limb and tissue perfusion may ensue that can only be managed by performing an escharotomy to the extremity and/or digits. In larger burns of the abdomen and chest wall, a compartment syndrome may develop whereby cardiovascular and respiratory compromise may mandate torso escharotomies or abdominal decompression. Surgical consultation should be sought immediately for any of these problems.

F. Carbon Monoxide Exposure

A fire in an enclosed space mandates consideration of carbon monoxide poisoning. The typical oxygen saturation monitor will not detect carbon monoxide and can give artificially elevated oxygen saturation levels; therefore, if carbon monoxide poisoning is suspected, an arterial blood gas with a carboxyhemoglobin level will clarify the clinical picture. High-flow 100% oxygen will reduce the half-life of carbon monoxide in the plasma and is the primary treatment. Early use of hyperbaric oxygen for patients with high carboxyhemoglobin levels (>25%) or evidence of significant neurologic or cardiovascular toxicity has been recommended, but data supporting this recommendation are limited.

G. Burn Wound

Local wound care begins with serial debridement of nonviable tissue and blisters by appropriate surgical consultants. Little care is required for the burn wound before transfer to the burn center or surgical consultation. If gross contamination is present, a gentle washing and coverage with clean linen may be appropriate. If the patient cannot be rapidly transferred to a burn center, it may be necessary to apply silver sulfadiazine (or appropriate antibiotic ointment) and occlusive dressings to help prevent evaporative heat loss.

H. Other Considerations

Placement of a nasogastric tube is indicated if the patient vomits, requires intubation, or has a burn >20% of TBSA. Intravenous opiates should be given for pain. Rings and bracelets should be removed as they may cause constriction early in resuscitation. Burns are tetanus-prone injuries, and tetanus prophylaxis should be reviewed (**Appendix 10**).

I. Special Considerations

1. Chemical Burns

Chemical burns may be caused by acid (eg, cleaning products, industrial applications), alkali (eg, hydrides of sodium, potassium, and sodas of ammonia), or organic compounds (eg, petroleum products). Severity of injury relates to the agent involved, its concentration, and the duration of contact. Initial care requires removing the patient from the source of chemical injury immediately. In general, removal of clothing is essential. Dry substances should be brushed off and the area irrigated copiously with water. Do not use neutralizing agents as they may increase the severity of burn.

Contact with petroleum products (such as spilled gasoline at the scene of a motor vehicle crash) is associated with rapid skin penetration and late multiple-organ failure. Again, rapid removal of the patient from the source and vigorous irrigation of exposed surfaces are warranted. Advice regarding chemical burns is available from regional burn centers.

2. Electrical Injury

Electrical injury is a syndrome with a variety of presentations. Exposure to an electrical source <1,000 volts produces a low voltage injury similar to other cutaneous burns. When exposure exceeds 1,000 volts, a greater potential for deep as well as cutaneous injury exists.

Three types of skin injury can occur with electrocution:

1. Entrance and exit wounds, typically circumscribed, deep lesions, occur at points of contact with the electrical source or ground (usually hands and feet).
2. Cutaneous burns may be caused by arc injury from the primary site to the patient, a flash injury, or an actual flame injury if clothing catches fire.
3. Deep soft tissue injuries involve muscle, nerve, or the vascular bed as current passes through the tissue.

Beware of pneumothorax, airway compromise, cardiac arrest, and blunt injury secondary to falls and violent muscle contraction. Muscle compartment pressures may increase, necessitating fasciotomy, not just escharotomy. If myoglobin is present in the urine or creatine kinase concentrations are elevated, provide adequate intravascular fluid to increase the urine output to 3 to 4 mL/kg/h until resolution of the rhabdomyolysis. Patients may develop ileus after electrocution. The ECG should be reviewed in electrical injury.

The initial priority in the management of electrocution is removal of necrotic tissue and decompression of compromised deep tissue compartments, particularly muscle. Resuscitation is begun at 4 mL/kg/% TBSA cutaneous injury and titrated to maintain urine output of 0.5 to 1 mL/kg/h unless rhabdomyolysis is present and higher urine output is desirable. Aggressive fluid resuscitation potentiates filtering of pigment and dilution of iron (nephrotoxic). Alkalinization of the urine may be considered to decrease the nephrotoxic potential despite lack of supportive evidence. If large areas of soft-tissue injury are present, surgical consultation should be requested. As with other burns, infection is the chief risk, but other potential problems are myocardial and vascular injury, encephalopathy, cataracts, and gut perforation.

Lightning injury may be thought of as massive exposure to direct current. Most injury is topical because exposure times are extremely brief. Mortality rates associated with lightning relate to early cardiac and respiratory arrest. Aggressive basic and advanced life support may be lifesaving for these patients.

IV. REFERRAL AND TRANSFER CONSIDERATIONS

Early involvement of surgical expertise is important in the care of the injured patient. A surgeon should be summoned as soon as it is known that a seriously injured patient is arriving. Early neurosurgical consultation is advised for patients with head injury.

General guidelines for field triage and interfacility transfer have used physiologic, anatomic, and high-risk mechanistic criteria to suggest triggers for triage and transfer. One may extrapolate that these parameters can be used to initiate involvement of a trauma surgeon as well. Some triggers are suggested in **Table 9-3** and **Table 9-4**.

Table 9-3 American Burn Association Criteria for Patient Transfer to a Burn Center[a]

- Partial-thickness burns greater than 10% of total body surface area
- Third-degree burns in any age group
- Burns involving the face, hands, feet, genitalia, perineum, or major joints
- Patients at the extremes of age or those with significant comorbid disease
- Electric burns and chemical burns
- Smoke-inhalation injury
- Patients with combined trauma and significant burn injury
- Children at hospitals with no expertise in caring for pediatric burn patients
- Burns suspected to be due to child or elder abuse
- Burn patients with a delayed presentation or evidence of burn wound infection

[a]Adapted with permission from the American College of Surgeons.[3] American College of Surgeons Committee on Trauma. Guidelines for the operation of burn centers. In: *Resources for Optimal Care of the Injured Patient.* Chicago, IL: American College of Surgeons; 2006:79-86.

Table 9-4 Indications for Field Triage and Interfacility Transfer

Physiologic Triggers

- Glasgow Coma Score <14
- Systolic blood pressure <90 mm Hg
- Respiratory rate <10/min or >29/min

Anatomic/Injury Triggers

- Penetrating injuries to head, neck, torso, and proximal extremities
- Deteriorating Glasgow Coma Scale score or lateralizing signs
- Paralysis, spinal cord injury
- Major chest trauma, flail chest, pulmonary contusion
- Widened mediastinum or other signs of great vessel injury
- Cardiac injury
- Solid organ injury, open or unstable pelvic ring fracture
- Fracture/dislocation with loss of distal pulse or open long bone fractures
- Crush injuries with limb ischemia
- Major burns >20% total body surface area or associated with trauma

Patient Triggers

- Age <5 y or >55 y
- Known cardiopulmonary or metabolic diseases
- Pregnancy
- Immunosuppression

Mechanism of Injury Triggers

- Falls
  - Adults: >20 ft (one story is equal to 10 ft)
  - Children: >10 ft or 2-3 times the child's height
- High-risk auto crash
  - Intrusion: >12 inches occupant side; >18 inches any side
  - Ejection (partial or complete) from auto
  - Death in same passenger compartment
  - Vehicle telemetry data consistent with high risk of injury
- Auto vs. pedestrian/bicyclist: thrown, run over, or with significant (>20 mph) impact
- Motorcycle crash >20 mph

If appropriate surgical services are unavailable, early transfer to the closest trauma or burn center should be initiated. This should not be delayed for additional radiologic studies if surgical resources are unavailable, unless those studies are requested by the accepting physician. The trauma center should be contacted for advice and to discuss potential problems or concerns with transport personnel.

Common pitfalls in the transfer of seriously ill patients include failure to intubate before transfer, failure to recognize the need for transfer to a higher level of care, and a general failure to stabilize the patient adequately before transport. Unrecognized ongoing hemorrhage, delayed onset of tension pneumothorax, and reversible/preventable causes of secondary brain injury must be considered.

Key Points

Basic Trauma and Burn Support

- The first goal in trauma management is to identify and treat immediately life-threatening injuries by following the ABCDE sequence of priorities.
- After blunt trauma, airway control should proceed on the assumption that an unstable cervical spine injury exists.
- A diagnosis of tension pneumothorax should be based on clinical criteria and not on a chest radiograph.
- Hemorrhage is the most likely cause of shock after injury, and initial empiric treatment consists of crystalloid infusion to normalize blood pressure, reverse tachycardia, and maintain adequate organ perfusion.
- In general, blood should be added to resuscitation fluids when crystalloid infusion is >50 mL/kg. Uncrossmatched, type-specific blood can be administered safely.
- A secondary assessment includes a head-to-toe examination to identify and treat potentially life-threatening injuries.
- Computed tomographic scanning is essential for the initial evaluation of head-injured patients with a depressed level of consciousness.
- Burn resuscitation is proportional to the area sustaining second- and third-degree burns and is titrated to signs of perfusion, including urine output.
- Closed-space smoke inhalation injury places the patient at high risk for upper airway and lung injury that may not be obvious at the initial presentation.
- Surgical expertise should be secured early and transfer considered for those patients who require higher level of care.
- Transfer to a specialized care setting should not be delayed for additional radiologic studies unless the accepting physician requests the studies.

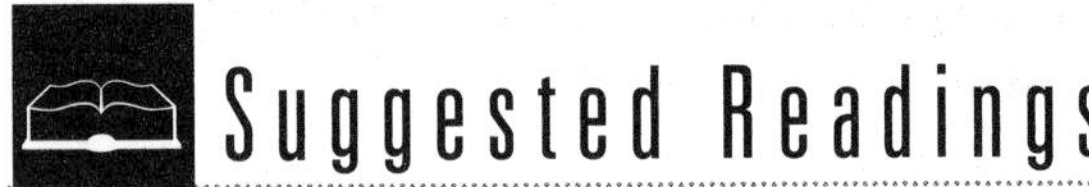

Suggested Readings

1. American College of Surgeons Committee on Trauma. *Advanced Trauma Life Support for Doctors (ATLS).* 8th ed. Chicago, IL: American College of Surgeons; 2008.

2. American College of Surgeons Committee on Trauma. *Advanced Trauma Life Support for Doctors (ATLS): Student Course Manual.* 8th ed. Chicago, IL: American College of Surgeons; 2008.

3. American College of Surgeons Committee on Trauma. Guidelines for the operation of burn centers. In: *Resources for Optimal Care of the Injured Patient.* Chicago, IL: American College of Surgeons; 2006:79-86.

4. Bagley LJ. Imaging of spinal trauma. *Radiol Clin North Am.* 2006;44:1-12.

5. Brain Trauma Foundation. Management and prognosis of severe traumatic brain injury. *J Neurotrauma.* 2007;24 (Suppl 1):i-S106.

6. Chan O, Wilson A, Walsh M. Major trauma. *BMJ.* 2005;330:1136-1138.

7. Cheatham ML, Malbrain ML, Kirkpatrick A, et al. Results from the International Conference of Experts on Intra-abdominal Hypertension and Abdominal Compartment Syndrome, II: Recommendations. *Intensive Care Med.* 2007;33:951-962.

8. Elliott DC. An evaluation of the end points of resuscitation. *J Am Coll Surg.* 1998;187:536-547.

9. Herndon DN, ed. *Total Burn Care.* 3rd ed. Philadelphia, PA: Saunders-Elsevier Inc; 2007.

10. Johnson JW, Gracias VH, Schwab CW, et al. Evolution in damage control for exsanguinating penetrating abdominal injury. *J Trauma.* 2001;51:261-271.

11. Holcomb JB, Jenkins D, Rhee P, et al. Damage control resuscitation: Directly addressing the early coagulopathy of trauma. *J Trauma.* 2007;62:307-310.

12. Moore EE, Feliciano DV, Mattox KL, eds. *Trauma.* 6th ed. New York, NY: McGraw-Hill; 2008.

13. Morrison CA, Carrick MM, Norman MA, et al. Hypotensive resuscitation strategy reduces transfusion requirements and severe postoperative coagulopathy in trauma patients with hemorrhagic shock: Preliminary results of a randomized controlled trial. *J Trauma.* 2011;70:652-663.

14. Pryor JP, Braslow B, Reilly PM, et al. The evolving role of interventional radiology in trauma care. *J Trauma.* 2005;59:102-104.

15. Rhee P, Nunley MK, Demetriades D, et al. Tetanus and trauma: A review and recommendations. *J Trauma.* 2005;58:1082-1088.

16. Rossaint R, Bouillon B, Cerny V, et al. Management of bleeding following major trauma: An updated European guideline. *Crit Care.* 2010;14(2):R52.

17. Sarrafzadeh AS, Peltonen EE, Kaisers U, et al. Secondary insults in severe head injury: Do multiply injured patients do worse? *Crit Care Med.* 2001;29:1116-1123.

18. Sheridan RL. Burns. *Crit Care Med.* 2002;30(suppl):S500-S514.

19. Society of Critical Care Medicine. *Fundamental Disaster Management.* 3rd ed. Mount Prospect, IL: Society of Critical Care Medicine; 2009.

20. Stengel D, Bauwens K, Sehouli J, et al. Emergency ultrasound-based algorithms for diagnosing blunt abdominal trauma. *Cochrane Database of Syst Rev.* 2005;(2):CD004446. doi: 10.1002/14651858.CD004446.pub2.

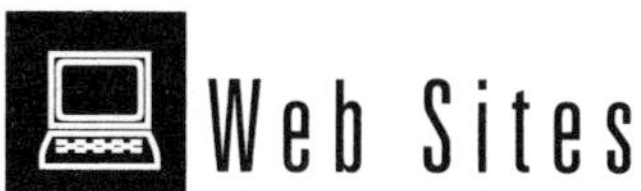

Web Sites

1. American Burn Association. www.ameriburn.org

2. American Burn Association. Advanced Burn Life Support Course (ABLS). 2nd ed. www.ameriburn.org/ablscoursedescriptions.php.

3. Burn Surgery. www.burnsurgery.org

4. American Association for the Surgery of Trauma. www.aast.org

5. Centers for Disease Control and Prevention – Data & Statistics. www.cdc.gov/injury/wisqars/

6. Eastern Association for the Surgery of Trauma. Resuscitation Endpoints. www.east.org/research/treatment-guidelines/resuscitation-endpoints. *Best site for evidence-based trauma care guidelines.*

7. Trauma.org. http://www.trauma.org. *Image bank and links.*

8. World Society of the Abdominal Compartment Syndrome. http://www.wsacs.org. *Consensus information on abdominal compartment syndrome.*

9. Eastern Association for the Surgery of Trauma. Appropriate Triage of the Victim of Trauma. http://www.east.org/research/treatment-guidelines/triage-of-the-victim-of-trauma

10. Centers for Disease Control. Injury Prevention and Control, Field Triage Decision Scheme. http://www.cdc.gov/ncipc/dir/FLD_TRIAGE.doc

11. Interfacility Transfer of Injured Patients; Guidelines for Rural Communities. http://www.facs.org/trauma/publications/ruralguidelines.pdf

Chapter 10

ACUTE CORONARY SYNDROMES

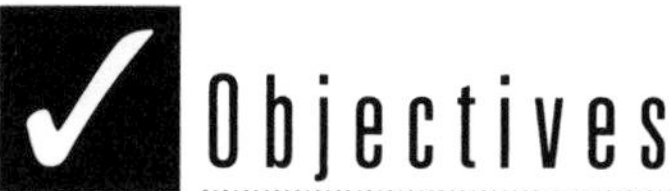

Objectives

- Identify patients with acute coronary syndromes with various electrocardiographic and clinical presentations.
- Outline diagnostic procedures and the acute management of unstable angina (UA), non–ST-segment elevation myocardial infarction (NSTEMI), and ST-segment elevation myocardial infarction (STEMI).
- Identify appropriate reperfusion interventions for patients with STEMI and high-risk patients with UA and NSTEMI.
- Recognize the complications of myocardial infarction and outline appropriate management.

Case Study

A 64-year-old man with type 2 diabetes and hypertension awoke with chest pressure. One hour later, when the pain failed to resolve, his wife drove him to the local emergency department. His vital signs on arrival are blood pressure 158/94 mm Hg, heart rate 98/min, respiratory rate 28/min, and Spo_2 97% on room air. His physical examination is remarkable only for a fourth heart sound (S_4) and mild diaphoresis.

- What information is needed to determine the type of acute coronary syndrome this patient may have?
- What immediate interventions should be performed

I. INTRODUCTION

Acute coronary syndromes (ACS) encompass overlapping clinical conditions of myocardial ischemia that include unstable angina (UA) and acute myocardial infarction (MI), both non-ST-segment elevation myocardial infarction (NSTEMI) and ST-segment elevation myocardial infarction (STEMI) (**Figure 10-1**). An important distinction is made clinically between patients with ACS that have ST-segment elevation on an electrocardiogram (ECG) and those who do not. Patients with ST-segment elevation should be considered for immediate reperfusion.

Figure 10-1. Overlapping Spectrum of Acute Coronary Syndromes

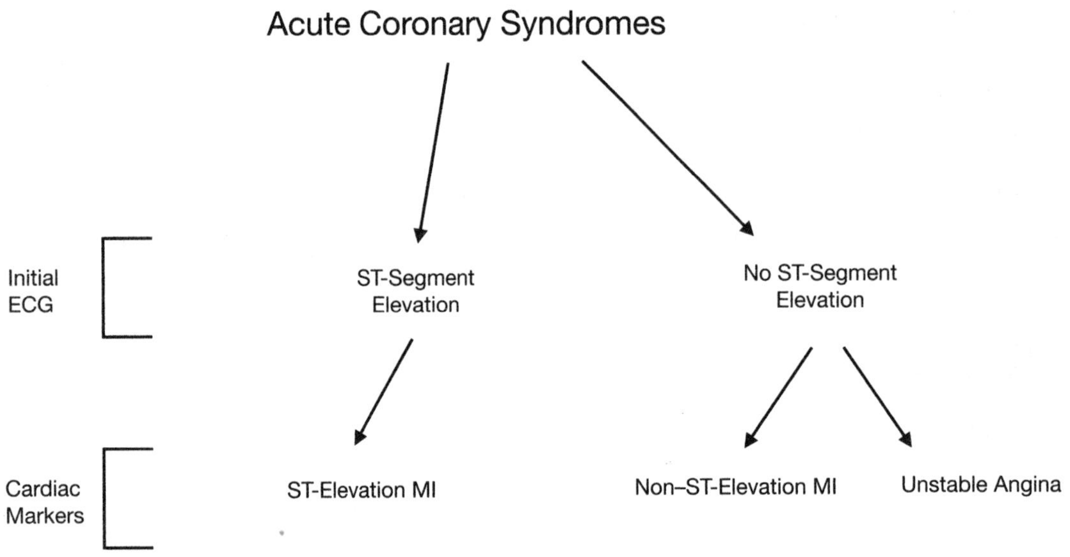

Abbreviations: ECG, electrocardiogram; MI, myocardial infarction
Acute coronary syndromes are distinguished by initial ECG findings and cardiac markers.

Unstable angina and NSTEMI are grouped together as unstable coronary syndromes that differ in the severity of ischemia and myocardial damage. Myocardial damage resulting in elevation of biochemical markers of myocardial injury establishes the diagnosis of NSTEMI. Although UA and NSTEMI are managed initially with pharmacologic interventions, high-risk patients may also require an invasive strategy with urgent reperfusion. Unstable angina and NSTEMI are characterized pathologically by various degrees of coronary artery occlusion that result in decreased myocardial oxygen supply relative to myocardial oxygen demand. Rupture or erosion of atherosclerotic plaques leads to a complex process of inflammation, platelet activation and aggregation, thrombus formation, and microembolization to distal vasculature. The patient's specific syndrome depends on the severity and duration of occlusion. Myocardial ischemia less commonly results from severe anemia or hypoxemia that limits myocardial oxygen delivery.

> *Be aware of changes in management of ACS as new evidence becomes available.*

Hospitals should establish multiprofessional teams (including primary care physicians, emergency medicine physicians, cardiologists, nurses, and others) to develop evidence-based protocols for triaging and managing patients with symptoms suggestive of ACS. The care of these patients continually evolves as information from clinical trials becomes available. Protocols for caring for such patients must be updated periodically based on the best current evidence.

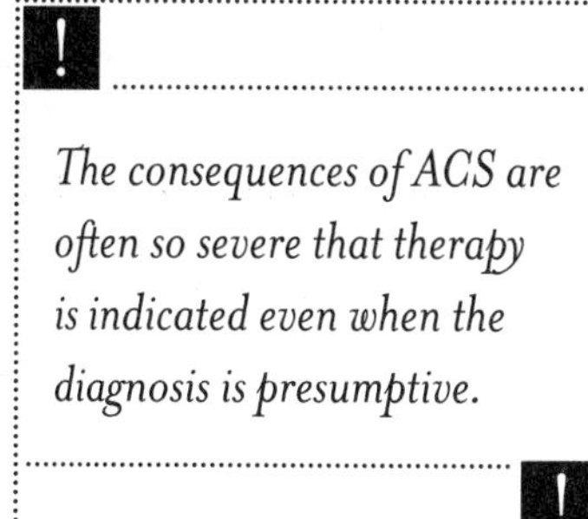

Identification of patients at risk for ACS includes an assessment of risk factors for coronary artery disease (**Table 10-1**) and identification of previous myocardial ischemia. Patients with other critical illness or injury have increased risk for ACS and frequently have atypical presentations. Definitive diagnosis of ACS often is not possible on initial evaluation and requires continuous observation, ECG monitoring, and/or laboratory confirmation. A brief history and physical examination may promote rapid triage, whereas a more detailed examination aids in the differential diagnosis and evaluation for possible complications. A brief physical examination should include vital signs and general observation, assessment of jugular venous distension, auscultation of the lungs and heart, evaluation of peripheral pulses, detection of neurologic deficits, and assessment for evidence of systemic hypoperfusion.

Table 10-1 Risk Factors for Coronary Artery Disease

Family history of myocardial infarction	Obesity
Hypertension	Diabetes mellitus
Smoking history	Other vascular disease
Hyperlipidemia	Sedentary lifestyle
Increasing age	Cocaine/amphetamine use
Postmenopausal state	

II. UNSTABLE ANGINA AND NON–ST-SEGMENT ELEVATION MYOCARDIAL INFARCTION

At presentation, patients with ischemic-type chest pain and an ECG with no ST-segment elevation are often presumed to have UA. Other causes of prolonged chest pain (**Table 10-2**) should also be considered. UA can present as rest angina, new-onset angina, or increasing angina (change in predictability of pain, such as pain that is more frequent, of longer duration, or induced by less effort). Based on serial ECGs and elevated levels of biochemical markers of cardiac injury, some patients with UA subsequently are found to have an NSTEMI. The initial evaluation and management of patients with UA and NSTEMI are similar. Pathologic correlates include a partially or intermittently occluding thrombus and microemboli from the thrombus to the distal vasculature.

Table 10-2 Differential Diagnosis of Prolonged Chest Pain

Acute myocardial ischemia
Aortic dissection/aortic aneurysm
Myocarditis
Pericarditis
Pain associated with hypertrophic cardiomyopathy or esophageal and gastrointestinal disorders
Pulmonary diseases such as pneumothorax, pulmonary embolism, and pleuritis
Hyperventilation syndrome
Aortic stenosis
Musculoskeletal or chest wall diseases, costochondral pain
Psychogenic pain

A. Diagnosis

> **!** *New-onset shortness of breath and/or new left branch bundle block should be considered evidence of ACS, particularly in women and diabetic patients, who may have atypical presentations.* **!**

The most important factors in a patient's history that suggest the likelihood of myocardial ischemia are the character of the pain, prior history of coronary artery disease, age, and number of risk factors. Results of physical examination are usually normal, although a fourth heart sound (S_4) may be heard during episodes of pain. When possible, a 12-lead ECG should be obtained and interpreted as soon as possible by prehospital personnel to facilitate diagnosis, triage, and treatment. If not obtained in the prehospital setting, a 12-lead ECG should be obtained and interpreted within 10 minutes of the patient's arrival at the hospital. The ECG is most helpful if it shows transient ST-segment depression (**Figure 10-2**) during anginal episodes. However, the ECG may be normal, or it may reveal nondiagnostic T-wave inversions or peaked T waves. The history, findings from physical examination, ECG interpretation, and cardiac markers should be used to assess the patient's short-term risk of an adverse outcome, such as death or nonfatal myocardial ischemia (**Table 10-3**).

Figure 10-2. Electrocardiogram of a Patient With Unstable Angina[a]

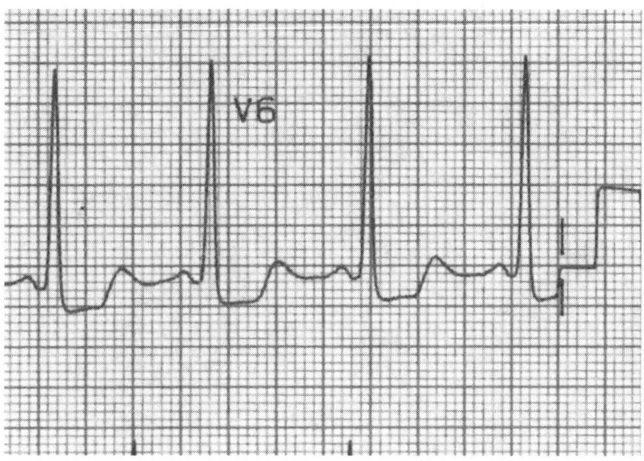

The ST-segment depression in lead V_6 is characteristic of unstable angina.
[a] Reproduced with permission of Shih-Chung Lin, MD.

Table 10-3 Risk Factors for Death or Nonfatal Myocardial Ischemia[a]

High Risk (1 or more of the following)	Intermediate Risk (No high risk factors and 1 of the following)	Low Risk (no high or intermediate risk factors and 1 of the following)
• Ongoing pain at rest (>20 min) • Pulmonary edema, S_3, or rales • Hypotension • Bradycardia, tachycardia • Age >75 y • Rest angina with dynamic ST-segment changes >0.05 mV • Elevated troponin (>0.1 ng/mL)	• Prolonged rest pain (>20 min) now resolved • Rest pain <20 min or relieved with nitroglycerin • Age >70 y • T-wave inversions >0.2 mV • Pathologic Q waves • Slightly elevated troponin (<0.1 ng/mL)	• Increasing frequency, severity, or duration of pain • Lower threshold for pain • Normal or unchanged electrocardiogram during pain • Normal troponin

[a]Adapted with permission from the Agency for Healthcare Research and Quality.[5] Braunwald E, Mark DB, Jones RH, et al. *Unstable Angina: Diagnosis and Management.* Rockville, MD: Agency for Health Care Policy and Research and National Heart, Lung, and Blood Institute. US Public Health Service, US Department of Health and Human Services; 1994. AHCPR Publication 94-0602.

Several risk stratification scores have been developed and validated to assist in predicting the risk of death and ischemic events in UA/NSTEMI. The GRACE (Global Registry for Acute Cardiac Events) score (http://www.outcomes-umassmed.org/grace/acs_risk/acs_risk_content.html) requires computer software or a web-based calculator, whereas the TIMI (Thrombolysis in Myocardial Infarction) risk score (http://www.mdcalc.com/timi-risk-score-for-uanstemi) can be easily determined at the bedside (**Table 10-4**). High-risk patients are considered to have a >6% risk of dying within 6 months and intermediate-risk patients have a 6-month mortality rate of 3% to

6%. This risk assessment has implications for location of care, selection of medical therapy, and use of reperfusion interventions. Serial cardiac markers (MB fraction of creatine phosphokinase [CK-MB], cardiac-specific troponins) along with serial ECGs should be obtained to determine if an NSTEMI is present. Cardiac-specific troponins (cTnT, cTnI) also provide useful prognostic information. Certain tests, such as hemoglobin/hematocrit, electrolytes, thyroid function, and arterial oxygen saturation, may be helpful in identifying a precipitating factor.

Table 10-4 TIMI Risk Score for Adverse Cardiac Events

1 point for each:

- Age ≥65 years
- Prior coronary stenosis ≥50%
- ST-segment deviation on electrocardiogram at presentation
- At least two anginal events in prior 24 hours
- Use of aspirin in prior 7 days
- At least three risk factors for coronary artery disease (family history, male gender, hypertension, hyperlipidemia, diabetes, smoking, obesity)
- Elevated serum cardiac markers

Risk Level	Score	Risk of Adverse Cardiac Event
Low	0-2	5% to 8%
Intermediate	3-4	13% to 20%
High	5-7	26% to 41%

Abbreviation: TIMI, Thrombolysis in Myocardial Infarction

If equipment and expertise are available, the use of transthoracic echocardiography allows bedside assessment of wall motion abnormalities as a marker for current or past ischemia and detection and follow-up of new abnormalities. This procedure also provides an estimate of left ventricular function and identification of valvular dysfunction and/or pericardial fluid. Echocardiography may allow assessment of other nonischemic causes of acute chest pain, such as myocarditis, pulmonary embolism, and thoracic aortic dissection (although the window for visualization may be poor).

B. Management

Management of the patient with chest pain includes increasing myocardial oxygen delivery by improving perfusion and decreasing myocardial oxygen demand. Reversing myocardial ischemia and confirming the diagnosis of ACS is the essential priority. Patients with UA should be admitted to a unit with cardiac monitoring (eg, telemetry unit, chest pain or observation unit) and placed at bed or chair rest (see treatment algorithm in **Figure 10-3**). Oxygen (2-4 L/min by nasal cannula) should be administered to patients with dyspnea, hypoxemia (Spo_2 <90% to 92% on room air), or evidence of heart failure or shock. Although oxygen is often administered to virtually all patients suspected of having acute myocardial ischemia, it is not known whether this therapy limits myocardial damage or reduces the morbidity or mortality rate. If precipitating, reversible causes — such as fever, anemia, hypoxemia, infection, hypertension, anxiety, hyperthyroidism, arrhythmias, or sympathomimetic drug ingestion (eg, cocaine, ephedrine) — can be identified, they should be treated aggressively. Further management includes relief of pain and anti-ischemic therapy, therapy for platelet aggregation/thrombosis, ongoing risk stratification, and consideration of invasive reperfusion procedures.

Figure 10-3. Treatment Algorithm for Unstable Angina

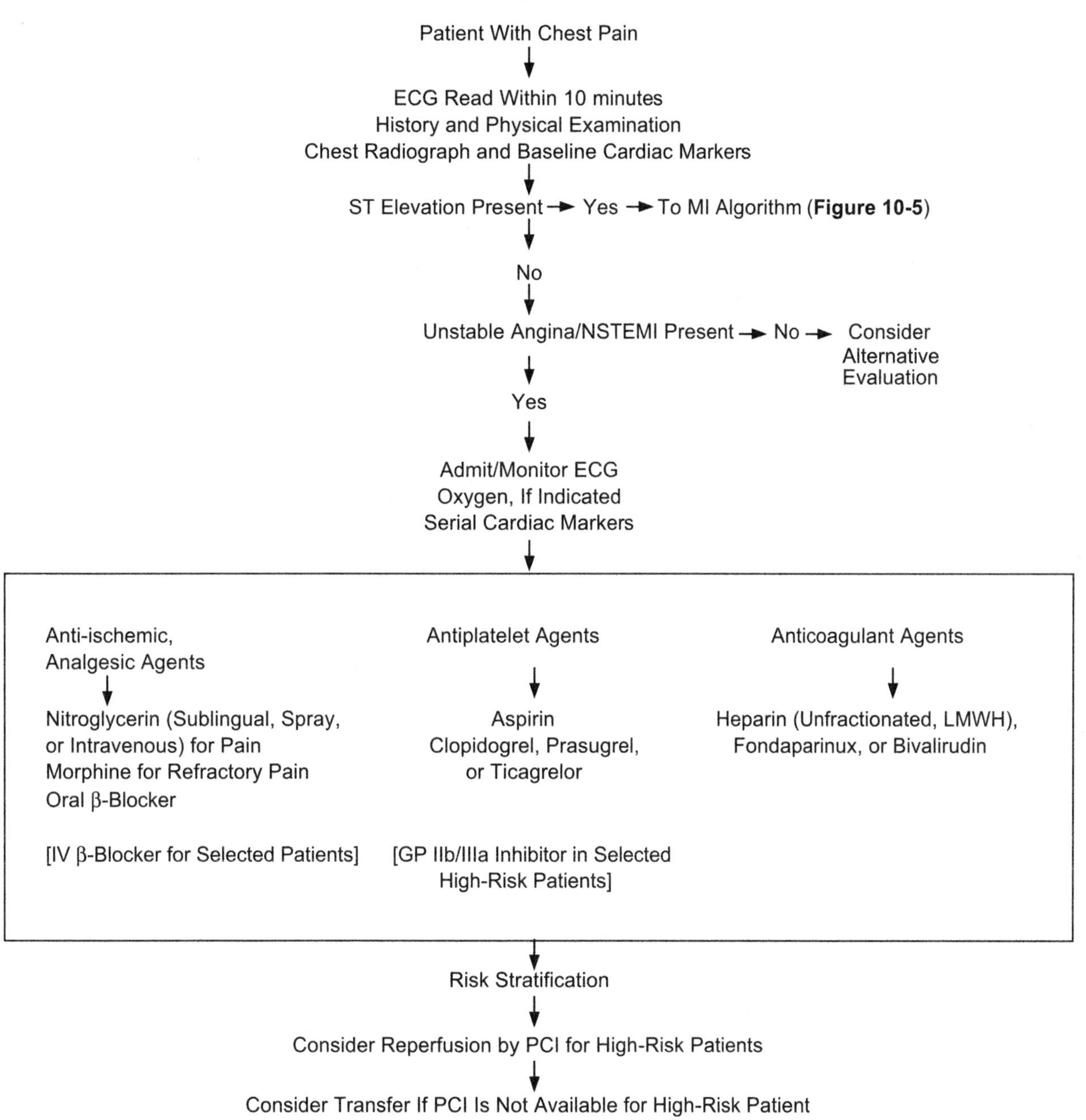

Abbreviations: ECG, electrocardiogram; MI, myocardial infarction; NSTEMI, non–ST-segment elevation myocardial infarction; LMWH, low-molecular-weight heparin; GP, glycoprotein; PCI, percutaneous coronary intervention

Pain relief is an important element in the early management of the patient with ACS. Pain management should be directed toward acute relief of symptoms of ongoing myocardial ischemia and general relief of anxiety and apprehension. Immediate control of ischemic pain is typically accomplished with a combination of nitrates and opiate agents. Antianginal medications that are effective in stabilizing patients with unstable angina are listed in **Table 10-5**. The goal is to reduce ischemia without causing hypotension or reflex tachycardia. Patients with ongoing ischemic discomfort should receive up to three doses of sublingual or spray nitroglycerin. Nitrates should not be administered if the systolic blood pressure is <90 mm Hg or ≥30 mm Hg below the patient's baseline blood pressure. Additional contraindications to nitrate administration are heart rate <50 beats/min, tachycardia >100 beats/min in the absence of heart failure symptoms, or suspected right ventricular infarction. If sublingual or spray nitroglycerin does not relieve pain, an assessment should be made about the need for intravenous nitroglycerin. Excessive decreases in blood pressure with nitroglycerin are predominantly due to increased venous capacitance and can often be treated with careful intravenous crystalloid infusion. If the mean arterial pressure

> **!** *Because nitroglycerin reduces the efficacy of heparin, unfractionated heparin infusion rates require adjustment when intravenous nitroglycerin is used.*

Table 10-5 Anti-ischemic Therapy

Agent	Oral Dose	Spray Dose	Intravenous Dose
Nitroglycerin	0.3-0.4 mg tablet sublingually to a maximum of 3 doses; contraindicated when systolic blood pressure <90 mm Hg	0.4 mg spray every 5 min to a maximum of 3 doses; contraindicated when systolic blood pressure <90 mm Hg	Initial infusion rate 10 µg/min; with increases of 10 µg/min every 3-5 min as needed to control pain; discontinue rate increases for significant drops in blood pressure or maximum of 200 µg/min
Morphine sulfate			1-5 mg every 5-30 min as needed for pain
β-blockers			
Propranolol	20-80 mg every 6-8 h		0.5-1 mg as a single dose
Metoprolol	50-100 mg every 12 h		5 mg every 5 min to a total dose of 15 mg
Atenolol	50-200 mg every 24 h		5 mg every 10 min to a total dose of 10 mg
Carvedilol	6.25 mg every 12 h titrated to maximum 25 mg every 12 h		
Diltiazem	30-60 mg every 6-8 h		

decreases by more than 25% when hypertension is present or if the systolic pressure decreases to <110 mm Hg in normotensive patients, the nitroglycerin dose should not be increased. Instead, a second antianginal agent should be administered. Tolerance to the hemodynamic effects of nitroglycerin becomes important after 24 hours of continuous infusion, and efforts should be made to switch to other dosing regimens. The dose of intravenous nitrates should be reduced and changed to an oral regimen when ischemic manifestations have resolved for 12 to 24 hours. Nitrates are contraindicated in patients who have received a phosphodiesterase inhibitor for erectile dysfunction in the previous 24 hours (48 hours for tadalafil). Morphine sulfate is the analgesic of choice for management of pain associated with myocardial ischemia that is refractory to initial antianginal therapy. Nonsteroidal anti-inflammatory drugs, other than aspirin, and COX-2 inhibitors may be harmful in patients with ACS and should not be administered.

Oral β-blockers should be initiated within the first 24 hours in patients without contraindications to their use (**Table 10-6**). Routine use of intravenous β-blockers in the initial management of patients with suspected ACS is not supported by current evidence, but they may be considered in patients with ongoing chest pain, especially with concomitant hypertension or tachycardia, and should be followed by oral administration. Caution is advised with the use of intravenous β-blockers in patients at higher risk of cardiogenic shock (older age, higher heart rate, lower blood pressure, or evidence of heart failure).

Table 10-6 Contraindications to β-Blocker Use in Acute Coronary Syndromes

Heart rate <50/min
Moderate to severe left ventricular dysfunction (uncompensated)
Shock or increased risk for cardiogenic shock
Marked first-degree atrioventricular block (with PR interval >0.24 s)
Second-degree or third-degree atrioventricular block
Systolic blood pressure <90 mm Hg
Peripheral hypoperfusion
Active bronchospastic disease (asthma or chronic obstructive pulmonary disease)

Non-dihydropyridine calcium channel blockers (eg, diltiazem or verapamil) do not reduce the risk of MI. In the absence of contraindications (such as significant left ventricular dysfunction), they may be considered only if patients cannot tolerate a β-blocker or symptoms are not controlled with nitroglycerin and β-blockers together.

Antiplatelet and anticoagulant agents (**Table 10-7**) are important interventions in UA and NSTEMI because of the contribution of platelet activation/aggregation and the coagulation system to platelet-rich thrombus formation. Three classes of antiplatelet drugs may be of benefit in myocardial ischemia: aspirin, adenosine diphosphate inhibitors (clopidogrel, prasugrel, and ticagrelor), and glycoprotein (GP) IIb/IIIa inhibitors. The intensity of therapy with these agents is often tailored to the patient's risk assessment

> !
> *Aspirin improves survival and reduces the incidence of MI.*
> !

and to plans for early invasive procedures. Non-enteric-coated aspirin at a dose of 162 to 325 mg should be administered (and chewed) as soon as possible to all patients with UA/NSTEMI. Aspirin should be administered indefinitely, as well as in the prehospital setting if no aspirin allergy is suspected. Clopidogrel or prasugrel should be considered as an alternative antiplatelet agent if aspirin is contraindicated. If a noninterventional conservative approach is planned for the patient, clopidogrel should be added to aspirin to decrease the risk of cardiovascular death, MI, and stroke. Clopidogrel, prasugrel, or ticagrelor should be administered in patients undergoing percutaneous coronary interventions (PCIs). Therapy with an adenosine diphosphate inhibitor is recommended for at least 1 month and up to 12 months, but the optimum duration has not been determined.

Table 10-7 Antiplatelet and Glycoprotein Receptor Inhibitor Drugs Used in Acute Coronary Syndromes

Drug	Dose
Antiplatelet Agents	
Aspirin	162-325 mg chewed and swallowed initially, then 75-325 mg as a minimum oral dose daily
Adenosine diphosphate inhibitors (thienopyridines)	
Clopidogrel	Loading dose of 300 mg orally can be used with a noninvasive approach or thrombolysis; loading dose of 300 to 600 mg orally with PCI; maintenance dose 75 mg orally daily
Prasugrel	Loading dose 60 mg orally may substitute for clopidogrel in patients with STEMI or UA/NSTEMI managed with early PCI who are not at high risk of bleeding; followed by maintenance dose 10 mg daily (consider 5 mg daily if weight <60 kg); not recommended for STEMI treated with thrombolysis
Ticagrelor	Loading dose 180 mg orally may be an option instead of clopidogrel in NSTEMI or STEMI managed with early PCI; maintenance dose 90 mg twice daily
Glycoprotein IIb/IIIa Inhibitors	
Abciximab	For planned PCI: loading dose 0.25 mg/kg intravenous bolus (10- 60 min before procedure), then maintenance dose 0.125 µg/kg/min intravenously (maximum 10 µg/min) for 12-24 h
Eptifibatide	ACS: 180 µg/kg intravenous bolus, then 2 µg/kg/min intravenous infusion for 72-96 h PCI: loading dose 180 µg/kg intravenous bolus followed by repeat bolus in 10 min; begin maintenance dose 2 µg/kg/min intravenous infusion after first bolus for 12-18 h (reduce maintenance infusion dose by 50% if creatinine clearance <50 mL/min)
Tirofiban	ACS or PCI: loading dose 25 µg/kg intravenous bolus, then maintenance dose 0.1 µg/kg intravenous infusion for up to 18 h (reduce maintenance infusion dose by 50% if creatinine clearance <30 mL/min)

Abbreviations: PCI, percutaneous coronary intervention; STEMI, ST-segment elevation myocardial infarction; UA, unstable angina; NSTEMI, non–ST-segment elevation myocardial infarction; ACS, acute coronary syndrome

Selected high-risk patients (with continuing ischemia, elevated troponin levels) may be candidates for additional antiplatelet therapy with GP IIb/IIIa inhibitors when a noninvasive strategy is chosen. However, the benefit of GP IIb/IIIa inhibitors may be limited when dual antiplatelet therapy (aspirin and an adenosine diphosphate inhibitor) and anticoagulation are instituted. GP IIb/IIIa inhibitors may also be utilized if a PCI is planned, but they may be given just before the intervention. The selection of a specific agent may depend on availability and the preferences of the interventional cardiologist. Coagulation and platelet baseline studies should be completed before the administration of GP IIb/IIIa inhibitors.

The combination of aspirin and an anticoagulant agent is more beneficial than aspirin alone in ACS. The selection of a specific agent should take into account the risks of ischemia and bleeding complications as well as the presence of renal dysfunction. In ACS patients treated with a conservative approach, unfractionated heparin (**Appendix 11**) or low-molecular-weight heparin should be administered as soon as possible unless there are significant contraindications. Fondaparinux is an alternative thrombin inhibitor equivalent to unfractionated heparin that can be used in patients managed with a noninvasive strategy. Patients managed with fondaparinux require an additional anticoagulant if PCI is subsequently performed. Low-molecular-weight heparin (enoxaparin) or fondaparinux are preferred over unfractionated heparin in UA/NSTEMI, unless surgical revascularization is planned within 24 hours. More bleeding complications occur with use of enoxaparin compared to unfractionated heparin and less bleeding occurs with fondaparinux compared to unfractionated heparin. Unfractionated heparin is continued at least 48 hours, and enoxaparin or fondaparinux for the duration of hospital stay (up to 8 days), in patients managed with medical therapy. Serial platelet counts are required to monitor for heparin-induced thrombocytopenia. If an urgent invasive strategy is planned, unfractionated heparin, enoxaparin, or bivalirudin should be initiated as soon as possible. Bivalirudin is equivalent to unfractionated heparin in patients treated with an invasive strategy and may be considered particularly as an alternative in patients with renal insufficiency. Bivalirudin also has fewer bleeding complications than unfractionated heparin and may be useful for patients at increased risk of bleeding. Patients who are adequately anticoagulated with warfarin still require antiplatelet therapy, but anticoagulation with heparin or alternative agents is generally not needed unless the international normalized ratio is less than 2.0.

An angiotensin-converting enzyme (ACE) inhibitor or angiotensin receptor blocker (ARB) should be administered in the first 24 hours to UA/NSTEMI patients with evidence of pulmonary congestion or left ventricular ejection fraction <40% unless contraindications are present. Thrombolytic agents have no proven efficacy in UA or NSTEMI. Most patients with UA can be medically stabilized, and consultation can then be obtained for further risk stratification and/or invasive strategies (cardiac catheterization laboratory). An early invasive strategy is indicated for patients with UA/NSTEMI without serious comorbidity when there are high-risk indicators (**Table 10-8**). Immediate expert consultation should be obtained for patients who cannot be medically stabilized or have serious comorbidity. Patients with UA/NSTEMI and shock benefit from early reperfusion with PCI or coronary artery bypass graft (CABG) and should be triaged to the catheterization laboratory as soon as possible. Risk-factor modification, including the use of lipid-lowering agents (statins), weight reduction, and information about smoking cessation, is recommended in all cases of ACS.

Table 10-8 High-Risk Indicators for an Early Invasive Strategy in UA/NSTEMI

Recurrent angina at rest or with minimal exertion despite therapy
Elevated troponin level
New ST-segment depression
Signs of heart failure
Depressed left ventricular function (ejection fraction <40%)
Hemodynamic instability
High-risk findings on noninvasive stress testing
Prior coronary artery bypass graft
Percutaneous coronary intervention within 6 months
Sustained ventricular tachycardia

Abbreviations: UA, unstable angina; NSTEMI, non–ST-segment elevation myocardial infarction

III. ST-SEGMENT ELEVATION MYOCARDIAL INFARCTION

Patients with STEMI have a high likelihood that a thrombus will totally occlude a coronary artery, resulting in a wave front of myocardial necrosis that begins at the endocardial surface within 15 minutes. The infarction progresses outward to the epicardium over approximately 6 hours unless collateral flow, spontaneous reperfusion, or reperfusion via an intervention is established. The progression of infarction may be modulated by the extent of collateral flow and determinants of myocardial oxygen consumption, which affords an opportunity for myocardial salvage. As with the patient with UA/NSTEMI, prompt diagnosis and early treatment of the patient with STEMI have great influence on morbidity and mortality rates.

A. Diagnosis

Patients with STEMI typically present with prolonged chest pain and associated symptoms, but some patients have MIs that are painless (silent infarction/ischemia) or have other related symptoms, such as dyspnea and fatigue. In the critically ill patient population, STEMIs may not be associated with classic symptoms and are often suspected when complications occur or ECG changes are noted. The findings from physical examination are nonspecific.

The most common finding in patients with normal sinus rhythm is the S_4 heart sound, indicating decreased left ventricular compliance at the end of ventricular filling. Bibasilar crackles may be present and are helpful in defining the hemodynamic status. A brief, focused physical examination aids in the diagnosis and assessment of possible complications of STEMI. A limited neurological examination for evidence of prior stroke or cognitive deficits also should be conducted.

A prehospital 12-lead ECG should be obtained and interpreted when possible to facilitate diagnosis, triage, and treatment on arrival at the medical facility. Otherwise, a patient with chest discomfort or symptoms suggestive of ACS should have a 12-lead ECG performed and read within 10 minutes of arrival. The ECG is diagnostic of STEMI in the absence of QRS confounders (ie, bundle branch block, pacing, left ventricular hypertrophy, Wolff-Parkinson-White syndrome) if it shows >1-mm ST-segment elevation in two or more contiguous leads (**Figure 10-4**).

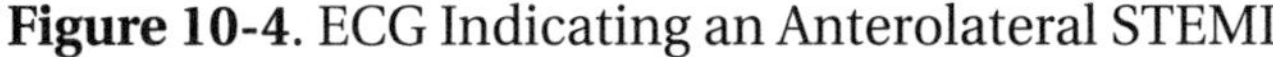

Figure 10-4. ECG Indicating an Anterolateral STEMI

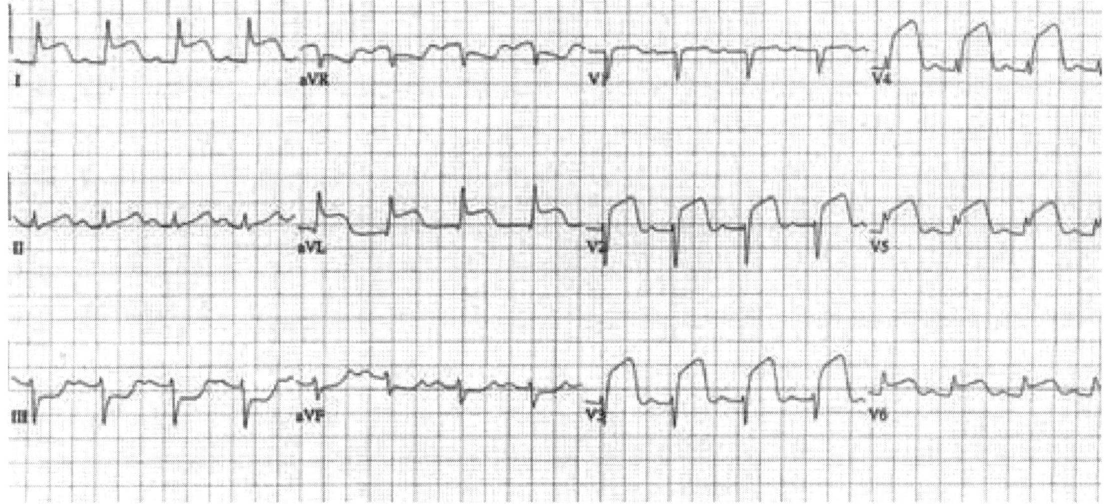

This electrocardiogram (ECG) shows classic findings of ST-segment elevation in the anterior (V_2 through V_4) and lateral (I, aVL, V_5, V_6) leads, indicating an anterolateral ST-segment elevation myocardial infarction (STEMI).
Reproduced with permission from Barbara McLean.

A right-sided ECG should be obtained in patients with an inferior STEMI to determine if ST-segment elevation suggesting right ventricular infarction is present. Patients with ECG findings of new or undiagnosed left bundle branch block and chest pain compatible with myocardial ischemia are treated similarly to those with ST-segment elevation. If the initial ECG is not diagnostic but the patient remains symptomatic with a high clinical suspicion for STEMI, serial ECGs at 5- to 10-minute intervals or continuous 12-lead ST-segment monitoring (if available) may be performed to detect the development of ST-segment elevation.

If the diagnosis is in doubt, echocardiography may add helpful information. The diagnosis is confirmed by detecting elevated serum levels of CK-MB or cardiac-specific troponins. The delay in elevation of these markers, however, prevents their use to determine reperfusion therapy. Cardiac-specific troponins are the optimum cardiac markers for the evaluation of patients with STEMI who have coexistent skeletal muscle injury.

B. General Management

Once STEMI is suspected or diagnosed, the immediate concerns are to ensure the patient's stability and to intervene to limit infarct size by restoring blood flow to the infarct artery as soon as possible (**Figure 10-5**). Treatment of STEMI in the patient with other critical illness requires careful individualization. Absolute and relative contraindications to therapies must be considered and relative risk assessed. Choices may be limited by the availability of specialized procedures, the need to transport the patient to another facility, significant comorbidities, bleeding risk, or the unavailability of the oral route for administering medication.

Figure 10-5. Treatment Algorithm for Myocardial Infarction With ST Elevation

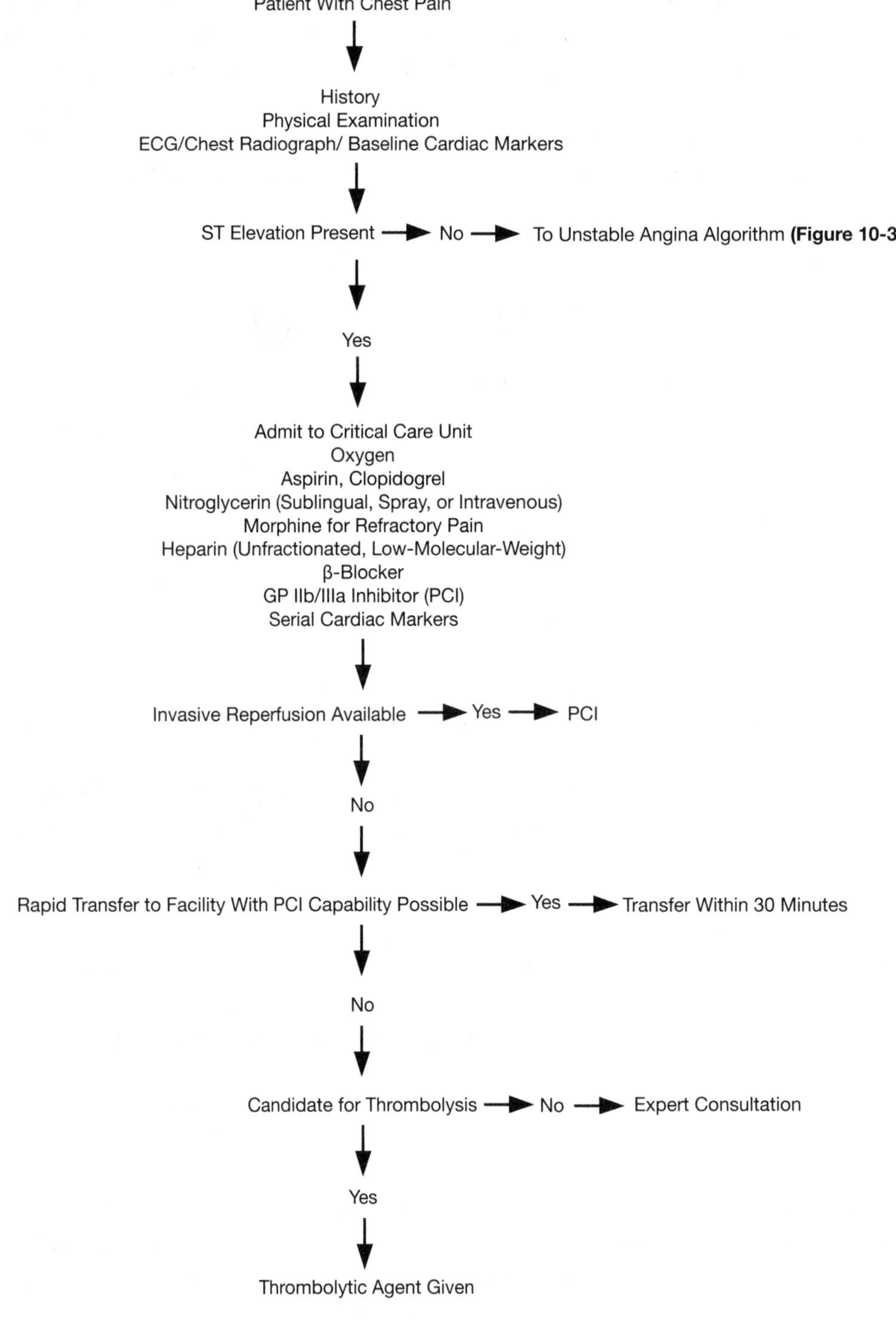

Abbreviations: ECG, electrocardiogram; GP, glycoprotein; PCI, percutaneous coronary intervention.

1. Early Therapy

Early therapy in STEMI is similar to the management of UA and NSTEMI. Immediate 12-lead ECG, cardiac markers, and related laboratory tests should be completed. Immediate therapy includes the administration of supplemental oxygen in the presence of dyspnea, hypoxemia, heart failure, or shock; the control of pain; and consideration of reperfusion therapy. Aspirin should be administered immediately. The addition of clopidogrel, prasugrel, or ticagrelor as part of dual antiplatelet therapy decreases the rates of mortality and major vascular events. An anticoagulant agent should also be administered. Because of its multiple salutary effects on myocardial oxygen demand and supply, nitroglycerin is indicated for the first 48 hours for treatment of persistent ischemia, hypertension, or heart failure, unless systolic blood pressure is <90 mm Hg. Intravenous β-blockers are not routinely administered but may be considered in patients with STEMI if tachyarrhythmia or hypertension is present when there are no contraindications.

2. Acute Reperfusion Therapy

Early reperfusion of the infarct-related coronary artery is associated with improved survival in patients with STEMI. Prompt restoration of flow in the infarct artery can be achieved by noninvasive pharmacological means (thrombolysis), invasive primary PCI, or surgical intervention. A plan for early reperfusion of patients with STEMI should be developed based on resources available in the facility and community.

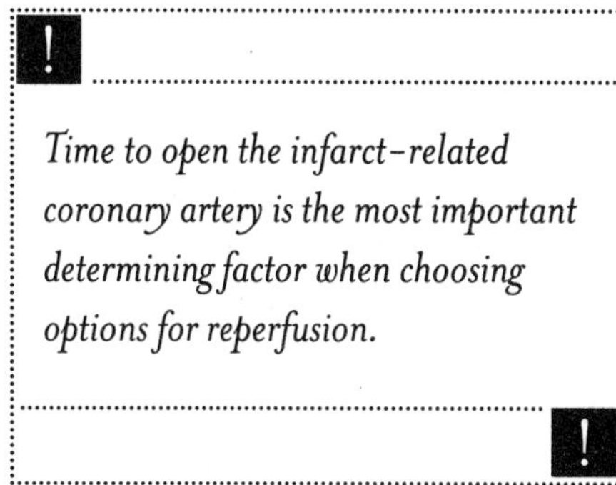

a. Percutaneous Coronary Interventions

PCIs include angioplasty, with or without deployment of an intracoronary bare-metal or drug-eluting stent, with support of pharmacologic measures to prevent thrombosis. Primary PCI is the preferred reperfusion technique if the procedure can be performed by experienced personnel within 12 hours of symptom onset. Primary PCI is also preferred with clinical or electrocardiographic evidence of ongoing ischemia, even if more than 12 hours have elapsed since symptom onset. A goal of 90 minutes or less from hospital presentation to balloon inflation is optimal.

Primary PCI is particularly preferred over thrombolysis for patients with contraindications to thrombolysis or a high risk of bleeding, for patients with severe heart failure or cardiogenic shock (within 18 hours of onset), and for patients in whom the diagnosis of MI is in doubt. If primary PCI is not available, transfer to a facility with invasive reperfusion capability should be initiated as soon as possible (preferably within 30 minutes).

In other patients, the choice of reperfusion strategy depends on available resources, factors specific to the patient, and transport time to another facility. The higher the patient's mortality risk (as with large infarctions, heart failure or hemodynamic instability, previous infarctions, or acute left bundle branch block), the more primary PCI is preferred. Similarly, the higher the risk of thrombolysis, the more primary PCI is preferred. Conversely, the longer the time required for performance of PCI or transfer to another facility, the more thrombolysis may be preferred. Patients presenting within 3 hours of the onset of symptoms who have a low risk of bleeding appear to derive particular benefit from prompt reperfusion with thrombolytic therapy. Transfer for PCI is preferred over thrombolysis in patients who present 3 to 12 hours after onset of symptoms if transfer can be accomplished in a timely manner. In patients with clinical failure to reperfuse after thrombolytic therapy, PCI is recommended, even if it requires transfer to another institution.

Pre-procedure management should include all of the strategies for ACS outlined previously. The use of an adenosine diphosphate inhibitor and an intravenous anticoagulant agent (unfractionated heparin, enoxaparin, or bivalirudin) before PCI is recommended. Clopidogrel (at a higher dose, 300-600 mg orally), prasugrel, or ticagrelor should be dosed appropriately as soon as the decision for PCI has been made. Prasugrel should not be used in STEMI patients with a prior history of stroke or transient ischemic attacks because of the higher risk of bleeding. Additional boluses of unfractionated heparin may be needed during PCI. An intravenous dose of enoxaparin (0.3 mg/kg) should be administered if the last dose of enoxaparin was 8 to 12 hours before PCI. Bivalirudin may be used with or without prior unfractionated heparin administration. If fondaparinux was used prior to PCI, an additional intravenous anticoagulant agent should be administered. GP IIb/IIIa inhibitors may be useful in selected patients but are no longer considered routine therapy when dual antiplatelet therapy and anticoagulation are instituted. Potential complications of an invasive strategy for treating STEMI include problems with the arterial access site; adverse reactions to volume loading, contrast medium, and antithrombotic medications; technical complications; and reperfusion events.

Regardless of the reperfusion strategy chosen, timely implementation by experienced personnel is optimal. Routine, early use of PCI for patients who reperfuse with thrombolysis increases patient risk and is not recommended.

b. Fibrinolysis/Thrombolysis

Optimal limitation of infarct size when administering thrombolytics requires intervention within 6 hours of symptom onset, but thrombolytics may have some benefit as long as 12 hours after symptoms begin (**Table 10-9**). If the diagnosis is uncertain, the patient has contraindications to thrombolytic therapy, or the presentation is more than 3 hours after symptom onset, invasive reperfusion with PCI is preferred. The physician must weigh potential risks against the benefits of thrombolysis for each patient. For those with definite indications for thrombolysis and no absolute contraindications, intravenous thrombolytic therapy should be administered expeditiously. Several agents are now available, and all are effective (**Table 10-10**). Findings that suggest reperfusion include relief of symptoms, maintenance or restoration of hemodynamic and/or electrical stability, reduction of at least 50% of

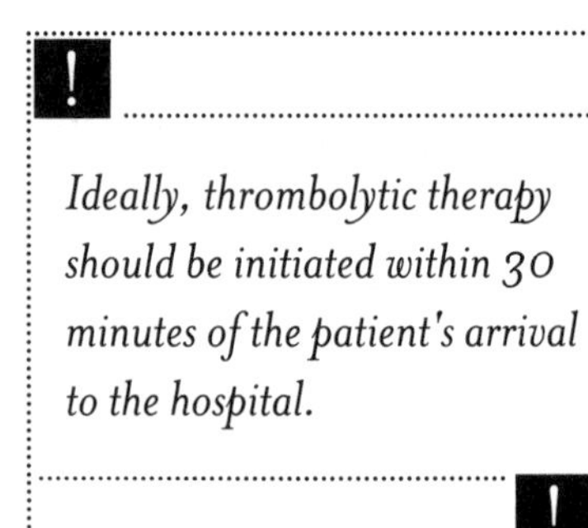

the initial ST-segment elevation injury pattern on a follow-up ECG 60 to 90 minutes after initiation of therapy, and an early peak in the level of CK-MB (12-18 hours). STEMI patients who have evidence of reperfusion failure or high-risk features after treatment with thrombolytics benefit from transfer to PCI-capable facilities as soon as possible. High-risk features may include persistent ST-segment elevation ≥2 mm in two anterior leads, systolic blood pressure <100 mm Hg, heart rate >100 beats/min, Killip class II to III (**Table 10-11**), ST-segment depression of ≥2 mm in the anterior leads, or ST-segment elevation ≥1 mm in right-sided lead V_4, which is indicative of right ventricular involvement for inferior MIs. Patients with STEMI who are not at high risk also may be considered for transfer to a PCI-capable facility. Antiplatelet and anticoagulant therapy should be continued before transfer.

Table 10-9 Identification of Candidates for Thrombolytic Therapy

Definite Indications

Consistent clinical syndrome: chest pain, new arrhythmia, unexplained hypotension, or pulmonary edema

Diagnostic ECG: ST-segment elevation ≥1 mm in ≥2 contiguous precordial leads or ≥2 adjacent limb leads, or new or presumed-to-be new left bundle branch block

Time course: less than 12 hours since onset of pain

Relative Indications

Consistent clinical syndrome

Nondiagnostic ECG: left bundle branch block of unknown duration

Absolute Contraindications

Prior intracranial hemorrhage

Known cerebral vascular lesion

Ischemic stroke within past 3 months

Allergy to the agent

Significant head or facial trauma within past 3 months

Known intracranial neoplasm

Suspected aortic dissection

Active internal bleeding or bleeding diathesis (except menstruation)

Relative Contraindications

Severe uncontrolled hypertension on presentation (blood pressure >180/110 mm Hg)

History of chronic severe hypertension

Ischemic stroke >3 months ago or intracerebral pathology

Current use of anticoagulants

Traumatic or prolonged (>10 min) CPR or major surgery within past 3 weeks

Previous use of streptokinase/anistreplase: allergy or prior exposure (>5 days ago)

Active peptic ulcer disease

Recent internal bleeding (within past 2-4 weeks)

Bleeding diathesis (hepatic dysfunction, use of anticoagulants)

Noncompressible arterial or central venous puncture

Abbreviations: ECG, electrocardiogram; CPR, cardiopulmonary resuscitation

Table 10-10 Thrombolytic Agents Used in ST-Segment Elevation Myocardial Infarction

Streptokinase	1.5 million units intravenously over 30-60 min
Alteplase	15 mg intravenous bolus, then 0.75 mg/kg (maximum 50 mg) intravenously over 30 min, then 0.50 mg/kg (maximum 35 mg) intravenously over 60 min
Reteplase	10 units intravenously over 2 min followed in 30 min by 10 units intravenously again over 2 min
Tenecteplase	Intravenous bolus adjusted for weight (30 mg if <60 kg; 35 mg if 60-70 kg; 40 mg if 70-80 kg; 45 mg if 80-90 kg; 50 mg if >90 kg)

Table 10-11 Killip-Kimball Hemodynamic Subsets

Class	Description
I	No dyspnea; physical examination results are normal
II	No dyspnea; bibasilar crackles or S_3 on examination
III	Dyspnea present; bibasilar crackles or S_3 on examination; no hypotension
IV	Cardiogenic shock

3. Continuing Therapy

Patients who undergo PCI with angioplasty, with or without stent placement, should be treated with aspirin, an adenosine diphosphate inhibitor (clopidogrel, prasugrel, or ticagrelor), and an anticoagulant agent. Administration of clopidogrel or an alternative agent should be discussed with the cardiologist because the optimum duration may vary with the type of stent used (bare metal vs drug-eluting). Anticoagulation with heparin is continued. Although fondaparinux reduces the bleeding risk in STEMI patients undergoing PCI, the risk of catheter thrombi is increased when fondaparinux is used alone. An increased risk of stent thrombosis occurs with use of bivalirudin after PCI. After thrombolysis with a plasminogen activator, heparin should be used to maintain vessel patency for at least 48 hours. Enoxaparin is preferred over unfractionated heparin following thrombolysis. Infusion rates of unfractionated heparin should be adjusted to keep the partial thromboplastin time at 1.5 to 2 times the control value. Heparin anticoagulation after use of streptokinase is not necessary; fondaparinux can be considered in these situations. Patients with large anterior infarctions who do not receive thrombolysis or PCI and patients who have intramural thrombus detected or suspected on echocardiography should receive heparin. Aspirin (162-325 mg/day) should be continued. Clopidogrel is the antiplatelet agent of choice in patients treated with thrombolytics who undergo delayed invasive reperfusion interventions. Intravenous nitroglycerin, if tolerated, is recommended for 48 hours post-MI in patients with hypertension, recurrent ischemia, or heart failure. In the absence of recurrent ischemia, heart failure, or arrhythmias, bed rest should not be continued beyond 12 to 24 hours.

Long-term use of oral β-blockers is helpful in all patients who are at risk for recurrent cardiovascular events and who have no contraindications to their use (**Table 10-6**). Oral β-blockers in STEMI can be initiated after the patient has stabilized.

Longer-acting calcium channel blockers may be a useful secondary therapy for recurrent myocardial ischemia but are not appropriate for first-line treatment. Immediate-release nifedipine is contraindicated in treatment of an acute MI. Diltiazem and verapamil are contraindicated in patients with STEMI and left ventricular dysfunction and heart failure.

Use of ACE inhibitors decreases the risk of mortality in all patients with STEMI. The greatest benefit is seen in patients with left ventricular dysfunction (ejection fraction <40%), anterior infarction, or pulmonary congestion. ACE inhibition should be started within the first 24 hours of the infarction with low doses of oral agents unless hypotension (systolic blood pressure <100 mm Hg) or other contraindications are present. An ARB may be administered if the patient cannot tolerate an ACE inhibitor. Statin therapy should be initiated early after hospital admission.

Expert consultation and/or transfer to another facility is indicated for patients who have persistent angina after MI, who develop cardiogenic shock, who have congestive heart failure despite aggressive therapy, or who have recurrent ventricular fibrillation or tachycardia despite aggressive antiarrhythmic therapy.

C. Risk Stratification for Patients With MI

It is crucial to identify high-risk patients with MI in whom severe or lethal complications may develop during the course of treatment. The following characteristics suggest high-risk patients who should be considered for aggressive therapy:

- Persistent ischemic symptoms after initial management
- Extensive infarction or ischemia
- Recurrent ischemia
- History of MI, CABG, or PCI
- Left ventricular dysfunction
- Angiographic findings compatible with high-risk coronary artery anatomy (eg, left main lesions)

The GRACE and TIMI (http://www.mdcalc.com/timi-risk-score-for-stemi) scores have also been used to identify high-risk STEMI patients. A GRACE score >140 is an indication for transfer to a PCI-capable facility after use of thrombolytics.

D. Complications

Common early complications of MI are heart failure and cardiogenic shock, recurrent ischemia and/or infarction, and arrhythmias.

1. Heart Failure and Cardiogenic Shock

Bedside evaluation allows accurate determination of a patient's hemodynamic status (**Table 10-10**) and the need for hemodynamic monitoring and intervention. Patients with Killip classes I and II heart failure can be managed without advanced hemodynamic monitoring. Class III patients should be considered for advanced hemodynamic monitoring if they do not respond promptly to medical therapy. Class IV patients generally require advanced hemodynamic monitoring. Expert consultation should be sought and/or transfer arranged for patients with class III or IV findings. Advanced hemodynamic monitoring may also be warranted for those with suspected mechanical complications resulting in shock, such as papillary muscle rupture or dysfunction, ventricular septal defect, or cardiac tamponade.

Pharmacologic treatment for heart failure should be tailored to the patient's clinical and hemodynamic state. Patients with systolic arterial pressure >100 mm Hg (pulmonary artery occlusion pressure >15 mm Hg, if available) and cardiac index <2.5 L/min/m^2 should be treated initially with a vasodilator, either intravenous nitroglycerin or intravenous nitroprusside (doses of 0.3 to 1 µg/kg/min, titrated up in increments of 0.5 µg/kg/min every 10 minutes). If arterial pressure decreases or the increase in cardiac output is inadequate, inotropic support with dobutamine should be initiated at 1 to 2 µg/kg/min and titrated to ≤15 µg/kg/min. Milrinone is an alternative inotropic agent. Loop diuretics, such as furosemide (20-40 mg intravenously or orally every 2-4 hours), should be used to reduce pulmonary congestion. Diuretics should be used with caution in hypotensive patients.

Patients with systolic arterial pressure <90 mm Hg (pulmonary arterial occlusion pressure >15 mm Hg, if available) and cardiac index <2.5 L/min/m^2 have cardiogenic shock. These patients should be treated as soon as possible with intra-aortic balloon counterpulsation. Hypotensive patients (systolic arterial pressure <90 mm Hg) should be treated with norepinephrine to raise the systolic arterial pressure. Once the systolic blood pressure has stabilized to at least 90 mm Hg, dobutamine can be added to further increase cardiac output and reduce the dosage of vasopressor.

Interventional therapy with intra-aortic balloon counterpulsation may be indicated in patients with pump failure who do not respond promptly to medical therapy. It has several potential benefits in these patients. During inflation, the balloon augments coronary blood flow and forward cardiac output. During deflation, it decreases afterload and preload as well. Intra-aortic balloon counterpulsation and other ventricular assist devices may stabilize the hemodynamic status sufficiently to allow PCI or coronary bypass surgery.

Evidence suggests that patients with STEMI who develop shock within 36 hours benefit from early invasive reperfusion performed within 18 hours of onset of shock. In patients with one- or two-vessel disease, PCI is preferred. Patients who remain symptomatic and have three-vessel disease or significant left main coronary artery disease should undergo urgent coronary bypass surgery. PCI should also be performed in patients with severe heart failure and/or pulmonary edema and onset of symptoms within 12 hours.

a. Right Ventricular Infarction/Ischemia

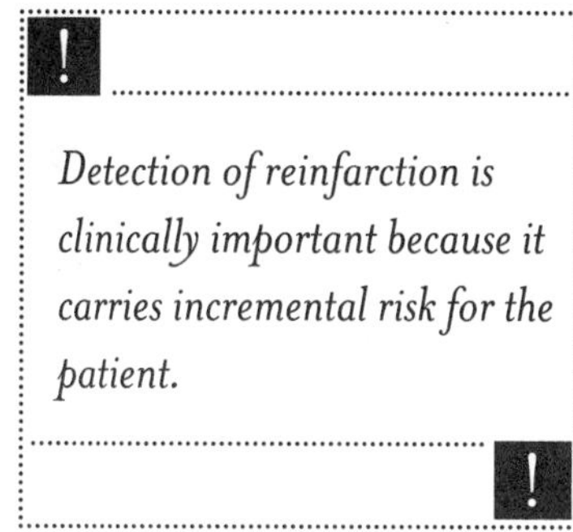

Some patients have heart failure from ischemia of the right ventricle, which results in elevation of right atrial and right ventricular end-diastolic pressures to >10 mm Hg, cardiac index <2.5 L/min/m^2, and systolic arterial pressure <100 mm Hg. These patients generally have clear lung fields, no third heart sound, and distended internal jugular veins. The ECG usually reveals an inferior infarction, and the ST segment in lead V_1 may be elevated in the absence of elevation in any other standard precordial lead. An ECG tracing of the right precordial leads should be obtained and may reveal characteristic ST-segment elevation, especially in V_4R. Initial therapy includes volume expansion until the blood pressure is stabilized, pulmonary arterial occlusion pressure is >20 mm Hg, or right atrial pressure is >20 mm Hg. Associated bradycardia or high-degree heart block may require chemical or electrical intervention. Agents such as morphine, nitrates, ACE inhibitors/ARBs, and diuretics that reduce preload should be avoided. If volume expansion is inadequate to stabilize the patient, dobutamine can be administered. Intra-aortic balloon counterpulsation should be considered for refractory hypotension.

2. Recurrent Ischemia or Infarction

Recurrent ischemia or infarction occurs in ≤20% of patients treated with thrombolytic therapy for MI. Patients treated with primary PCI have a lower incidence of recurrent ischemia. Ischemia after MI can be caused by residual stenosis in the infarct-related artery, by disease in another coronary artery, or by occlusion of a new stent. An ECG recorded during recurrent pain should be compared with those from the index MI event. Reinfarction may present special diagnostic difficulties because cardiac troponin levels can be elevated for 5 to 14 days. If the first blood sample reveals an elevated cardiac troponin value when recurrent ischemia is suspected, then serial levels of a cardiac marker with a shorter time course of returning to normal, such as CK-MB or myoglobin, could be analyzed to clarify the possibility of recurrent infarction. No cardiac marker is reliable for diagnosis of reinfarction in the first 18 hours after onset of STEMI. Pericarditis should also be considered as a potential cause of recurrent chest pain after an MI.

Medical treatment of post-MI ischemia is similar to management of UA but also includes cardiac catheterization and reperfusion, if possible and not recently accomplished. Recurrent infarction with ST-segment elevation on ECG can be treated with repeat thrombolysis. Streptokinase-based drugs should not be used a second time because of the risk of allergic reactions. Plasminogen activator-based regimens can be repeated. Acute reperfusion with PCI or CABG may be required for stabilization.

3. Arrhythmias

Arrhythmias associated with ACS and reperfusion include atrial bradycardias, atrial tachyarrhythmias, atrioventricular (AV) blocks, ventricular tachyarrhythmias, and asystole. Hemodynamically significant atrial bradycardia or AV block can be treated initially with intravenous atropine in a dose of 0.5 mg every 3-5 minutes to a total dose of 3 mg while preparing for transcutaneous pacing. Atropine rarely corrects complete heart block or type II second-degree AV block. Temporary transvenous pacing is indicated for complete heart block, bilateral bundle branch block, new or indeterminate-age bifascicular block with first-degree AV block, type II second-degree AV block, and symptomatic sinus bradycardia that is unresponsive to atropine. Transcutaneous pacing should be initiated for patients who have indications for emergent temporary pacing until transvenous pacing can be instituted (**Appendix 7**).

Atrial tachyarrhythmias, such as atrial fibrillation, may cause hemodynamic instability and precipitate myocardial ischemia, or may be clinically insignificant and transient. Immediate cardioversion is indicated in unstable patients. Depending upon the specific arrhythmia, intravenous adenosine, β-blockers, diltiazem, digoxin, or amiodarone may be effective (**Appendix 4**). Careful attention must be given to contraindications for any of these agents.

Ventricular tachycardia and ventricular fibrillation should be treated according to current advanced cardiac life support guidelines. After defibrillation and if indicated, amiodarone is the drug of choice in patients with an acute MI. Patients with new-onset, symptomatic ventricular ectopy may also benefit from treatment with amiodarone. Antiarrhythmic drugs are not recommended as prophylaxis for ventricular arrhythmias in the setting of acute MI.

E. Special Considerations

1. Perioperative MI

Perioperative MI can occur before surgery, intraoperatively, and during the postoperative period. The latter is the most common, with the peak incidence on the third postoperative day. Perioperative MI is often associated with atypical presentations and is frequently painless. New onset, or an increase in, atrial or ventricular arrhythmias is often the presenting finding, as is postoperative pulmonary edema. The diagnosis can be confirmed with serial ECG and cardiac marker determinations. Treatment is similar to standard treatment, except that thrombolytic therapy may be contraindicated depending on the type of surgery. Primary PCI should be considered for these patients.

2. Effects of Coexisting Diseases

Many, if not most, critically ill patients suffer from more than one medical condition that may require significant alterations in the standard therapeutic approach. Some have relative or absolute contraindications to standard medications or procedures. Patients with stress ulceration or gastritis may not be candidates for aspirin therapy. Postoperative patients or those with a bleeding diathesis may not be candidates for clopidogrel, heparin, thrombolytic therapy, GP IIb/

IIIa inhibitors, or aspirin. β-Blockers should be avoided in patients with significant bronchospasm or decompensated heart failure. Because dopamine can significantly elevate pulmonary artery pressures or increase heart rate, lower doses or an alternative drug may be necessary in patients with respiratory failure or atrial tachyarrhythmias. Certain drugs will need dose adjustments for renal or hepatic dysfunction.

Key Points

Acute Coronary Syndromes

- The preliminary diagnosis of UA/NSTEMI is based on the clinical symptoms, assessment of risk factors for coronary artery disease, and ECG interpretation.
- A 12-lead ECG should be obtained and interpreted within 10 minutes in patients with possible MI.
- Non–enteric-coated aspirin at a dose of 162 to 325 mg should be administered (and chewed) as soon as possible in all patients with suspected or diagnosed ACS.
- Antiplatelet and anticoagulant agents are important interventions in all patients with ACS.
- High-risk patients (continuing ischemia, elevated troponin levels) with UA/NSTEMI may be candidates for additional therapy with an early invasive strategy.
- Oral β-blockers should be initiated in the first 24 hours for all patients with ACS unless there are strong contraindications.
- A plan for early reperfusion of patients with STEMI should be developed based on resources available in the facility and community.
- A goal of 90 minutes or less from hospital presentation to balloon inflation is optimal for primary PCI for STEMI.
- Thrombolytic therapy for reperfusion in STEMI ideally should be initiated within 30 minutes of the patient's arrival to the hospital.
- Patients who undergo PCI with angioplasty with or without stent placement should be treated with aspirin and another antiplatelet agent such as clopidogrel, prasugrel, or ticagrelor.
- Use of ACE inhibitors decreases the mortality rate in all patients with STEMI.
- Evidence suggests that patients with STEMI who develop shock within 36 hours of MI benefit from early invasive reperfusion performed within 18 hours of onset of shock.

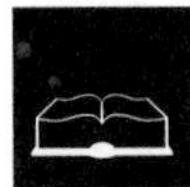

Suggested Readings

1. Anderson JL, Adams CD, Antman EM, et al. ACC/AHA 2007 guidelines for the management of patients with unstable angina/non-ST-elevation myocardial infarction: A report of the American College of Cardiology/American Heart Association Task Force on Practice Guidelines. *Circulation.* 2007;116:e148-304.

2. Antman E, Bassand J-P, Klein W, et al. Myocardial infarction redefined: A consensus document of the Joint European Society of Cardiology/American College of Cardiology Committee for the Redefinition of Myocardial Infarction. *J Am Coll Cardiol.* 2000;36:959-969.

3. Arntz HR, Bossaert LL, Danchin N, et al. European Resuscitation Council Guidelines for Resuscitation 2010, Section 5. Initial management of acute coronary syndromes. *Resuscitation.* 2010;81:1353-1363.

4. Bavry AA, Kumbhani DJ, Quiroz R, et al. Invasive therapy along with glycoprotein IIb/IIIa inhibitors and intracoronary stents improves survival in non–ST-segment elevation acute coronary syndromes: A meta-analysis and review of the literature. *Am J Cardiol.* 2004;93:830-835.

5. Braunwald E, Mark DB, Jones RH, et al. *Unstable Angina: Diagnosis and Management.* Rockville, MD: Agency for Health Care Policy and Research and National Heart, Lung, and Blood Institute. US Public Health Service, US Department of Health and Human Services; 1994. AHCPR Publication 94-0602.

6. Kushner FG, Hand M, Smith SC Jr., et al. 2009 Focused Updates: ACC/AHA guidelines for the management of patients with ST-elevation myocardial infarction (updating the 2004 guideline and 2007 focused update) and ACC/AHA/SCAI guidelines on percutaneous coronary intervention (updating the 2005 guideline and 2007 focused update): A report of the American College of Cardiology Foundation/American Heart Association Task Force on Practice Guidelines. *Circulation.* 2009;120:2271-2306.

7. O'Connor RE, Bossaert L, Arntz HR, et al. Part 9: Acute coronary syndromes: 2010 International Consensus on Cardiopulmonary Resuscitation and Emergency Cardiovascular Care Science With Treatment Recommendations. *Circulation.* 2010;122[Suppl 2]:S422-S465.

8. Task Force for the Diagnosis and Treatment of Non-ST-Segment Elevation Acute Coronary Syndromes of the European Society of Cardiology, Bassand JP, Hamm CW, et al. Guidelines for the diagnosis and treatment of non-ST-segment elevation acute coronary syndromes. *Eur Heart J.* 2007;28:1598-1660.

9. Ting HH, Yang EH, Rihal CS. Narrative review: Reperfusion strategies for ST-segment elevation myocardial infarction. *Ann Intern Med.* 2006;145:610-617.

10. Van de Werf F, Bax J, Task Force on the Management of ST-segment Elevation Acute Myocardial Infarction of the European Society of Cardiology, et al. Management of acute myocardial infarction in patients presenting with persistent ST-segment elevation. *Eur Heart J.* 2008;29:2909-2945.

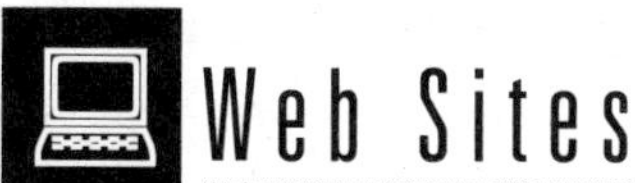

Web Sites

1. American College of Cardiology. http://www.acc.org. *Guidelines for management of acute coronary syndromes and related cardiovascular topics.*

2. American Heart Association. http://www.americanheart.org. *Guidelines for management of acute coronary syndromes and related cardiovascular topics.*

3. European Society of Cardiology. http://www.escardio.org. *Guidelines for management of acute coronary syndromes and additional cardiovascular information available in the section "Knowledge Centre."*

4. Global Registry of Acute Cardiac Events (GRACE). http://www.outcomes-umassmed.org/GRACE/default.aspx. *Additional information and resources from the international database.*

5. National Institute for Health and Clinical Excellence. http://www.nice.org.uk. *Guidelines for management of chest pain and UA/NSTEMI from an independent organization in the United Kingdom.*

Chapter 11

LIFE-THREATENING INFECTIONS: DIAGNOSIS AND ANTIMICROBIAL THERAPY SELECTION

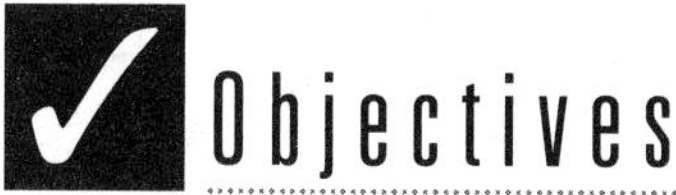

Objectives

- Understand and apply the terminology specific to life-threatening infections.
- List the risk factors for the development of infection.
- Identify systemic and site-specific clinical manifestations of life-threatening infections, and understand the diagnostic use of clinical laboratory testing.
- Describe the different clinical and epidemiologic variables used to guide the selection of antimicrobial therapy.
- Outline antimicrobial treatment for empiric therapy and for specific infections.

Case Study

A 75-year-old man presents to the emergency department with altered mental status. His family reports that he has had a productive cough for the last 2 days. His vital signs are: blood pressure 110/70 mm Hg, heart rate 110/min, temperature 102.2°F (39°C), respiratory rate 20/min, and pulse oximetry 92% while receiving 2 L/min oxygen by nasal cannula. You are the primary physician and are called to admit him to the hospital.

- Does this patient have sepsis or severe sepsis?
- What level of care is needed for this patient?
- What initial interventions should be instituted immediately?

I. INTRODUCTION

Life-threatening infections are both a cause and a consequence of critical illness. The incidence of life-threatening infections or sepsis is increasing as a reflection of the growing population of patients at risk, for example, the elderly; immunocompromised patients; those with malignancy, chronic illness, or multiple trauma. Septic shock, the most severe form of systemic response to infection, is a common cause of death in critically ill adults and children. Early recognition and appropriate management of infections and their sequelae can decrease the mortality rate.

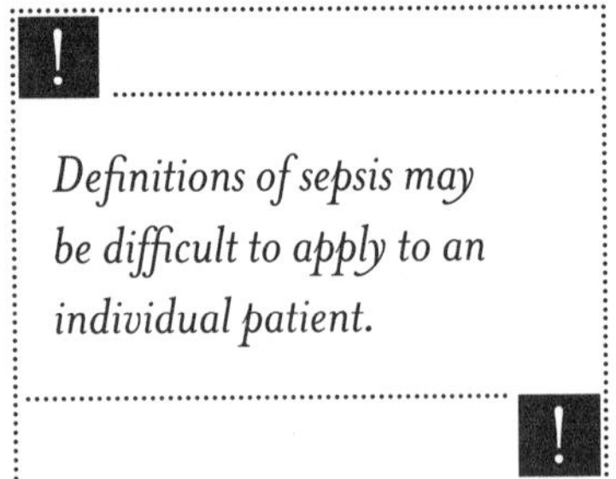

Definitions of sepsis may be difficult to apply to an individual patient.

Sepsis is defined as systemic manifestations of infection. *Severe sepsis* is sepsis associated with organ dysfunction, hypoperfusion, or hypotension. Abnormalities that suggest hypoperfusion and organ dysfunction may include, but are not limited to, lactic acidosis, oliguria, coagulation disorders, and an acute alteration in mental status. These abnormalities are not specific for sepsis and may be present in other conditions. *Septic shock* is sepsis with arterial hypotension, defined as a systolic blood pressure <90 mm Hg or a decrease of >40 mm Hg from the patient's baseline systolic blood pressure despite adequate fluid resuscitation, with concomitant organ dysfunction. Patients receiving inotropic or vasopressor agents may not be hypotensive when perfusion abnormalities are measured.

Initial considerations in resuscitation and infection management are described in **Table 11-1**. Additional details are found in this chapter and in **Chapters 6** and **7**.

II. DIAGNOSIS OF INFECTION

The diagnosis of serious or life-threatening infection is based on a careful and complete assessment of the patient's history, including risk factors, and the presence of characteristic clinical manifestations. Atypical presentations that may occur, particularly in the elderly and in the immunocompromised patient, must also be considered. Laboratory, microbiologic, and imaging results also support the diagnosis of documented or suspected infection.

A. Evaluation of New Fever in Critically Ill Adult Patients

In some ICUs, the measurement of a newly elevated temperature triggers an automatic order set that includes many tests that are time consuming, costly, and disruptive to the patient and staff. Moreover, the patient may experience discomfort, be exposed to unneeded radiation, require transport outside the controlled environment of the ICU, or lose considerable blood to this testing, which is often repeated several times within 24 hours and daily thereafter. In an era when utilization of hospital and patient resources is under intensive scrutiny, such fevers should be evaluated in a prudent and cost-effective manner. A new fever in a patient in the ICU should trigger a careful clinical assessment rather than automatic orders for laboratory and radiologic tests. The goal of such an approach is to determine, in a directed manner, whether infection is present so that additional testing can be avoided and therapeutic decisions can be made. Recommendations for the evaluation of new fever are listed in **Table 11-2**.

Table 11-1 Initial Resuscitation and Infection Issues[a,b]

Initial Resuscitation (first 6 hours)

- Begin resuscitation immediately in patients with hypotension or elevated serum lactate >4 mmol/L; do not delay pending ICU admission
- Follow resuscitation goals:

  CVP 8-12 mm Hg

  Mean arterial pressure ≥65 mm Hg

  Urine output ≥0.5 mL/kg^{-1}/h^{-1}

  Central venous (superior vena cava) oxygen saturation ≥70%

Diagnosis

- Obtain appropriate cultures before starting antibiotics provided this does not significantly delay antimicrobial administration
- Obtain two or more blood cultures **(Table 11-2)**
- Cultures other sites as clinically indicated
- Perform imaging studies promptly to confirm and sample any source of infection, if safe to do so

Antibiotic Therapy

- Begin intravenous antibiotics as early as possible and always within the first hour of recognizing severe sepsis and septic shock
- Choose broad-spectrum agent(s): one or more agents active against likely bacterial/fungal pathogens and with good penetration into presumed source
- Reassess antimicrobial regimen daily to optimize efficacy, prevent resistance, avoid toxicity, and minimize costs

Source Identification and Control

- Establish specific anatomic site of infection as rapidly as possible
- Implement source control measures as soon as possible
- Remove intravascular access devices if potentially infected

Abbreviation: CVP, central venous pressure
[a]See **Chapters 6** and **7**.
[b]Adapted with permission from Lippincott, Williams & Wilkins.[4] Dellinger RP, Levy MM, Carlet JM, et al. Surviving Sepsis Campaign: International guidelines for management of severe sepsis and septic shock: 2008. *Crit Care Med.* 36(1):296-327.

Table 11-2 Evaluation of Fever in the Critically Ill Adults[a]

Measuring Temperature	1. Temperature in the ICU is most accurately measured by an intravascular, esophageal, or bladder thermistor, followed by rectal, oral, and tympanic membrane measurements. 2. Axillary measurements, temporal artery estimates, and chemical dot thermometers should not be used in the ICU. Rectal thermometers should be avoided in neutropenic patients. 3. Any device used to measure temperature must be maintained and calibrated appropriately, and must be used in a manner that does not facilitate spread of pathogens. 4. A new onset of temperature ≥100.9°F (38.3°C) or ≤96.8°F (36°C) in the absence of a known cause of hypothermia (eg, hypothyroidism, cooling blanket, etc.) is a reasonable trigger for a clinical assessment but not necessarily a laboratory or radiologic evaluation for infection.
Obtaining Blood Cultures	1. Three to four blood cultures should be obtained within the first 24 h of the onset of fever. Draw the first cultures before the initiation of antimicrobial therapy. They can be drawn consecutively or simultaneously, unless there is suspicion of an endovascular infection, in which case separate venipunctures by timed intervals can be drawn to demonstrate continuous bacteremia. 2. Additional blood cultures are indicated when there is clinical suspicion of continuing or recurrent bacteremia or fungemia or for test of cure, 48-96 h after initiation of appropriate therapy. 3. For patients without an indwelling vascular catheter, obtain at least two blood cultures by separate venipunctures, using strict aseptic technique from peripheral sites. 4. If the patient has an intravascular catheter, one blood culture should be drawn by venipuncture and at least one culture should be drawn through an intravascular catheter. 5. Each blood culture requires 20-30 mL of blood.
Management of Intravascular Catheters	1. Examine the patient at least daily for inflammation or purulence at the exit site or along the tunnel, and assess the patient for signs of venous thrombosis or evidence of embolic phenomena. Gram stain and culture indicated for any expressed purulence from the insertion site. 2. If there is evidence of a tunnel infection, embolic phenomenon, vascular compromise, or septic shock, the catheter should be removed and cultured, and a new catheter inserted at a different site. 3. Short-term temporary catheters, peripheral venous catheters, noncuffed central venous catheters, or arterial catheters should be removed and a catheter segment cultured. Blood cultures should be obtained as well. 4. At least two blood cultures should be obtained, one peripherally by venipuncture, and one from the suspected catheter. If a quantitative culture system is available, it should be used to determine if the catheter is the source of bacteremia/fungemia. 5. All catheters removed from ICU patients do not require culture, only those suspected of being the source of infection. 6. It is not necessary to routinely culture infusate specimens unless there is clinical suspicion that they are infected.
Evaluation of Pulmonary Infections	1. A chest imaging study should be obtained. In most cases, an upright portable anteroposterior chest radiograph is the most feasible study to obtain. Posterior-anterior chest radiographs with lateral view or CT scans offer more information and should be obtained when clinically indicated, especially to rule out opportunistic infections in immunocompromised patients. 2. One sample of lower respiratory tract secretions should be obtained for direct examination and culture before initiation of or change in antibiotics. Expectorated sputum, induced sputum, tracheal secretions, or bronchoscopic or nonbronchoscopic alveolar lavage material can be used effectively. 3. Respiratory secretions obtained for microbiologic evaluation should be transported to the laboratory and processed in 2 h. 4. Pleural fluid should be obtained for Gram stain and routine culture (with other studies as clinically indicated) if there is an adjacent infiltrate or another reason to suspect infection and if the fluid can be safely aspirated.

Table 11-2 Evaluation of Fever in the Critically Ill Adults[a] (continued)

Evaluation of the Gastrointestinal Tract	1. Testing for *Clostridium difficile* or its toxins should be performed only on diarrheal (unformed) stool, unless ileus due to *C difficile* is suspected. Testing of stool from asymptomatic patients is not clinically useful. 2. One stool sample is sent for *C difficile* common antigen, EIA for toxin A and B, or tissue culture assay. 3. PCR testing appears to be rapid, sensitive, and specific. 4. If severe illness is present and rapid tests for *C difficile* are negative or unavailable, consider flexible sigmoidoscopy. 5. If severe illness is present, consider empirical therapy with vancomycin while awaiting diagnostic studies. Empirical therapy generally is not recommended if two stool evaluations are negative. 6. Stool cultures for other enteric pathogens are rarely indicated in a patient who did not present to the hospital with diarrhea or in patients who are not infected with HIV.
Evaluation of the Urinary Tract	1. For patients at high risk for urinary tract infection (kidney transplant patients, granulocytopenic patients, or those with recent urologic surgery or obstruction), a laboratory evaluation is necessary if infection is suspected. 2. Patients who have urinary catheters in place should have urine collected from the sampling port of the catheter and not from the drainage bag. 3. Urine should be transported to the laboratory and processed within 1 h to avoid bacterial multiplication. 4. Cultures from catheterized patients showing 10^3 CFU/mL represent true bacteriuria or candiduria, but neither higher counts nor the presence of pyuria alone are of much value in determining if the catheter-associated bacteriuria or candiduria is the cause of fever. 5. Gram stains of centrifuged urine are reliable in detection of the infecting organisms. 6. In the analysis of possible catheter-associated infection, rapid dipstick tests are not recommended for patients with urinary catheters.
Evaluation of the Sinuses	1. If sinusitis is suspected to be a cause of fever, a CT scan of the facial sinuses should be obtained. 2. If the patient has not responded to empirical therapy, puncture and aspiration of the involved sinuses should be performed under antiseptic conditions. Aspirated fluid should be sent for Gram stain and culture for aerobic and anaerobic bacteria and fungi.
Evaluation of Fever Within 72 Hours of Surgery	1. A chest radiograph and urinalysis are not mandatory during the initial 72 h after surgery if fever is the only indication. 2. Urinalysis and culture should be performed for those febrile patients having indwelling bladder catheters for ≥72 h. 3. Surgical wounds should be examined daily for infection. They should not be cultured if there is no suggestion of infection. 4. A high level of suspicion should be maintained for deep venous thrombosis, superficial thrombophlebitis, and pulmonary embolism, especially in patients who are sedentary, have lower limb immobility, have a malignant neoplasm, or are taking an oral contraceptive.
Evaluation of Surgical Site Infection	1. Examine the surgical incision at least once daily for erythema, purulence, or tenderness as part of the fever evaluation. If there is suspicion of infection, the incision should be opened and cultured. Tissue biopsies or aspirates are preferable to swabs. 2. Drainage from superficial surgical site infections may not require Gram stain and culture because incision, drainage, and local care may be sufficient treatment. Antibiotic therapy may not be required. Superficial swab cultures are likely to be contaminated with commensal skin flora and are not recommended.

Table 11-2 Evaluation of Fever in the Critically Ill Adults[a] (continued)

Evaluation of Central Nervous System Infections	1. If altered consciousness or focal neurologic signs are unexplained, lumbar puncture should be considered in any patient with a new fever and no contraindication to the procedure. 2. For a patient with a new fever and new focal neurologic findings suggesting disease above the foramen magnum, an imaging study is usually required before lumbar puncture. 3. In febrile patients with an intracranial device, CSF from the reservoir should be obtained for analysis. The device should be removed and cultured (eg. ventriculostomy). 4. CSF should be evaluated by Gram stain and culture, glucose, protein, and cell count with differential. Additional tests (eg, tuberculosis, viral and fungal disease, neoplasia) should be performed as dictated by the clinical situation.
Recognizing Noninfectious Causes of Fever	1. All of the patient's new medications and blood products should be considered. Ideally, the new drug should be stopped or a similar agent substituted. 2. Fever induced by drugs may take several days to resolve.

Abbreviations: CT, computerized tomography; EIA, enzyme immunoassay; PCR, polymerase chain reaction; CFU, colony-forming units; CSF, cerebrospinal fluid

[a]Adapted with permission from Lippincott, Williams & Wilkins.[9] O'Grady NP, Barie PS, Bartlett JG, et al. Guidelines for evaluation of new fever in critically ill adult patients: 2008 update from the American College of Critical Care Medicine and the Infectious Diseases Society of America. *Crit Care Med.* 36(4):1330–1349.

B. Epidemiologic Factors

Serious or life-threatening infections may occur in patients from the community, long-term care facilities (ie, nursing homes), or hospital settings. Serious or life-threatening community-acquired infections include bacterial pneumonia, central nervous system (CNS) infections or meningitis, urosepsis, intra-abdominal sepsis due to a ruptured or obstructed viscus, or sporadic uncommon infections, such as necrotizing fasciitis. Patients from long-term care facilities share this spectrum but often have infections with more resistant pathogens and may develop different device-related infections. Finally, hospitalized patients are exposed to antimicrobial-resistant flora and numerous invasive devices, and they have more comorbidities and greater severity of illness than the other populations.

C. Predisposing Conditions

The presence of predisposing conditions should alert the care team to patients at higher risk of developing infections (**Table 11-3**). Permanent prosthetic implants, such as heart valves, intravascular grafts, or orthopedic devices, may become infected in either the early or the late postoperative period. Invasive procedures (eg, surgery, vascular catheterization, placement of urinary catheters, and endotracheal intubation) breech the normal mucosal defense barriers and predispose patients to infection. The lack of predisposing conditions does not eliminate the possibility that a serious infection is present, particularly in patients admitted directly to the ICU from the community.

Table 11-3 Conditions Predisposing to Infection

Extremes of age	Diabetes
Transplant recipients	Hepatic failure
Multiple trauma	Malnutrition
Alcoholism	Malignancy
HIV	Corticosteroid use
Chemotherapy/radiotherapy	Burns
Absence of spleen	Prosthetic implants
Invasive procedures	

D. Clinical Manifestations

The clinical manifestations of life-threatening infections are diverse, and they may be subtle or overt and localized or systemic. An awareness of the signs and symptoms associated with specific infections allows early recognition and prompt institution of appropriate empiric antimicrobial and supportive management. However, most of the clinical manifestations are not specific.

1. Systemic Signs and Symptoms

Fever is the most frequent systemic manifestation of infection, but patients with serious infection may be normothermic or even hypothermic, particularly if they are elderly or if antipyretic medications, alcoholism, or renal or hepatic failure are involved. Temperature probes on a urinary catheter, when available, are the most reliable methods to measure the core temperature. Temperature measurement is most practically obtained via the oral or rectal routes, although the limitations of each method should be considered. Axillary temperatures are unreliable, and tympanic measurements have not been validated in the critically ill.

> ! *Hypothermia is a poor prognostic sign in serious infections.* !

Other systemic manifestations include chills, rigors, hypotension, tachypnea, dyspnea, tachycardia, and nausea and vomiting. Tachycardia is almost always present but may be absent in the presence of cardiac conduction disturbances, autonomic dysfunction, β-blockers or calcium channel blockers, and drug fever. Hypotension may be due to dehydration and hypovolemia but may also indicate septic shock, particularly if the blood pressure does not respond to volume resuscitation. Hypoperfusion of the kidneys may result in oliguria or anuria. Encephalopathy is a common clinical manifestation and ranges from lethargy/irritability to delirium and coma. Petechiae and/or ecchymosis may be present, particularly on distal extremities.

2. Site-Specific Signs and Symptoms

Some signs and symptoms of infection could be associated with the specific source of infection:

- Infections of the CNS may be associated with headache, seizures, meningismus, or focal neurologic findings. Altered mental status is often present but not specific for CNS infections.

- Diffuse or localized respiratory tract infections may be associated with dyspnea, tachypnea, cough, sputum production, or (rarely) hemoptysis. Chest auscultation findings, such as crackles, rhonchi, or tubular breath sounds, indicate whether the process is localized or diffuse. Diminished breath sounds and dullness on percussion are suggestive of a pleural effusion.

- Intra-abdominal infections may cause abdominal pain, abdominal distension, nausea and/or vomiting, diarrhea, and anorexia. Diaphragmatic irritation can be perceived as pain in the side of the neck and proximal shoulder area or may cause hiccups. Findings on examination may include diffuse or local tenderness, rebound tenderness, ileus, or guaiac-positive stool. A wound infection with evidence of fascial disruption may signal an intra-abdominal infection below the fascia.

- Urinary tract infections may produce flank pain or abdominal pain, tenderness, dysuria, hematuria, and oliguria. Typically, a urinary catheter–associated infection does not produce localized symptoms.

- Cutaneous manifestations may result from a primary infection of the skin or skin structures (eg, pain, erythema, and induration due to cellulitis; wound margin erythema; tenderness or purulent discharge; vesicular lesions due to herpes infection) or be a consequence of disseminated systemic infection (eg, erythematous indurated papules or nodules of ecthyma gangrenosum due to bacteremia, septic emboli due to infective endocarditis, diffuse macular erythema due to toxic shock syndrome, distal symmetric purpura fulminans due to meningococcemia).

E. Laboratory Manifestations

Routine laboratory tests are not specific in the diagnosis of life-threatening infections but may be suggestive and allow assessment of organ function. The white blood cell count is usually elevated with a shift to more immature forms (called a left shift). Leukocytosis is commonly observed in noninfectious processes such as the early postoperative period, corticosteroid therapy, massive transfusions, and polytrauma. Conversely, a normal leukocyte count may be observed despite active infection in the elderly and in patients with hypersplenism or chronic myelosuppressive disorders. Neutropenia may result from overwhelming infection (especially in neonates and AIDS patients), severe viral infection, typhoid fever, brucellosis, and other infections. Toxic granulation within neutrophils may also be noted.

The most common coagulation abnormality in sepsis is isolated thrombocytopenia. A decline in platelet count may be a subtle, early clue to the presence of infection. Disseminated intravascular coagulation is a less common finding but is a poor prognostic sign. It is characterized by elevations in prothrombin time, partial thromboplastin time, fibrin split products, and/or D-dimer, and decreased fibrinogen.

Sepsis causes relative insulin resistance, usually resulting in hyperglycemia, whereas hypoglycemia is less frequent and often reflects low hepatic glycogen stores. Arterial blood gas measurements usually reflect metabolic acidosis, a low Pa_{CO_2} due to respiratory compensation and often hypoxemia. An elevated serum lactate level is a significant sign of compromised peripheral perfusion and oxygen balance due to severe sepsis or septic shock. Hepatic dysfunction is usually not severe but presents as a cholestatic picture with elevated bilirubin and mild elevation of transaminases. Renal insufficiency often occurs due to multiple factors such as hypotension and hypovolemia. Other possible nonspecific markers of inflammation/infection include procalcitonin and C-reactive protein.

F. Microbiologic Studies

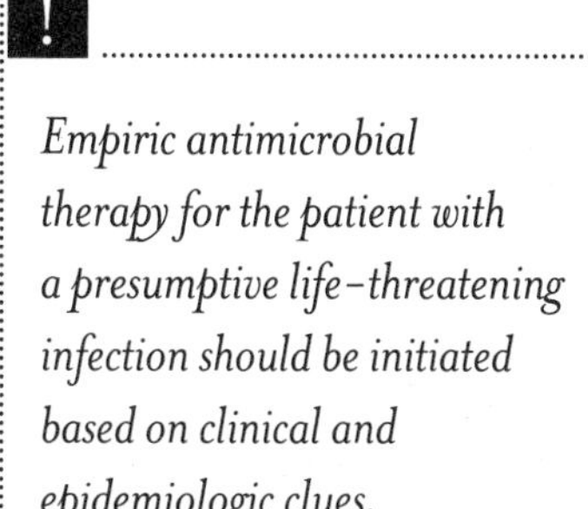

Microbiologic studies are divided into those with immediately available results (minutes to a few hours) and those requiring a period for incubation or laboratory determinations. Among the studies with quickly available results is Gram stain of body fluids. Special stains (such as fungal and acid-fast stains), immunoassays (such as urine *Legionella* antigen and *Clostridium difficile* toxins), and counterimmunoelectrophoresis panels require time to process.

Ideally, all cultures should be obtained before initiation or modification of antimicrobial therapy, but this may not be possible in the rapidly deteriorating patient. The selection of culture site(s) should be guided by clinical manifestations. Indiscriminate sampling from many sites not only may yield misleading results due to culture contamination or site colonization, but is also not cost-effective and may pose additional risks to the patient. Repeat cultures may be appropriate to assess for changes in the type of organism or resistance patterns.

At least two sets of peripheral blood cultures (aerobic and anaerobic bottle) should be obtained either from different anatomic sites or from the same site but separated by 30 minutes. A blood volume of 10 to 15 mL per culture set is optimal in adults. Obtaining blood cultures from indwelling peripheral or central intravascular catheters may yield false-positive results because of microbial contamination of the catheter hub. Isolator blood cultures may improve the diagnostic yield for some organisms (eg, *Candida, Mycobacterium*) or in patients already receiving antimicrobial therapy.

Respiratory tract cultures require expectorated sputum from the nonintubated patient and tracheal suction or bronchoscopic specimens from an intubated patient. Many microbiology laboratories will screen the specimen for the number of epithelial cells and neutrophils to determine adequacy for culture. Quantitative cultures of lower respiratory tract secretions may discriminate between colonizing and pathogenic bacteria.

In the absence of catheterization, urine cultures should be clean-catch voided specimens; in catheterized patients, specimens should be aspirated from the urinary catheter tubing. Semiquantitative culture is needed; however, thresholds for significance differ for clean-catch urine (>10^5 organisms/mL) and catheter-obtained urine (>10^3 organisms/mL). Urinalysis for the detection of pyuria will help to discriminate bacteriuria from cystitis or upper tract infection.

Intravascular catheters should be removed in aseptic fashion (by applying chlorhexidine to the surrounding skin and external part of the catheter adjacent to the skin exit) and the intradermal segment should be sent for semiquantitative culture. However, clinical correlation between the catheter culture result, blood culture(s), and appearance of the catheter exit site is required to discriminate between catheter-related bacteremia, local catheter-related infection, and simple colonization of the catheter itself. The best method for diagnosis of intravascular catheter-related bloodstream infections is the testing of paired cultures from peripheral and catheter blood samples.

G. Additional Studies

A complete description of additional studies for all infections is beyond the scope of this chapter. However, some of the studies specific for the chest, CNS, and abdomen/retroperitoneum are summarized in **Table 11-4**.

Table 11-4 Selected Additional Studies

Chest

- An upright posterior-anterior and lateral chest radiograph
- A lateral decubitus chest radiograph or ultrasound to evaluate for possible pleural fluid
- CT scan of chest to evaluate the mediastinum, lung parenchyma, and pleural-based lesions
- Thoracentesis if fluid is present
- Transthoracic and/or transesophageal echocardiogram

Central Nervous System

- Lumbar puncture for patients with possible central nervous system infection, including patients with evidence of meningismus and/or altered mental status for which no other cause is readily apparent. A lumbar puncture is mandatory in febrile neonates, because of the high incidence of sepsis with meningitis in these patients. Contraindications to lumbar puncture are severe thrombocytopenia and coagulopathy, suspected intracranial mass lesion, or severe respiratory compromise that precludes adequate positioning. If a significant delay of 1 h or longer is anticipated before performing the lumbar puncture, empiric antimicrobials should be initiated immediately, before the procedure.
- CT or MRI of the head or spine
- Electroencephalogram

Abdomen/Retroperitoneum

- Supine, upright, or supine decubitus films to assess for free air
- CT scan, usually with intravenous and oral contrast
- Hepatobiliary ultrasound
- Renal ultrasound

Abbreviations: CT, computed tomography; MRI, magnetic resonance imaging

III. ANTIMICROBIAL THERAPY

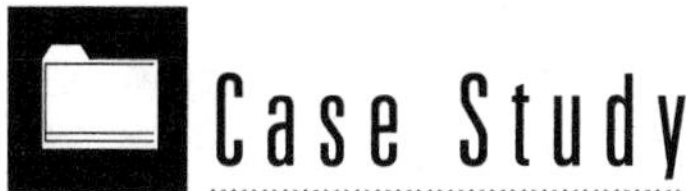

Case Study

A 23-year-old woman who had been in a motor vehicle accident was transferred to the floor from the ICU. She had been intubated for 4 days due to pulmonary contusions. After 1 day on the floor, she develops fever, an elevated white blood cell count, and worsening hypoxemia. You are called to evaluate her.

- What is the likely source of this patient's infection?
- What factors would influence your choice of antimicrobial agent?

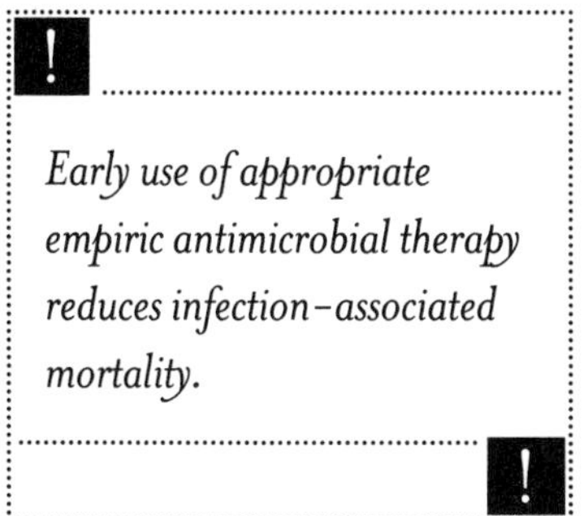

Early use of appropriate empiric antimicrobial therapy reduces infection-associated mortality.

The first priority in managing a hemodynamically unstable patient with a severe or life-threatening infection is resuscitation (**Chapters 6** and **7**). After evaluation of the patient by history, physical examination, and auxiliary tests (laboratory and imaging studies), antimicrobial agents should be instituted promptly.

Early source control (suspected source of infection) is paramount to favorable outcomes and is an essential adjunct to adequate antimicrobial therapy. Examples of source control include wound debridement, percutaneous or surgical drainage of a closed-space infection, foreign body removal, and surgery. The antimicrobial therapy recommendations found in this chapter are general guidelines only. For each clinical scenario, antimicrobial choices must be individualized to match the clinical manifestations and the available epidemiologic and microbiologic information, including the patterns of microbial prevalence and resistance in the institution or local community.

The selection of appropriate antimicrobial therapy depends on the following factors:

1. **The suspected microbial pathogen(s) and site of infection:** The most common sites for life-threatening infections in adult patients involve the lower respiratory tract, the intra-abdominal cavity, and the bloodstream. Rapidly progressive soft tissue infections and CNS infections should also be considered and are often clinically obvious. Antimicrobial penetration to the site of infection should also be considered. The CNS and lungs are two sites that allow limited penetration of certain antimicrobials; therefore, the pharmacokinetic characteristics of the selected agents must be understood to ensure maximal antimicrobial activity at those sites.

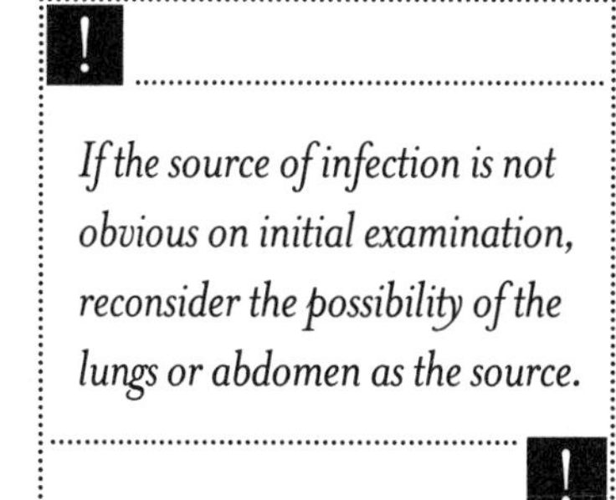

If the source of infection is not obvious on initial examination, reconsider the possibility of the lungs or abdomen as the source.

2. **Gram stain results of available specimens from the suspected site:** The description of early stain results direct the clinician to the broad categories of organism(s) that should be covered.

Examples include gram-positive cocci in clusters (staphylococci) or pairs and chains (enterococci, streptococci), lancet-shaped diplococci (pneumococcus), gram-positive bacilli *(Corynebacterium, Nocardia)*, gram-negative bacilli *(Escherichia coli, Klebsiella, Pseudomonas)*, small pleomorphic gram-negative bacilli *(Bacteroides* spp*)*, gram-negative coccobacilli *(Haemophilus* spp, *Moraxella, Acinetobacter)*, and yeast *(Candida)*. However, the clinician should wait for final culture results to make changes to initial antimicrobial therapy.

3. **Assessment for antimicrobial resistance:** Factors predicting that a particular bacterial pathogen may be resistant to a wider range of antimicrobials include the following:

   - Prior isolation of resistant strains from the same patient
   - Prior antimicrobial therapy (broad-spectrum antimicrobial therapy such as antipseudomonal penicillin/β-lactamase inhibitor combinations, third- and fourth-generation cephalosporins, fluoroquinolones, carbapenems, vancomycin, etc)
   - Extended hospital or ICU stay
   - High endemic rate of multidrug-resistant bacteria in the institution or ICU (eg, methicillin-resistant *Staphylococcus aureus*, vancomycin-resistant *Enterococcus*, multidrug-resistant *Pseudomonas, Stenotrophomonas*)
   - Ongoing epidemic outbreak in the hospital or ICU
   - Long-term dialysis
   - Residence in a nursing home or extended-care facility
   - Immunosuppressive diseases or therapy

   Certain common organisms have become increasingly resistant to formerly effective antimicrobials. This category includes *Streptococcus pneumoniae* with intermediate and high-level resistance to penicillin and ceftriaxone, *Enterococcus faecium* strains resistant to ampicillin and vancomycin, *Staphylococcus aureus* resistant to oxacillin/methicillin (MRSA), gram-negative bacilli *(E coli, Klebsiella pneumoniae)* with extended-spectrum β-lactamase or chromosomal-mediated β-lactamase production observed in strains of *Pseudomonas aeruginosa*, or other mechanisms of multiple resistance to broad-spectrum antimicrobial therapy. It is vital to know and update the resistance pattern of the different bacterial pathogens in each institution and each ICU.

4. **Comorbid conditions:** Less nephrotoxic antimicrobials may be preferable in patients with diminished renal function or patients at risk for renal failure unless the benefit of use outweighs the risk of renal dysfunction. Other comorbidities to consider include bone marrow suppression, chronic or acute liver failure, prior hearing deficits, pregnancy, and a history of major hypersensitivity or other strong adverse reactions to a specific antimicrobial.

IV. RECOMMENDED ANTIMICROBIAL THERAPY

The use of the antimicrobial therapies recommended here is based on the suspected site of infection in the absence of culture results. The clinician should always consider the dose, dose adjustments, possible interactions, and side effects of selected agents. Antimicrobial therapy should be given in maximum appropriate therapeutic doses. In critically ill patients, intravenous administration is preferred to intramuscular or oral routes. Oral dosing of antimicrobials with similar bioequivalence (eg, quinolones) and adequate gastrointestinal absorption may be substituted after the patient stabilizes. Dosage adjustments must be made for the elderly, neonates, children, and patients with renal or hepatic dysfunction. Antimicrobial de-escalation should be implemented in appropriate clinical situations once cultures are negative. In the treatment of infection, antimicrobial agents must be used appropriately and responsibly.

!

Prudent antimicrobial therapy involves early initiation as well as suitable de-escalation.

!

A. Central Nervous System

1. Meningitis

Of all infectious diseases, bacterial meningitis causes one of the crucial emergencies. When bacterial meningitis is suspected clinically, antimicrobial therapy should be instituted immediately, without waiting for the results of lumbar puncture. Community-acquired acute bacterial meningitis in adults is most commonly caused by *S pneumoniae* or *Neisseria meningitidis,* and initial empiric therapy with a third-generation cephalosporin (ceftriaxone or cefotaxime) provides adequate empiric coverage, with vancomycin added if penicillin-resistant *S pneumoniae* is suspected or confirmed. If *S pneumoniae* is isolated, a third-generation cephalosporin should be continued until penicillin sensitivity is confirmed, at which point the patient should be switched to high-dose penicillin G. *N meningitidis* in cerebrospinal fluid (CSF) or blood culture should be treated with high-dose parenteral penicillin G. If *N meningitidis* is isolated, healthcare workers with significant exposure will require antimicrobial prophylaxis. In addition to antimicrobial therapy, adjunctive dexamethasone (0.15 mg/kg intravenously q 6 hours for 2-4 days) is also recommended to decrease morbidity and mortality, particularly in pneumococcal meningitis.

Special circumstances require different empiric antimicrobial coverage. *Listeria monocytogenes* may be a cause of bacterial meningitis in extremes of age (neonates, infants, and the elderly) and in patients with T-lymphocyte defects, usually due to diabetes, corticosteroid use, and immunosuppressive therapy (eg, organ recipients and patients with autoimmune disease). Patients with suspected *Listeria* meningitis should receive ampicillin (trimethoprim-sulfamethoxazole in the penicillin-allergic patient). Those who have undergone recent neurosurgical procedures or placement of CSF shunts are at increased risk for *S aureus,* coagulase-negative staphylococci, and gram-negative bacilli *(Pseudomonas, Klebsiella).* Therefore, such patients require initial empiric antimicrobial coverage with high-dose vancomycin and a third- or fourth-generation cephalosporin. If methicillin-susceptible *S aureus* is confirmed, nafcillin is the drug of choice.

Meningitis presenting in a subacute fashion over several weeks or longer, with predominance of CSF lymphocytes, is more likely to occur in immunocompromised patients. Pathogens such as *Mycobacterium tuberculosis, Toxoplasma gondii,* and *Cryptococcus neoformans* should be considered in this setting.

2. Encephalitis or Meningoencephalitis

Many viral agents can cause encephalitis or meningoencephalitis, but only herpes simplex (HSV) and cytomegalovirus (CMV) encephalitis are amenable to therapy. Herpes simplex encephalitis usually occurs in immunocompetent individuals presenting from the community. This is considered an emergency. Fever, lethargy, confusion, and seizures are the most common presenting complaints. Hemorrhagic CSF and temporal lobe involvement on imaging studies (computed tomography or magnetic resonance imaging) or electroencephalography are suggestive of HSV encephalitis. Polymerase chain reaction testing of CSF is sensitive for diagnosis of this infection. If HSV encephalitis is suspected or confirmed, a 14- to 21-day course of parenteral acyclovir should be initiated promptly, pending further studies. CMV encephalitis usually occurs in patients with suppressed immune status (HIV and transplant patients) and could have the same clinical manifestations as HSV encephalitis. Polymerase chain reaction testing of CSF for CMV is also highly sensitive, and therapy should include ganciclovir or foscarnet.

3. Brain Abscess

Brain abscess is an uncommon infection but should be suspected in patients with chronic infections of parameningeal structures, left-sided endocarditis, or congenital cyanotic heart disease. Brain abscesses also have been associated with immunosuppression, as in AIDS patients, intravenous drug abusers, or transplant recipients. Infections are often polymicrobial, and etiologic organisms include aerobic and anaerobic streptococci, staphylococci, gram-negative bacteria, and anaerobes. Initial antimicrobial therapy should include vancomycin, high-dose metronidazole, and a third-generation cephalosporin (ceftriaxone). In patients at high risk for toxoplasmosis (eg, those with AIDS, cardiac transplant recipients), pyrimethamine/sulfadiazine should be part of the initial antimicrobial regimen. Less common causes of brain abscess include tuberculosis, nocardiosis, syphilis, amoeba, and other parasites. The diagnostic yield of CSF cultures for brain abscess is extremely low, and brain biopsy may be needed in patients who fail to respond to empiric therapy.

B. Respiratory Tract

1. Severe Community-Acquired Pneumonia (Immunocompetent Host)

The most common organism resulting in hospitalization for community-acquired pneumonia is *S pneumoniae,* but other causative organisms include *Legionella, Mycoplasma,* and *Chlamydia. Haemophilus influenzae* is an uncommon pathogen in the United States since the introduction of the vaccine against *H influenzae* type B in children. A β-lactam (ceftriaxone, cefotaxime, ampicillin-sulbactam) plus either a macrolide (azithromycin) or a respiratory fluoroquinolone are recommended in patients admitted to the ICU. If the patient is allergic to penicillin, a respiratory fluoroquinolone and aztreonam are recommended. If aspiration pneumonia is suspected (alcoholics, presence of poor dentition), the addition of clindamycin is warranted unless a β-lactam/β-lactamase inhibitor combination is utilized. If *Pseudomonas* is a consideration, an antipseudomonal β-lactam (piperacillin-tazobactam, cefepime, imipenem, or meropenem) should be used. Vancomycin or linezolid may be added if community-acquired MRSA is suspected.

2. Community-Acquired Pneumonia (Immunocompromised Host)

Immunocompromised patients with pneumonia may have the same pathogens as an immunocompetent host but with more severe infection. Radiographic evidence of interstitial pneumonia or a normal chest radiograph in a patient with prominent respiratory symptoms who has T-cell deficiency (AIDS, chronic steroid use) should prompt the addition of trimethoprim-sulfamethoxazole in appropriate doses for possible *Pneumocystis carinii* infection. Consider the addition of steroids in *P carinii* pneumonia associated with significant hypoxemia. Focal lesions (eg, abscess, nodules) are suggestive of fungal infections, *M tuberculosis*, or *Nocardia;* empiric coverage with antifungal agents, antimycobacterial agents, and trimethoprim-sulfamethoxazole may be warranted in these circumstances. Patients with suspected *M tuberculosis* infection also require respiratory isolation. CMV or other viral infection also should be considered in the differential of an interstitial pneumonitis.

3. Nosocomial and Ventilator-Associated Pneumonia

Gram-negative organisms and *S aureus* are frequent causes of pneumonia in hospitalized patients or those who require mechanical ventilation. Nosocomial organisms tend to be more resistant and are more likely to be present in patients with extended hospital stays, prior antimicrobial therapy, and comorbidities. If possible, attempts should be made to obtain lower respiratory tract samples for quantitative microbiologic evaluation in mechanically ventilated patients. Adequate antimicrobial coverage can usually be provided with a third- or fourth-generation cephalosporin, β-lactam/β-lactamase inhibitor combinations, or a carbapenem, plus a fluoroquinolone or an aminoglycoside. If *Pseudomonas* is a consideration, an antipseudomonal β-lactam (piperacillin-tazobactam, cefepime, imipenem, or meropenem) should be used. Therapy with trimethoprim-sulfamethoxazole should be included if the possibility of *Stenotrophomonas maltophilia* is suspected or confirmed. Vancomycin should be considered if methicillin-resistant *S aureus* is a possible pathogen. Pneumonia due to methicillin-sensitive strains of *S aureus* should be treated with an antistaphylococcal penicillin as these agents are superior to vancomycin. Patients with methicillin-resistant *S aureus* who are vancomycin-intolerant or are not responding to vancomycin may be treated with linezolid. If vancomycin is utilized, serum trough levels should be maintained no lower than 15 to 20 μg/mL as lung penetration of this agent is limited. Shorter courses (8 days) of therapy may be appropriate as long as non-lactose-fermenting organisms are not isolated.

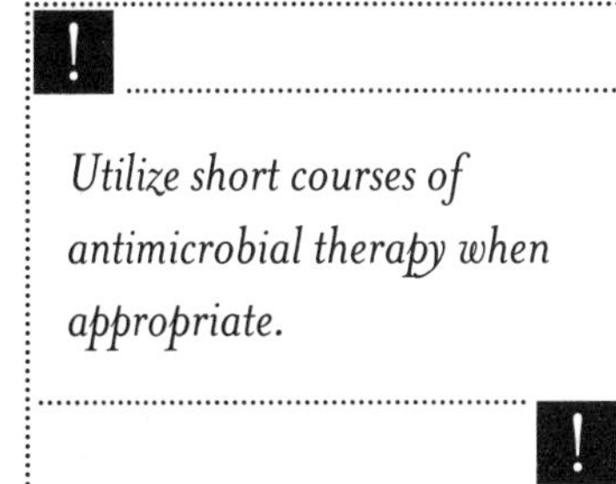

C. Heart

Infections of the heart are usually severe and life-threatening and require coordinated medical care with a cardiologist and sometimes also with a cardiovascular surgeon. Microbiologic studies and echocardiography (transthoracic or transesophageal) are the cornerstones for the diagnosis and management of any infection in the heart.

Infective endocarditis, or infection of the endocardial surface of the heart, most frequently involves the heart valves. Intravenous drug abuse, prosthetic valves, sclerosing of natural valves due to aging, hospital-acquired infections, and newly identified pathogens *(Bartonella* spp, *Coxiella burnetii, Tropheryma whipplei,* fungi) are the main risk factors for this condition. Demonstration of bloodstream infection and positive echocardiographic evidence of valvular vegetations are key to making the diagnosis, although peripheral embolic phenomena and other findings are strongly suggestive. Gram-positive cocci, mainly *Staphylococcus* and *Streptococcus,* but also *Enterococcus,* are the most common microorganisms isolated in infective endocarditis in the general population and in specific risk groups (intravenous drug users and prosthetic valve endocarditis), but gram-negative, polymicrobial, fungal, and culture-negative endocarditis are becoming more common. Bactericidal antimicrobial therapy (eg, penicillins/third-generation cephalosporins with or without an aminoglycoside, glycopeptides, linezolid, daptomycin), high drug concentrations, the resistance pattern of the microorganism, and long-term therapy are the cornerstones of treatment.

D. Intravascular Catheters

In patients with confirmed or suspected intravascular catheter infection associated with organ dysfunction, systemic emboli, or cardiovascular instability, the intravascular catheter should be removed promptly. In addition, local changes at the catheter site (purulence, erythema) mandate catheter removal. In the absence of local changes or sepsis, an option is to insert a new catheter in the existing site over a guidewire; however, this approach needs to be supported with negative blood cultures as well as negative culture of the intradermal portion of the removed catheter.

Coagulase-negative *Staphylococcus* and *S aureus* are the most common pathogens in catheter-related bloodstream infections. In the immunocompetent patient who has a coagulase-negative staphylococcal line infection but no systemic symptoms, the removal of the infected catheter line may be sufficient. Vancomycin is recommended in immunocompromised patients with coagulase-negative staphylococcal line infections, patients with systemic manifestations, or those with prosthetic devices at risk for becoming secondarily infected. If *S aureus* is the infecting organism, nafcillin is recommended; however, if there is a high rate of MRSA in the hospital or MRSA is confirmed, vancomycin should be used. A third- or fourth-generation cephalosporin or fluoroquinolone should be added if a nosocomial gram-negative organism is suspected.

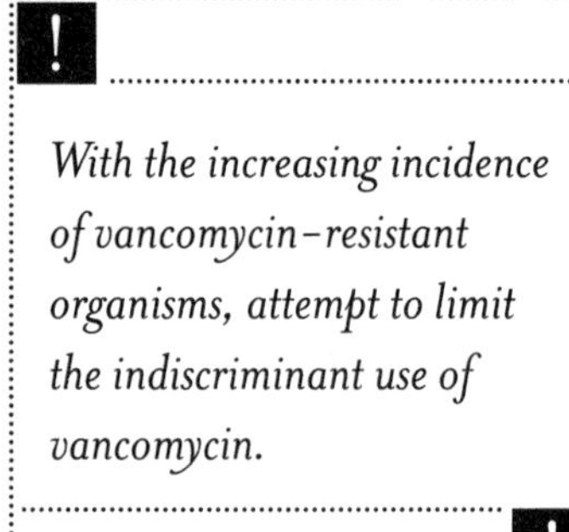

Candida is occasionally isolated from catheter tips and should increase the suspicion that occult candidemia may have been recently present. The treatment of choice is fluconazole, or if there is a possibility of resistant *Candida,* such as *Torulopsis glabrata* or *Candida krusei,* caspofungin should be used. When a fungal microorganism is identified in an intravascular catheter-related bloodstream infection, a non-tunneled catheter always should be removed, whereas the removal of a tunneled catheter should be based on the likelihood of catheter-related candidemia rather than candidemia from another source. Antimicrobial-impregnated catheters appear to have a lower rate of bloodstream infection, but the maximum longevity of such catheters is still under investigation.

E. Abdomen

When an intra-abdominal infection is suspected, a surgeon must be involved in the evaluation of the patient. Both the infecting flora and the antimicrobial therapy are related to whether the infection is community-acquired or healthcare-associated. For community-acquired infections, location of a possible perforation determines the probable organism, with gram-positive, facultative, and aerobic gram-negative bacteria beyond the proximal small bowel and anaerobes beyond the proximal ileum. Recommended therapies include β-lactam/β-lactamase inhibitor combinations and carbapenems as monotherapy or cephalosporins/fluoroquinolones with metronidazole. Antimicrobial therapy should be continued until clinical resolution, which typically occurs in 5 to 7 days. Further diagnostic workup should be pursued in patients with persistent or recurrent symptoms. Flora isolated from healthcare-associated intra-abdominal infections resembles that of other nosocomial infections. Antimicrobial therapy should be based on knowledge of the flora and antimicrobial susceptibilities of the institution. Anti-enterococcal therapy is indicated only when enterococci are isolated from patients with healthcare-associated infections. Antifungal therapy is indicated only in those who have isolated fungi and comorbid conditions – like recent immunosuppressive therapy for neoplasms, transplantation, and inflammatory disease – or have postoperative or recurrent infections.

F. Urinary Tract

The most common pathogens in urinary tract infections are gram-negative enteric bacteria. Hospitalized patients with urinary catheters commonly have bacteriuria yet exhibit no pyuria or localized symptoms. Such patients (in the absence of urologic obstruction) rarely develop sepsis or bacteremia arising from the urinary tract, and removal of the catheter may allow resolution of the bacteriuria. Patients who develop upper urinary tract infection always merit antimicrobial therapy. More serious complications may be seen in diabetic patients or other immunocompromised individuals, including those with emphysematous pyelonephritis, papillary necrosis, or perinephric abscess, which may require surgical intervention. Empiric antimicrobial options for gram-negative urinary tract infections are dictated by susceptibility testing and include the following:

- Third-generation cephalosporins
- Fluoroquinolones

- Aminoglycosides
- Piperacillin-tazobactam
- Trimethoprim-sulfamethoxazole

Enterococcal infection in the urinary system should be suspected in patients who have long-term urinary catheters or who have had recent manipulation of the urinary tract. Therapy should include ampicillin, piperacillin, or vancomycin.

Candiduria is not uncommon and usually occurs in patients who have long-term urinary catheters and are receiving broad-spectrum antimicrobial therapy or patients with glycosuria. Therapeutic options include a short course of fluconazole (not effective against *T glabrata* or *C krusei*) or continuous amphotericin bladder irrigation. Relapse rates, however, are quite significant with either treatment. If candiduria is treated in a patient with an indwelling catheter, the catheter should be changed or removed during the treatment course.

G. Cutaneous Infection

Staphylococcus aureus or group A β-hemolytic streptococci are the most likely etiologic organisms in cellulitis or cutaneous abscess. *H influenzae* must also be considered in facial or orbital cellulitis. Onset of postoperative wound infections usually occurs 5 to 7 days after surgery. However, rapidly progressive wound infections occurring within 24 to 48 hours after surgery should prompt the consideration of *Clostridium perfringens* or group A β-hemolytic streptococci *(S pyogenes)*. This type of infection warrants surgical debridement and prompt antimicrobial therapy directed by Gram stain and culture. Antimicrobial choices include the following:

- Cefazolin or nafcillin if methicillin-resistant *S aureus* is unlikely
- Vancomycin or linezolid if there is a possibility of methicillin-resistant *S aureus*
- Penicillin G with or without clindamycin for wound infections developing within 48 hours to cover C *perfringens* and β-hemolytic streptococci

Wound toxic shock syndrome is a rare condition that can occur within 48 hours of a wound or surgical incision. The causes are toxin-producing S *aureus* or β-hemolytic streptococci, but often the wound does not appear infected. Presenting symptoms include fever, diarrhea, vomiting, hypotension, and uremia. Erythroderma and subsequent desquamation are characteristic but may be delayed for several days. Treatment involves opening the wound and prompt use of specific antimicrobial therapy.

H. Necrotizing Soft Tissue Infection

Infection of the subcutaneous tissue, fascia, and muscle may occur in any patient but may be more common in immunocompromised patients, particularly individuals with diabetes. If gas is present in the tissue, cutaneous gangrene or bullae are noted, or infection progresses rapidly, a necrotizing soft tissue infection must be considered. This condition requires prompt surgical debridement in addition to broad-spectrum antimicrobial therapy. These infections are usually polymicrobial, involving aerobic and anaerobic gram-positive and gram-negative organisms.

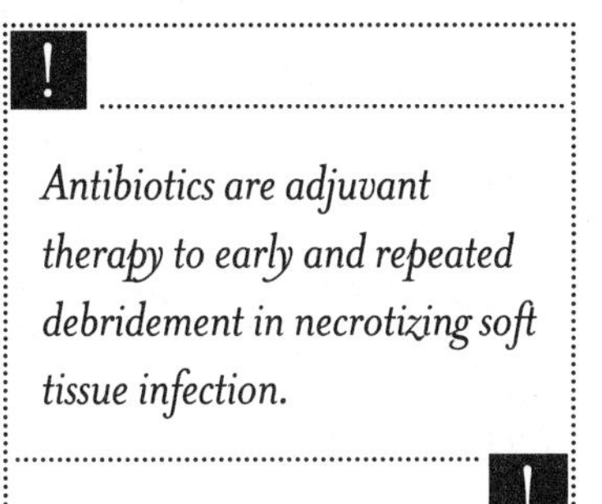

Adequate empiric therapy should include vancomycin and a β-lactam/β-lactamase inhibitor, a carbapenem and fluoroquinolone, or an aminoglycoside and clindamycin (the latter to reduce the amount of toxins).

I. Immunocompromised or Neutropenic Patients

In the absence of a specific source, pending culture results, broad-spectrum antimicrobial therapy is indicated in the immunocompromised or neutropenic patient with fever. Monotherapy can be effective, but combination therapy is indicated initially for more severely ill patients. To reduce the emergence of resistance, a third-generation cephalosporin as monotherapy should be avoided if *Pseudomonas* spp, *Acinetobacter* spp, *Enterobacter* spp, *Citrobacter* spp, or *Serratia* spp are prevalent.

Suggested antimicrobial regimens include the following:

- Third- or fourth-generation cephalosporin (ceftazidime or cefepime for *P aeruginosa* coverage) with an aminoglycoside or fluoroquinolones
- Carbapenems
- Piperacillin-tazobactam
- Addition of vancomycin if gram-positive organisms are likely

The use of white cell growth factors (ie, granulocyte colony-stimulating factor, granulocyte-macrophage colony-stimulating factor) may improve outcome by shortening the duration of neutropenia. These progenitor cell stimulants should be targeted for patients with an anticipated duration of neutropenia of 5 to 7 days and a high risk for serious infection.

J. Antibiotic-Associated Colitis

Antibiotic-associated diarrhea and colitis resulting from *C difficile* infection can complicate the course of treatment for many patients. Antimicrobials most commonly involved include clindamycin, penicillins, cephalosporins, and quinolones, although this infection has been described in association with almost all antimicrobials. Patients do not need to receive antimicrobial therapy to develop this condition.

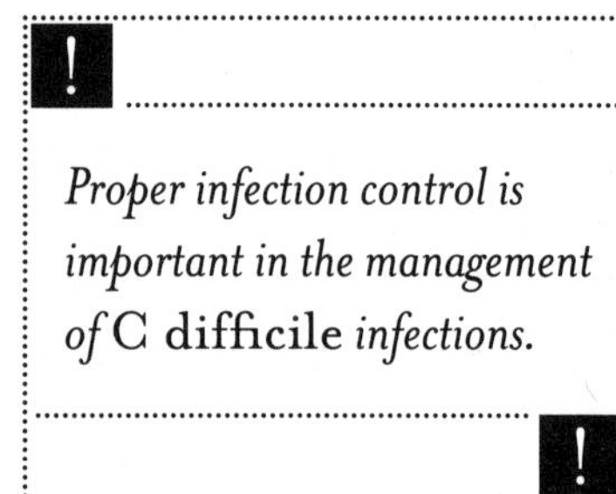

C difficile is also recognized as an important nosocomial pathogen capable of cross transmission to patients in adjacent areas. Diagnosis is usually done by identification of *C difficile* toxins and detection of cytotoxin activity in tissue culture. Treatment begins with discontinuation of the implicated antimicrobial therapy (if possible) and initiation of specific antimicrobial therapy against *C difficile* if symptoms are moderate, severe, or persistent. The preferred regimen is oral metronidazole, 250 to 500 mg three times daily for 10 days. Oral vancomycin, 125 to 500 mg four times daily for 10 days, is also effective, but its use is discouraged in an attempt to reduce development of resistant organisms. For patients who are unable to take oral medications, intraluminal vancomycin with or without intravenous metronidazole is recommended. Fulminant colitis unresponsive to these measures or progressing to toxic megacolon may require total colectomy.

Fidaxomicin is a first-in-class, narrow-spectrum macrocyclic antibiotic that acts by eradicating *C difficile* with minimal disruption of the normal intestinal flora. It is approved by the US Food and Drug Administration for use in treating and preventing the recurrence of *C difficile* in children under the age of 16 years, and is under consideration for use in adults.

K. Fungal Diseases

Life-threatening infections due to fungi may be extremely difficult to diagnose by routine physical examination or routine cultures. *Candida* albicans is the most common etiologic organism in critically ill patients. Non-albicans species of *Candida* and other fungi have increased significantly in recent years. Fungal infection should be considered in certain geographic regions and in the presence of predisposing factors, such as HIV, malignancy, neutropenia, long-term use of steroids, broad-spectrum antimicrobial therapy, parenteral nutrition, severe burns or organ transplantation, or in the presence of central venous vascular catheters.

The polyenes (amphotericin B and lipid preparations of amphotericin B) have been the most commonly utilized antifungal agents for serious infections. Newer agents (caspofungin, voriconazole) have shown comparable or superior clinical outcomes compared with the polyenes. All lipid formulations have less nephrotoxicity and their efficacy against *Candida* is equivalent to conventional amphotericin B. Fluconazole is still active against most *Candida* species and *Cryptococcus,* and itraconazole may be used for some of the mold infections. Both agents have an important role in primary or secondary prophylaxis. The newer agents, such as voriconazole, posaconazole, and caspofungin, have activity against resistant *Candida* strains and some of the mold infections resistant to other regimens. Recent studies suggest a role in the treatment of neutropenic fever and fungal infections in immunocompromised patients.

L. Other Therapy

In addition to antimicrobial therapy, surgical intervention must be considered in patients with life-threatening infections. Any abscess must be drained, and injured or ischemic organs must be repaired or removed. Vascular catheters that may be a source of infection should be removed. Early surgical consultation should be sought when the abdomen may be a source of infection in the critically ill patient. Guidelines for tetanus prophylaxis are found in **Appendix 10**. Further management of the patient with septic shock is discussed in **Chapter 7**.

M. Healthcare-Associated Infection Control

Recent data estimate that one of every 10 to 20 (5%-10%) hospitalized patients experience a healthcare-associated infection (HAI) each year. HAI are associated with almost 100,000 deaths annually in the United States. Many studies show that HAI increase hospital length of stay, and morbidity and mortality rates. Strategies have been proposed to prevent HAI. In **Appendix 10**, some of the important guidelines for prevention of HAI are summarized. More details are available in the Web sites listed at the conclusion of this chapter. Guidelines cannot always account for individual variation among patients and are not intended to supplant physician judgment with respect to individual patients or special clinical situations.

Key Points

Life-Threatening Infections

- Fever is the most frequent systemic manifestation that raises the suspicion of infection.
- Ideally, appropriate cultures should be obtained before initiation of antibiotics in patients with suspected infection.
- Selection of appropriate empiric antimicrobial therapy depends on the suspected pathogen(s) and site of infection, Gram stain results of available specimens from the suspected site, assessment for antimicrobial resistance, and comorbid conditions.
- When bacterial meningitis is suspected clinically, antimicrobial therapy should be instituted immediately, without waiting for the results of lumbar puncture.
- The most common organism resulting in community-acquired, life-threatening pneumonia is *Streptococcus pneumoniae.*
- Resistant gram-negative organisms and *Staphylococcus aureus* are frequent causes of pneumonia in hospitalized patients or in those who require mechanical ventilation.
- Bactericidal antimicrobial therapy, high concentrations of the antimicrobial agent, the resistance pattern of the microorganism, and long-term therapy are the cornerstones of therapy for infective endocarditis.
- Suspicion of intra-abdominal infection requires the prompt involvement of a surgeon.
- Necrotizing soft tissue infection requires prompt surgical debridement in addition to broad-spectrum antimicrobial therapy.
- In the absence of a specific source and pending culture results, broad-spectrum antimicrobial therapy is indicated in the immunocompromised or neutropenic patient with fever.
- Fungal infection should be considered in the presence of predisposing factors, such as malignancy, neutropenia, broad-spectrum antimicrobial therapy, parenteral nutrition, severe burns, or organ transplantation, or if central venous vascular catheters are in place.

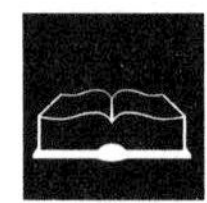

Suggested Readings

1. American Thoracic Society, Infectious Diseases Society of America. Guidelines for the management of hospital-acquired, ventilator-associated, and healthcare-associated pneumonia. *Am J Respir Crit Care Med.* 2005;171:388-416.

2. Avecillas JF, Mazzone P, Arroliga AC. A rational approach to the evaluation and treatment of the infected patient in the intensive care unit. *Clin Chest Med.* 2003;24:645-669.

3. Calandra T, Cohen J, International Sepsis Forum Definitions of Infection in the Intensive Care Unit Consensus Conference. The International Sepsis Forum Consensus Conference on Definitions of Infection in the Intensive Care Unit. *Crit Care Med.* 2005;33:1538-1548.

4. Dellinger RP, Levy MM, Carlet JM, et al. Surviving Sepsis Campaign: International guidelines for management of severe sepsis and septic shock: 2008. *Crit Care Med.* 2008;36:296-327.

5. Guerrant RL, Van Gilder T, Steiner TS, et al. Practice guidelines for the management of infectious diarrhea. *Clin Infect Dis.* 2001;32:331-351.

6. Leone M, Bourgoin A, Cambon S, et al. Empirical antimicrobial therapy of septic shock patients: Adequacy and impact on the outcomes. *Crit Care Med.* 2003;31:462-467.

7. Mandell LA, Wunderink RG, Anzueto A, et al. Infectious Diseases Society of America/ American Thoracic Society consensus guidelines on the management of community-acquired pneumonia in adults. *Clin Infect Dis.* 2007;44:S27-S72.

8. Mermel LA, Farr BM, Sherertz RJ, et al. Guidelines for management of intravascular catheter-related infections. *Clin Infect Dis.* 2001;32:1249-1272.

9. O'Grady NP, Barie PS, Bartlett JG, et al. Guidelines for evaluation of new fever in critically ill adult patients: 2008 update from the American College of Critical Care Medicine and the Infectious Diseases Society of America. *Crit Care Med.* 2008;36:1330–1349.

10. Pappas PG, Rex JH, Sobel JD, et al. Guidelines for treatment of candidiasis. *Clin Infect Dis.* 2004;38:161-189.

11. Solomkin JS, Mazuski JE, Baron EJ, et al. Guidelines for the selection of anti-infective agents for complicated intra-abdominal infections. *Clin Infect Dis.* 2003;37:997-1005.

12. Tunkel AR, Hartman BJ, Kaplan SL, et al. Practice guidelines for the management of bacterial meningitis. *Clin Infect Dis.* 2004;39:1267-1284.

13. Yokoe DS, Mermel LA, Anderson DJ, et al. A compendium of strategies to prevent healthcare-associated infections in acute care hospitals. *Infect Control Hosp Epidemiol.* 2008;29 Suppl 1:S12-S21.

Web Sites

1. Centers for Disease Control. http://www.cdc.gov. *This Web site contains regularly updated guidelines for management and prevention of specific infections.*

2. Infectious Diseases Society of America. http://www.idsociety.org. *This Web site contains regularly updated guidelines for management and prevention of specific infections.*

Chapter 12

MANAGEMENT OF LIFE-THREATENING ELECTROLYTE AND METABOLIC DISTURBANCES

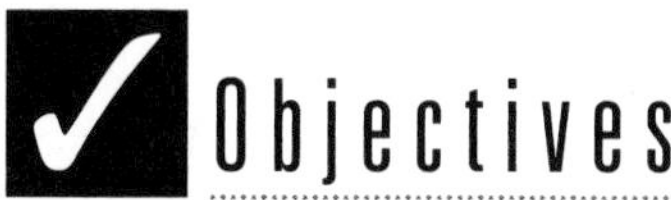

Objectives

- Review the emergent management of severe electrolyte disturbances.
- Recognize manifestations of acute adrenal insufficiency and initiate appropriate treatment.
- Describe the management of severe hyperglycemic syndromes.

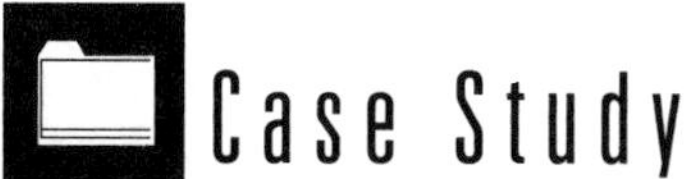

Case Study

An 80-year-old woman with hypertension, heart failure, and chronic renal insufficiency is admitted to the hospital with confusion, lethargy, poor oral intake, and weakness for the past 3 days. Her vital signs are blood pressure 108/70 mm Hg, heart rate 110/min, respiratory rate 18/min, and temperature 97.6°F (36.4°C). The electrocardiography monitor shows nonsustained episodes of ventricular tachycardia.

- What risk factors does this patient have for electrolyte disturbances?
- Which electrolyte abnormalities might contribute to her presentation?
- How would you initiate the evaluation and treatment of this patient?

I. INTRODUCTION

Electrolyte and metabolic disturbances are common in critically ill and injured patients. These abnormalities alter physiologic function and contribute to morbidity and mortality. The most common life-threatening electrolyte and metabolic disorders in critically ill patients are disturbances in potassium, sodium, calcium, magnesium, and phosphate levels, adrenal function, and glucose regulation. With early recognition and treatment of these abnormalities, life-threatening complications might be avoided and outcomes improved.

II. ELECTROLYTE DISTURBANCES

Electrolyte disturbances result from an underlying disease process, and it is important to seek the cause of the abnormality as well as to treat the electrolyte change. Many clinical manifestations are not specific to a particular electrolyte change and may be due to multiple abnormalities. The urgency of treatment depends on the clinical circumstances rather than the absolute electrolyte concentration. All severe electrolyte abnormalities require frequent reassessment during correction.

A. Potassium

Potassium is primarily an intracellular ion that is essential for maintenance of the electrical membrane potential. Approximately 2% of total body potassium is present in the extracellular compartment. Alterations in this ion primarily affect the cardiovascular, neuromuscular, and gastrointestinal systems.

1. Hypokalemia

Hypokalemia (potassium <3.5 mmol/L) results from renal or extrarenal losses, transcellular shifts, and decreased intake (**Table 12-1**). Life-threatening clinical manifestations of hypokalemia involve the cardiac and neuromuscular systems. Arrhythmias (ventricular and supraventricular, conduction delays, sinus bradycardia), electrocardiogram (ECG) abnormalities (U waves, QT interval prolongation, flat or inverted T waves), muscle weakness or paralysis, paresthesias, ileus, abdominal cramps, nausea, and vomiting are common manifestations.

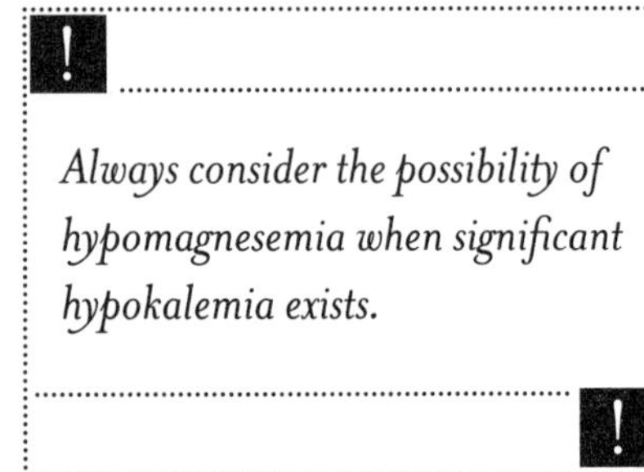

Treatment of hypokalemia is aimed at correcting the underlying cause and administering potassium (**Figure 12-1**). Discontinue offending drugs (if possible), correct hypomagnesemia and other electrolyte disturbances, and correct alkalosis. Because potassium is primarily an intracellular ion, an estimated deficit cannot be calculated from serum values. Therefore, administration must be titrated against periodic reassessment of the serum levels. Infusion of 10 mmol potassium in 100 mL fluid over 20 minutes, with additional doses administered sequentially, is recommended to avoid potential mishaps with more concentrated solutions. This must be administered through a central line. The infusion rate can be slowed after life-threatening symptoms resolve. Continuous ECG monitoring and close observation are necessary during parenteral administration of high concentrations of potassium chloride. Serum potassium levels must be monitored at frequent intervals during repletion (ie, every 1-2 hours during initial replacement). If acidemia is present, correct the potassium level before correcting the pH, since potassium shifts intracellularly as the pH increases.

Table 12-1 Causes of Hypokalemia

Transcellular Shifts	Renal Losses	Extrarenal Losses	Decreased Intake
Acute alkalosis	Diuresis	Diarrhea	Malnutrition
Hyperventilation	Metabolic alkalosis	Profuse sweating	Alcoholism
Insulin	Renal tubular defects	Nasogastric suction	Anorexia nervosa
β-Adrenergic agonists	Diabetic ketoacidosis		
	Drugs (diuretics, aminoglycosides, amphotericin B)		
	Hypomagnesemia		
	Vomiting		
	Hyperaldosteronism		
	Cushing's syndrome		

Figure 12-1. Treatment of Hypokalemia

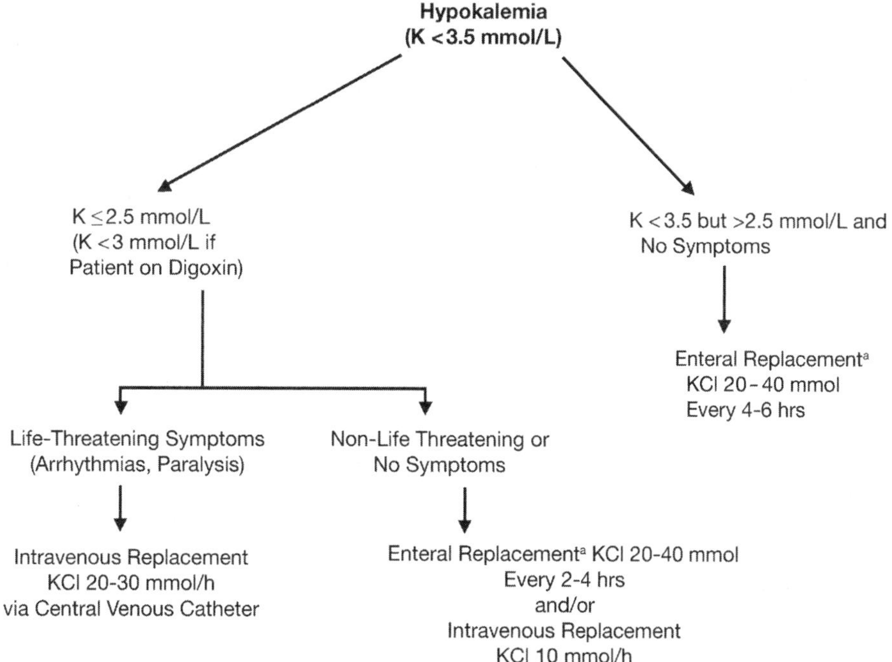

[a]Enteral replacement may be oral or via nasogastric tube; nausea and/or vomiting may preclude use of the enteral route.

2. Hyperkalemia

Hyperkalemia (potassium >5.5 mmol/L) in critically ill patients most often results from renal dysfunction. Other causes are listed in **Table 12-2**. Pseudohyperkalemia may result from a white blood cell count >100,000/mm^3 or platelet count >600,000/mm^3. Hemolysis secondary to phlebotomy technique must also be considered.

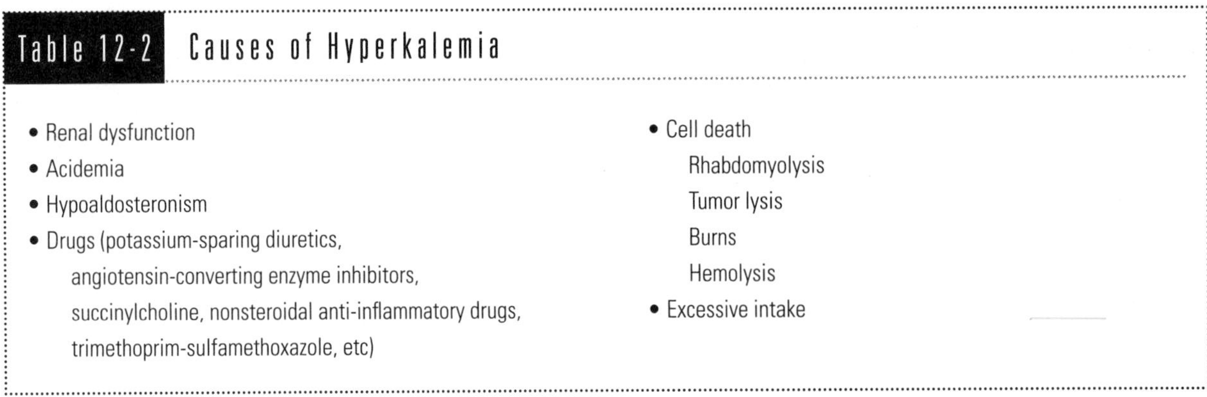

Table 12-2 Causes of Hyperkalemia

- Renal dysfunction
- Acidemia
- Hypoaldosteronism
- Drugs (potassium-sparing diuretics, angiotensin-converting enzyme inhibitors, succinylcholine, nonsteroidal anti-inflammatory drugs, trimethoprim-sulfamethoxazole, etc)
- Cell death
  - Rhabdomyolysis
  - Tumor lysis
  - Burns
  - Hemolysis
- Excessive intake

Clinical manifestations of hyperkalemia relate primarily to the heart and muscle (**Figure 12-2**). Arrhythmias, heart block, bradycardia, diminished conduction and contraction, ECG abnormalities (eg, diffuse peaked T waves, PR interval prolongation, QRS widening, diminished P waves, sine waves), muscle weakness, paralysis, paresthesias, and hypoactive reflexes are common manifestations.

Figure 12-2. Electrocardiographic Effects of Hyperkalemia

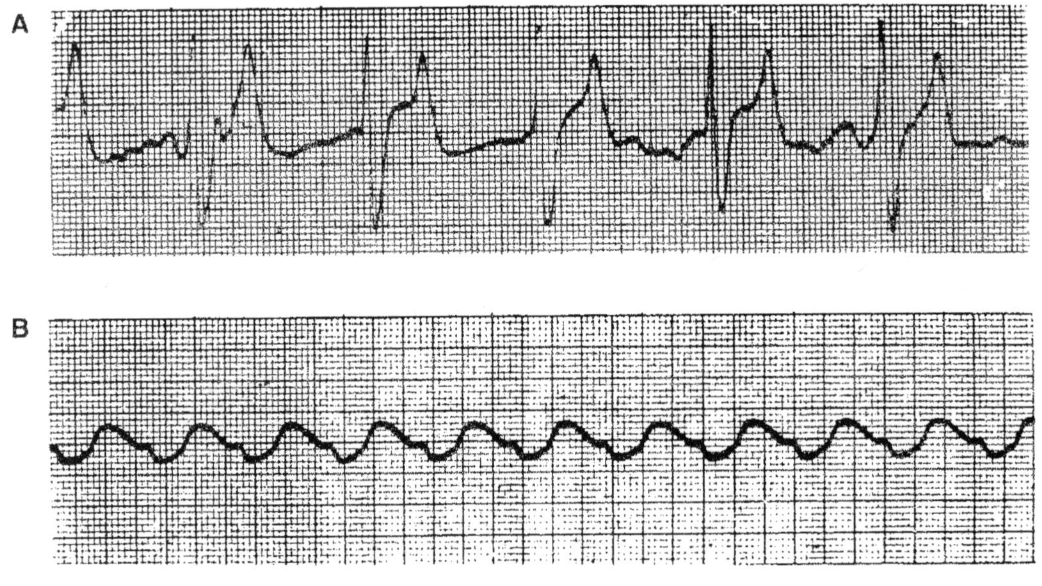

Two rhythm strips showing the electrocardiographic effects of hyperkalemia. **A**, peaked T waves and widened QRS complex. **B**, sine wave pattern.

Treatment of hyperkalemia involves the recognition and treatment of underlying diseases, the removal of offending drugs, the limitation of potassium intake, and the correction of acidemia or electrolyte abnormalities. Any serum potassium level >6 mmol/L should be addressed, but the urgency of treatment depends on the clinical manifestations and ECG findings. Options for treating hyperkalemia are summarized in **Table 12-3**. Serum potassium levels, continuous cardiac monitoring, and serial ECG tracings should be obtained during evaluation and treatment.

!

Hyperkalemia with significant ECG changes, such as widened QRS and sine wave, mandates immediate therapy.

!

Table 12-3 Options for Treating Hyperkalemia

If Significant Electrocardiographic Abnormalities Are Present

Administer calcium chloride, 5-10 mL of a 10% solution, intravenously over 5-10 minutes to stabilize the myocardial cell membrane and decrease the potential for arrhythmias. If calcium gluconate is used, 10-20 mL of a 10% solution is needed for treatment because of the lower elemental calcium content. The effect lasts only 30-60 minutes and should be followed by additional treatment.

For Redistribution of Potassium

1. Administer insulin and glucose (10 units of regular insulin with 50 g of 50% dextrose over 5-10 minutes intravenously). Glucose monitoring is necessary to avoid hypoglycemia.
2. Administer sodium bicarbonate (1 mmol/kg intravenously over 5-10 minutes). Be aware of the potential for sodium overload. Sodium bicarbonate is less effective than glucose and insulin for decreasing the potassium level in patients with end-stage renal failure.
3. Administer inhaled β_2-agonists in high doses (albuterol [salbutamol], 10-20 mg), which can decrease serum potassium by approximately 0.5 mmol/L.

For Removal of Potassium From the Body

1. Increase urine output with a loop diuretic (furosemide 1-2 mg/kg) and isotonic fluids.
2. Increase gastrointestinal potassium loss with sodium polystyrene sulfonate, 25-50 g in sorbitol, enterally or by enema. (Be aware of potential for sodium overload. This may not be a good option in critical illness.)
3. Initiate dialysis.

B. Sodium

Sodium functions as the primary determinant of blood osmolality in the body and is involved in the regulation of extracellular volume. Abnormalities in circulating sodium primarily affect neuronal and neuromuscular function.

1. Hyponatremia

The most common cause of hyponatremia (sodium <135 mmol/L) associated with a low serum osmolality (hypo-osmolar hyponatremia) is excess secretion of antidiuretic hormone (ie, euvolemic hyponatremia). Hypo-osmolar hyponatremia or dilutional hyponatremia can also be associated with hypovolemic and hypervolemic conditions. A common defect is impaired ability to excrete free water through the kidneys. Hyponatremia can also result less frequently from the presence of a nonsodium solute, such as glucose and mannitol. These causes are characterized by a normal or elevated serum osmolality. Pseudohyponatremia, a spurious form of iso-osmolar hyponatremia, may occur in the presence of severe hyperlipidemia, hyperproteinemia, or hyperglycemia when the sodium concentration is measured by flame photometry. **Figure 12-3** outlines a diagnostic approach to determining the etiology of hyponatremia.

Figure 12-3. Diagnostic Approach to the Etiology of Hyponatremia

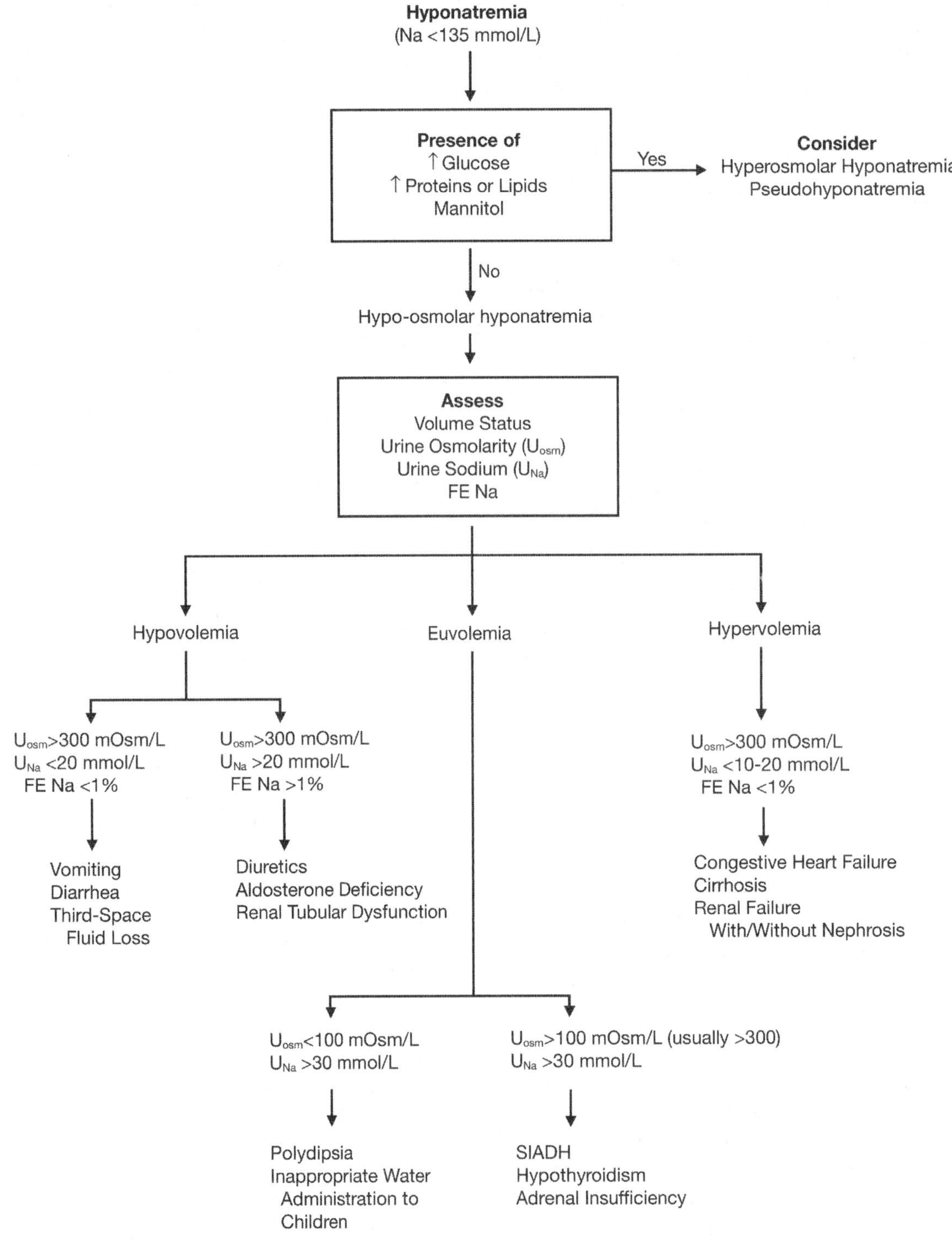

Abbreviations: FE Na, fractional excretion of sodium; SIADH, syndrome of inappropriate antidiuretic hormone

Clinical manifestations of hyponatremia involve the central nervous system (CNS) and muscular system and include disorientation, decreased mentation, irritability, seizures, lethargy, coma, nausea/vomiting, weakness, and respiratory arrest. Treatment requires identifying the type of hyponatremia, treating the underlying disease, removing offending drugs, and improving the circulating sodium level. Hypovolemic hyponatremia usually responds to intravascular volume repletion (ie, with normal saline). As volume is replaced, antidiuretic hormone is suppressed and the kidneys begin to excrete free water. Hypervolemic hyponatremia is usually not severe and improves with successful treatment of the underlying condition.

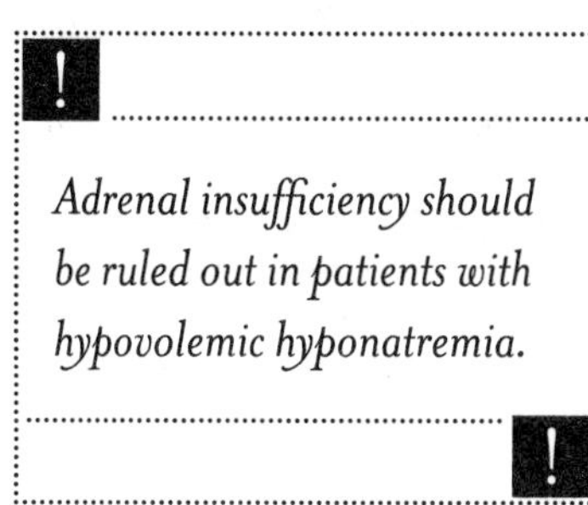

Euvolemic hyponatremia is almost always secondary to elevated levels of antidiuretic hormone. Diagnosis is facilitated by determining urine osmolality before treatment (especially with diuretics) to compare with a calculated serum osmolality [(2 × serum sodium) + glucose/18 + blood urea nitrogen/2.8]. The urine osmolality is inappropriately higher than serum osmolality (usually >300 mOsm). If the hyponatremia is acute or the patient is symptomatic, the serum sodium level should be increased by restricting free-water intake, increasing free-water clearance with loop diuretics, and replacing intravascular volume with normal saline (154 mmol/L) or hypertonic 3% saline (513 mmol/L). Hypertonic saline is indicated for treatment in the presence of severe symptoms, such as seizures, coma, or impending respiratory arrest. The goal of therapy in this situation is to remove free water and not sodium. The increase in serum sodium should be controlled, and although the precise rate of increase is controversial, the serum sodium increase should be limited to approximately 8 to 12 mmol/L in the first 24 hours. One option is to accelerate the rate of serum sodium elevation early in the treatment course in the presence of life-threatening symptoms, such as seizures, and to slow the rate of increase after resolution of the symptoms. If hypertonic saline is used, 1 mmol/kg sodium chloride should be infused initially (3% saline contains ~0.5 mmol/mL). The same amount can be administered in incremental doses to a maximum of 3 to 5 mmol/kg or until symptoms resolve. Alternatively, the change in serum sodium expected after administering 1 liter of fluid can be estimated by using the following formulas:

$$\text{Change in Serum Sodium} = \frac{\text{Infusate Sodium} - \text{Serum Sodium}}{\text{Total Body Water} + 1}$$

$$\text{Change in Serum Sodium} = \frac{(\text{Infusate Sodium} + \text{Infusate Potassium}) - \text{Serum Sodium}}{\text{Total Body Water} + 1}$$

$$\text{Total Body Water} = 0.6 \times \text{Weight (kg) for men; } 0.5 \times \text{Weight (kg) for women}$$

The sodium concentrations of various infusates are listed in **Table 12-4**. The formulas presented above do not take into account other fluid gains and losses (eg, urine output), and therefore, should serve only as guides to intervention. Serum sodium levels should be monitored at frequent intervals during therapy for hyponatremia. When serum sodium is greater than 125 to 130 mmol/L, restriction of free water alone allows for slower return of the sodium level to normal. Correction of the serum sodium level that is too rapid may result in CNS injury (ie, osmotic demyelinating syndrome), particularly in chronic hyponatremia. Osmotic demyelinating syndrome rarely occurs in patients whose serum sodium is greater than 120 mmol/L. Symptoms are typically seen after initial improvement in mentation. One to seven days after reversal of hyponatremia, patients may develop focal motor deficits, respiratory insufficiency and progressive loss of consciousness. Patients at greatest risk for osmotic demyelinating syndromes are those with alcohol abuse, malnutrition, hypokalemia, elderly women, and burned patients. If hyponatremia is chronic and asymptomatic, regardless of the magnitude of hyponatremia, free-water restriction alone may be sufficient to allow for slow return of serum sodium to normal.

Table 12-4 Sodium Concentrations of Selected Infusates

Infusate	Sodium Concentration (mmol/L)
5% sodium chloride	855
3% sodium chloride	513
0.9% sodium chloride	154
Ringer's lactate	130
0.45% sodium chloride	77
5% dextrose in water	0

2. Hypernatremia

Hypernatremia (sodium >145 mmol/L) indicates intracellular volume depletion with a loss of free water that exceeds sodium loss. Causes of hypernatremia are listed in **Table 12-5.**

Table 12-5 Causes of Hypernatremia

Water Loss	Reduced Water Intake	Excessive Sodium Intake
Diarrhea	Altered thirst	Salt tablets
Vomiting	Impaired access	Hypertonic saline
Excessive sweating		Sodium bicarbonate
Diuresis		
Diabetes insipidus		

The clinical manifestations of hypernatremia relate to CNS and muscle function. Manifestations of hypernatremia include altered mentation, lethargy, seizures, coma, and muscle weakness. Polyuria suggests the presence of diabetes insipidus or excess salt and water intake.

Treatment focuses on correcting the underlying cause of hypernatremia. Nearly all patients with hypernatremia require free-water repletion. The water deficit can be estimated by using the following equation:

Water Deficit (L) = 0.6 (0.5 for women) × weight (kg) [(measured Na/normal Na) – 1]

Example: Water deficit of a 70-kg man with sodium measurement of 160 mmol/L
0.6 × 70 [(160/140) – 1]
42 [1.14 – 1]
42 × 0.14 = 5.88 L water deficit

A portion of free water should be replaced initially at a speed commensurate with the severity of symptoms, and the patient should be reevaluated for subsequent replacement. If the patient is hemodynamically unstable (hypotensive, orthostatic, or significantly tachycardic), administer normal saline until the intravascular volume is corrected. When the patient is hemodynamically stable, replace water with 5% dextrose in water, 0.45% NaCl, or 0.2% NaCl with 5% dextrose. To estimate the change in serum sodium expected after administering 1 liter of fluid, use the same formulas as for hyponatremia:

$$\text{Change in Serum Sodium} = \frac{\text{Infusate Sodium} - \text{Serum Sodium}}{\text{Total Body Water} + 1}$$

$$\text{Change in Serum Sodium} = \frac{(\text{Infusate Sodium} + \text{Infusate Potassium}) - \text{Serum Sodium}}{\text{Total Body Water} + 1}$$

In stable patients, water may be replaced via the enteral route (ie, nasogastric tube). In the rare patient with sodium overload, sodium may be removed with loop diuretics or dialysis (provided intravascular volume is adequate). Administration of aqueous vasopressin or desmopressin should be considered for patients with central diabetes insipidus.

Sodium concentration should be measured frequently during treatment, and therapy should be adjusted for optimal correction of the sodium level. If hypernatremia developed over a period of hours, reducing the serum sodium by 1 mmol/L/h is appropriate. In hypernatremia of longer or unknown duration, a slower rate of correction (0.5 mmol/L/h) is recommended. Increasing free-water intake in maintenance fluids allows for a slow return to normal sodium levels.

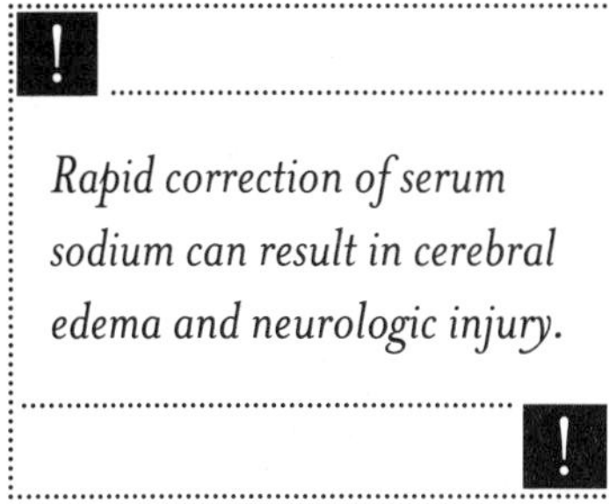

C. Other Electrolyte Abnormalities

1. Calcium

Calcium is required for muscle contraction, nerve impulse transmission, hormone secretion, blood clotting, cell division, cell motility, and wound healing. Effective calcium levels in a seriously ill patient are best assessed by using ionized calcium measurements, if available. If treatment decisions are based on total serum calcium, the albumin concentration must be considered as 40% of circulating calcium is protein bound, mainly to albumin. In general, for each increase or decrease in serum albumin of 1 g/dL, the serum calcium increases or decreases by 0.8 mg/dL (0.2 mmol/L). However, the relationship between albumin and serum calcium is less reliable in critically ill patients.

a. Hypocalcemia

Hypocalcemia (total calcium <8.5 mg/dL [<2.12 mmol/L], ionized calcium <1 mmol/L) is common in critically ill patients and results from impairment of the parathyroid and/or vitamin D systems (**Table 12-6**). Cardiovascular abnormalities, the most common clinical manifestations of hypocalcemia in critically ill patients, include hypotension, bradycardia, arrhythmias, heart failure, cardiac arrest, digitalis insensitivity, and QT-interval and ST-segment prolongation. Neuromuscular manifestations include weakness, muscle spasm, laryngospasm, hyperreflexia, seizures, tetany, and paresthesias.

Table 12-6 Causes of Hypocalcemia

Hypoparathyroidism	Pancreatitis	Calcium chelators
Sepsis	Malabsorption	Hypomagnesemia
Burns	Liver disease	Massive transfusion
Rhabdomyolysis	Renal disease	

Treatment is aimed at correcting the underlying disease process and any concomitant electrolyte abnormalities, and administering calcium. Mild hypocalcemia is well tolerated, and aggressive treatment may result in tissue injury (especially during ischemic and septic states). If the hypocalcemia is severe or if the patient is symptomatic, administer 100 mg calcium intravenously over 5 to 10 minutes (3-4 mL of 10% calcium chloride or 10 mL of 10% calcium gluconate), followed by calcium in the amount of 0.3- to 2 mg/kg/h. Calcium preparations vary in their content of elemental calcium: 1 g of 10% calcium chloride contained in 10 mL has 272 mg of calcium; 1 g of 10% calcium gluconate contained in 10 mL has 90 mg of calcium. When the circulating calcium concentration is stable, calcium may be replaced via the enteral route (ie, 500-1,000 mg every 6 hours).

Monitor ionized or total calcium levels frequently during treatment, and adjust repletion to maintain calcium in the lower normal range so as not to suppress parathyroid gland function. If calcium replacement alone fails to maintain the circulating calcium level, consider administration of vitamin D and confirm normal magnesium levels. Adverse effects of calcium administration include hypercalcemia, bradycardia, nausea/vomiting, flushing, and tissue calcium precipitation.

b. Hypercalcemia

The most common causes of hypercalcemia (total calcium >11 mg/dL [>2.75 mmol/L], ionized calcium >1.3 mmol/L) are the result of calcium release from bone (**Table 12-7**). The clinical manifestations of hypercalcemia relate primarily to the cardiovascular and neuromuscular systems and include hypertension, cardiac ischemia, arrhythmias, bradycardia, conduction abnormalities, digitalis toxicity, dehydration, hypotension,

Table 12-7 Causes of Hypercalcemia

Hyperparathyroidism	Excess intake of vitamin A or vitamin D
Malignancy	Thyrotoxicosis
Immobilization	Granulomatous disease

weakness, depressed mentation, coma, seizures, and sudden death. Gastrointestinal manifestations include nausea/vomiting, anorexia, abdominal pain, constipation, pancreatitis, and ulcer disease. Nephrogenic diabetes insipidus with polyuria may occur and contribute to volume depletion. Renal stones, nephrocalcinosis, and renal failure also may be encountered.

Treatment of hypercalcemia is aimed at controlling the underlying disease, rehydrating the patient, and lowering the calcium level. The circulating calcium level frequently needs to be lowered while the primary disease is being evaluated and treated. Intravascular volume should be restored with normal saline to ensure adequate tissue perfusion and renal blood flow (urine output 2-3 mL/kg/h). Saline also decreases renal tubular calcium reabsorption. Once adequate hydration is ensured, diuresis with a loop diuretic further increases renal calcium loss. Serum potassium and magnesium levels should be monitored and low levels corrected. In patients with renal failure, pulmonary edema, or life-threatening hypercalcemia, calcium levels may be lowered with dialysis. After initial stabilization, therapy with calcitonin and bisphosphonates can be considered.

2. Phosphorus

Phosphate is important in cellular energy metabolism. Hypophosphatemia (phosphate <2.5 mg/dL [0.81 mmol/L]) results from transcellular shifts, renal loss, gastrointestinal loss, or inadequate intake (**Table 12-8**). Phosphate depletion primarily affects the neuromuscular and central nervous systems. Clinical manifestations include muscle weakness, respiratory failure, rhabdomyolysis, paresthesias, lethargy, disorientation, obtundation, coma, and seizures. Other possible complications include impaired renal tubular function, impaired pressor responses, hepatic dysfunction, immune dysfunction, impaired protein synthesis, hemolysis, impaired platelet function, and impaired oxygen off-loading from hemoglobin.

Table 12-8 Causes of Hypophosphatemia

Transcellular Shift	Renal Loss	Gastrointestinal Loss	Decreased Intake
Acute alkalosis	Hyperparathyroidism	Malabsorption	Malnutrition
Carbohydrate administration	Diuretic use	Diarrhea	Parenteral nutrition
Drugs (insulin, epinephrine)	Hypokalemia	Intestinal fistulas	
	Hypomagnesemia	Antacids	
	Steroids		

Treatment of hypophosphatemia consists of controlling the underlying disease, removing offending drugs, correcting electrolyte abnormalities, and replacing phosphate. Phosphate levels <1 mg/dL (<0.32 mmol/L) associated with symptoms are considered life-threatening and require immediate treatment. For emergency treatment, administer phosphate at 0.6 to 0.9 mg/kg daily intravenously. When circulating levels are stable, maintenance replacement of phosphate is 1,000 mg/day intravenously plus excess losses (ie, in urine or stool). Phosphate may be administered as potassium phosphate (93 mg/mL phosphate, 1.1 mmol/mL potassium) or sodium phosphate (93 mg/mL). Enteral administration of phosphate is preferred in patients with serum phosphate levels >1.0 to 1.5 mg/dL (>0.32-0.48 mmol/L).

Serum phosphate should be monitored during repletion and therapy adjusted to achieve a circulating level of 3 to 4 mg/dL (0.97-1.29 mmol/L). Adverse effects of phosphate administration include hyperphosphatemia, hypocalcemia, tissue calcium precipitation, renal injury, and diarrhea (enteral phosphate).

Hyperphosphatemia is uncommon in critical illness except with renal failure. Increased bone metabolism secondary to tumors or increased gut absorption also may cause hyperphosphatemia. Symptoms are similar to those of hypocalcemia: ventricular arrhythmias, prolonged QT interval, seizures, paresthesias, and muscle cramps. Hyperphosphatemia is treated with intravenous calcium and enteral phosphorus binders. Dialysis may be initiated with renal failure.

3. Magnesium

Magnesium is important to the body for energy transfer and electrical stability. Causes of hypomagnesemia (magnesium <1.8 mg/dL or 1.5 mEq/dL [<0.75 mmol/L]) are listed in **Table 12-9**.

Table 12-9 Causes of Hypomagnesemia

Renal Loss	Gastrointestinal Loss	Transcellular Shift	Decreased Intake
Renal tubular dysfunction	Malabsorption	Refeeding	Malnutrition
Diuresis	Diarrhea	Recovery from hypothermia	Alcoholism
Hypokalemia	Nasogastric suction		Parenteral nutrition
Drugs (aminoglycosides, amphotericin, etc)			

Clinical manifestations of hypomagnesemia overlap those of hypokalemia and hypocalcemia, including cardiovascular abnormalities (eg, QT-interval prolongation, arrhythmias, vasospasm, myocardial ischemia), neuromuscular abnormalities (eg, weakness, tremor, seizures, tetany, obtundation, coma), and electrolyte abnormalities (eg, hypokalemia, hypocalcemia).

Treatment of hypomagnesemia consists of addressing the underlying disease, discontinuing problematic drugs, correcting concomitant electrolyte abnormalities, and replenishing magnesium. For emergency treatment (eg, arrhythmias), administer 1 to 2 g magnesium sulfate intravenously over 5 to 10 minutes. The agent can be administered over a longer interval (10-60 minutes) in less-urgent situations. Depending on the clinical situation, subsequent intravenous replacement ranges from 1 to 2 g magnesium sulfate every 4 to 6 hours. Once serum levels stabilize, intravenous maintenance doses are 0.1 to 0.2 mmol/kg daily (1 g magnesium sulfate = 8 mmol). Maintenance magnesium may be administered enterally. The dose should be reduced if renal failure is present. Magnesium levels should be monitored during repletion. Deep tendon reflexes can be used to assess for hypermagnesemia during replacement (ie, decreased at serum level 4-5 mg/dL [1.65 2.06 mmol/L]).

Hypermagnesemia is uncommon in critical illness but may be seen with renal failure or shifts in magnesium from intracellular fluid due to soft tissue injury as with crush, burn trauma, and rhabdomyolysis. Hyporeflexia, lethargy, and apnea may result. Treatment consists of administration of intravenous calcium, diuretic administration, and dialysis in severe cases.

III. METABOLIC DISTURBANCES

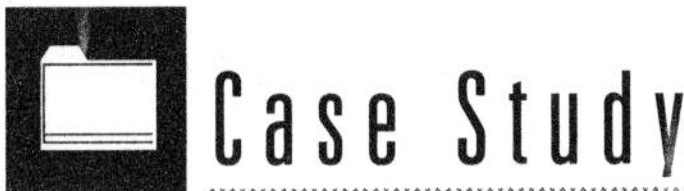

Case Study

A 34-year-old man presented to the emergency department with nonspecific complaints of a flu-like syndrome. His vital signs include respiratory rate 24/min, heart rate 126/min, blood pressure 96/48 mm Hg, and temperature 103.2°F (39.5°C). His laboratory results are remarkable for a white blood cell count 18,000/mm^3 with 14% bands. After blood cultures, antibiotics, and volume resuscitation, the patient feels better and is admitted to the floor. Two hours later, he is found to be lethargic with a palpable systolic blood pressure of 60 mm Hg. After transfer to the ICU, aggressive fluid resuscitation (40 mL/kg), and 10 µg/min of norepinephrine, he remains hypotensive.

- What metabolic disorders may contribute to the refractory hypotension?
- What testing is needed?
- What interventions should be considered?

A. Acute Adrenal Insufficiency

Acute adrenal insufficiency in the critically ill patient may result from preexisting or previously undiagnosed chronic disease of the adrenal glands or hypothalamic-pituitary axis, or acute conditions affecting these endocrine organs (**Table 12-10**). Patients with chronic disease may develop acute adrenal insufficiency precipitated by infection or other stressors. In addition, functional impairment during serious illness may result from relative or absolute insufficiency of glucocorticoid production, which usually reverses with recovery from the illness. Relative adrenal insufficiency occurs when cortisol response is normal or high, but is reduced in relation to the severity of illness.

Table 12-10 Etiologies of Adrenal Insufficiency

Etiologies of Adrenal Insufficiency
Chronic Conditions
Adrenal glands
Autoimmune destruction
Granulomatous disease (tuberculosis)
HIV infection
Other infection (cytomegalovirus, fungal)
Primary or metastatic malignancy
Drug effects (ie, ketoconazole)
Hypothalamic/pituitary axis
Withdrawal from exogenous glucocorticoid therapy
Hypopituitarism (tumors, infarction, radiation)
Sarcoidosis, histiocytosis
Head trauma
Acute Conditions
Critical illness (affects adrenal glands and hypothalamic-pituitary axis)
Hypoperfusion
Cytokine effects (alter cortisol metabolism, receptor affinity)
Acute adrenal hemorrhage
Meningococcemia
Disseminated intravascular coagulation
Anticoagulation (warfarin, heparin, etc)
Drug effects
Increased cortisol metabolism (phenytoin, phenobarbital, rifampin)
Interference with glucocorticoid synthesis (ketoconazole, etomidate)

Lack of specific signs and symptoms makes early recognition of acute adrenal insufficiency difficult in the critically ill patient. Clinical manifestations suggesting acute adrenal insufficiency include weakness, nausea and vomiting, abdominal pain, tachycardia, orthostatic hypotension, hypotension refractory to volume or vasopressor agents, and fever. Suggestive laboratory findings may include eosinophilia, hyponatremia, hyperkalemia, acidosis, hypoglycemia, and prerenal azotemia. Acute adrenal hemorrhage may cause abdominal, flank, or back pain. Clinical and laboratory manifestations overlap significantly with manifestations of other common critical illnesses such as sepsis.

> ! *Electrolyte abnormalities are less likely with acute adrenal insufficiency compared to chronic adrenal insufficiency.*

Important clues for possible adrenal insufficiency in seriously ill patients are vasopressor-dependent states and/or failure to respond to appropriate fluid administration, fever without apparent source, and discrepancy between the expected disease severity and the patient's condition.

The value of standard tests for hypothalamic-pituitary-adrenal axis function using baseline cortisol levels and/or the short adrenocorticotropic hormone (ACTH) stimulation test is limited in the critically ill patient due to variation in testing methodology and lack of consensus criteria for absolute or relative adrenal insufficiency. Thus, the decision to provide steroid therapy is made on clinical grounds. Proposed definitions of adrenal insufficiency in critical illness include a random cortisol level <10 μg/dL (others suggest <20 or 25 μg/dL). Cortisol levels generally reflect total cortisol rather than metabolically active free cortisol. Performance of commercially available assays is also inconsistent in the setting of critical illness, particularly sepsis. Improvement in hemodynamic status after administration of hydrocortisone may be an important physiologic indicator. If chronic adrenal insufficiency is suspected, ACTH stimulation testing may be appropriate after resolution of the acute illness. Emergent treatment is indicated in critically ill patients, even if the diagnosis is not firmly established. Treatment steps for adrenal insufficiency associated with critical illness are presented in **Table 12-11**. Note that high-dose steroid therapy, previously employed in trials of shock management, has been deemphasized.

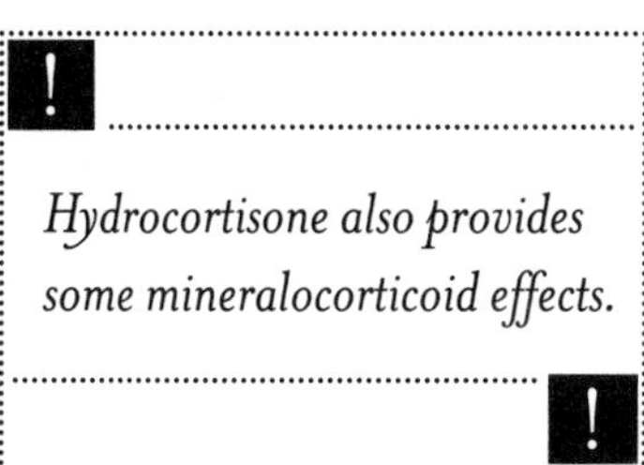

If a clinical response to glucocorticoid (hydrocortisone) administration is observed and relative adrenal insufficiency is suspected, treatment should be continued until resolution of the critical illness (7 days is recommended for steroid therapy in septic shock). Tapering of steroid therapy may avoid rebound effects associated with abrupt discontinuation. Patients with evidence of persistent adrenal insufficiency (chronic or newly diagnosed) should be converted to oral steroid therapy. Steroid therapy may have a role in the management of other shock states. Few data are available regarding these applications.

Table 12-11 Regimen for Corticosteroid Treatment in Critically Ill Patients[a]

Indications[b]
Vasopressor-dependent septic shock (dosage of norepinephrine or equivalent >0.05 to 0.1 µg/kg/min) within 12 h of onset, or
Progressive acute respiratory distress syndrome after 48 h of supportive care
Dosing Schedule
Hydrocortisone 50 mg IV every 6 h or 100-mg bolus then 10 mg/h continuous infusion for at least 7 d with option of treatment for 10-14 d. Vasopressors and ventilator should be stopped before taper
Hydrocortisone taper
Hydrocortisone 50 mg IV every 8 h for 3-4 d
Hydrocortisone 50 mg IV/po every 12 h for 3-4 d
Hydrocortisone 50 mg IV/po daily for 3-4 d
Reinstitution of full-dose hydrocortisone with recurrence of shock or worsening oxygenation
Fludrocortisone 50 µg po (optional)
Hydrocortisone and methylprednisolone are considered interchangeable
Limiting Complication of Corticosteroid Treatment
Infection surveillance: low threshold for performing blood cultures, mini-bronchoalveolar lavage, and other appropriate cultures
Hyperglycemia: monitor blood glucose, limit glycemic load, and treat with insulin as appropriate
Myopathy: monitor creatine phosphokinase and muscle strength, and avoid neuromuscular blocking agents

Abbreviation: po, by mouth

[a]Reproduced with permission from the American College of Chest Physicians.[8] Marik PE. Critical illness-related corticosteroid insufficiency. *Chest.* 2009; 135:181-193.

[b]A random cortisol or adrenocorticotropic hormone (ACTH) stimulation test is not required.

B. Hyperglycemic Syndromes

1. Diabetic Emergencies

Serious metabolic complications of diabetes result from a relative or absolute lack of insulin coupled with increased production of counterregulatory hormones such as glucagon, catecholamines, cortisol, epinephrine, and others. Life-threatening hyperglycemic syndromes include diabetic ketoacidosis (DKA) and hyperglycemic hyperosmolar state (HHS). These syndromes differ in the severity of dehydration and degree of acidosis (ketosis) but share many clinical manifestations and therapeutic interventions. In addition, patients may manifest components of both syndromes. **Table 12-12** lists characteristics that may distinguish the syndromes, but considerable variability is possible. Although DKA and HHS may be the initial presentation of diabetes, the most common precipitating factors are infection and medication noncompliance. Other precipitants include corticosteroid use, myocardial infarction, stroke, alcohol abuse, pancreatitis, trauma, and pregnancy.

> !
> *HHS develops over days to weeks and results in greater dehydration than does DKA, which usually evolves in <24 hours.*
> !

Table 12-12 Characteristics of Hyperglycemic Syndromes

	DKA	HHS
Glucose	>250 mg/dL	>600 mg/dL
Arterial/venous pH	<7.3	>7.3
Anion gap	Increased	Variable
Serum/urine ketones	Positive	Negative or small
Serum osmolality	Normal	Increased

Abbreviations: DKA, diabetic ketoacidosis; HHS, hyperglycemic hyperosmolar state

Clinical manifestations result from hyperglycemia in both syndromes and from excess ketone production in DKA. Hyperglycemia causes hyperosmolality, osmotic diuresis, fluid and electrolyte loss, dehydration, and volume depletion. Ketones cause acidosis and also contribute to the osmotic diuresis. Clinical features of both hyperglycemic syndromes may include weakness, dehydration, polyuria, polydipsia, tachycardia, hypotension, anorexia, nausea/vomiting, and ileus. Abdominal pain, hyperpnea (Kussmaul respirations), and fruity odor to the breath are more characteristic of DKA, whereas altered mental status (ranging from lethargy to coma) and arrhythmias are more common in HHS. Laboratory investigation may reveal hyperglycemia, hyperosmolality (more common in HHS), glucosuria, ketonemia/ketonuria (DKA), anion gap metabolic acidosis (DKA), hypokalemia or hyperkalemia, hypophosphatemia, hypomagnesemia, leukocytosis, and azotemia. Serum sodium concentrations may be decreased due to translocation of water to the extracellular space. An elevated serum sodium concentration suggests severe dehydration.

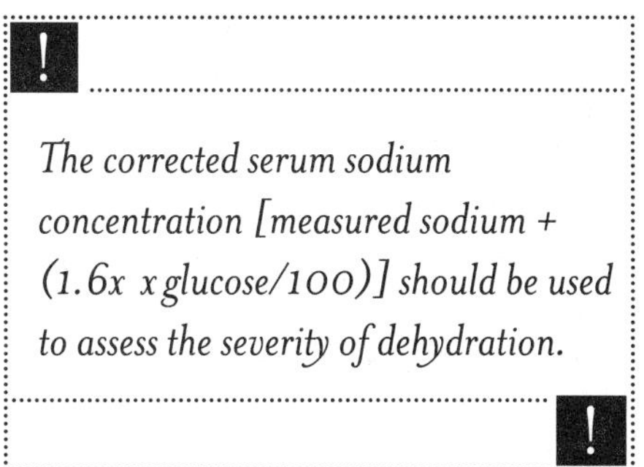
The corrected serum sodium concentration [measured sodium + (1.6x x glucose/100)] should be used to assess the severity of dehydration.

An initial rapid evaluation of the patient with possible hyperglycemic condition should include assessment of mental status, degree of dehydration (vital signs, orthostatic changes, urine output), and presence of infection. Laboratory studies should include complete blood count, electrolytes, renal function, glucose (plasma or fingerstick), urine or serum ketones, and arterial blood gas (or venous pH in hemodynamically stable patients). An electrocardiogram should be obtained to evaluate for ischemia and changes due to electrolyte abnormalities. If infection is suspected, appropriate cultures are indicated.

The goals for treatment of hyperglycemic syndromes are to restore the fluid and electrolyte balance, provide insulin, and identify precipitating factors. The initial management of DKA and HHS is outlined in **Table 12-13**. Volume deficits correlate with the severity of hyperglycemia and are usually greater in HHS. Urine output should be maintained at 1 to 3 mL/kg/h to ensure adequate tissue perfusion and clearance of glucose. Invasive hemodynamic monitoring (eg, arterial catheter, central venous catheter) may be required in patients with underlying cardiovascular disease.

Table 12-13 Initial Management of Hyperglycemic Syndromes

Fluids

1. Assess severity of dehydration.
2. Institute crystalloid resuscitation, initially with normal saline at approximately 15-20 mL/kg/h in the first hour in the absence of cardiac dysfunction to restore hemodynamic stability and renal perfusion. Subsequent fluid infusion rates should be guided by assessment of hydration and urine output, and 250-500 mL/h is often adequate.
3. After stabilization of the hemodynamic status, fluids with less chloride (eg, 0.45% saline) should be considered to avoid or minimize the development of hyperchloremic metabolic acidosis. The corrected serum sodium should also be used to guide fluid selection.
4. Add glucose to fluids when glucose is 250-300 mg/dL (13.9-16.7 mmol/L) in DKA. Administer 10% dextrose if necessary to maintain glucose >150 mg/dL (>8.3 mmol/L). In HHS, add glucose to fluids when glucose is 300 mg/dL (16.7 mmol/L) to maintain the glucose concentration between 250-300 mg/dL (13.9-16.7 mmol/L).

Insulin

1. Administer a regular insulin loading dose as an intravenous bolus (0.1-0.15 units/kg), followed by an infusion at 0.1 units/kg/h. Hold insulin if potassium concentration is <3.3 mmol/L until potassium is replaced.
2. If the glucose concentration does not fall by 50 mg/dL (2.8 mmol/L) in the first hour, consider increasing the insulin infusion rate or administering additional insulin boluses (10 units regular insulin hourly). Lack of response may also be due to inadequate volume resuscitation or serious infection.
3. In DKA, continue insulin infusion or decrease by 50% when the glucose reaches 250 mg/dL (13.9 mmol/L). Maintain the glucose concentration between 150 and 200 mg/dL (8.3 and 11.1 mmol/L) until acidosis and ketosis are resolved.
4. In HHS, decrease insulin infusion when the glucose concentration reaches 300 mg/dL (16.7 mmol/L) to maintain the glucose at 250-300 mg/dL (13.9-16.7 mmol/L) until the plasma osmolality is ≤315 mOsm/kg and the patient is alert.

Electrolytes

1. If serum potassium is <3.3 mmol/L, hold insulin and administer potassium 40 mmol/h as potassium chloride or potassium phosphate (or combination) until potassium is >3.3 mmol/L to avoid arrhythmias or severe weakness.
2. If serum potassium is >3.3 mmol/L but <5 mmol/L and urine output is adequate, administer potassium, 20-30 mmol, in each liter of fluids to maintain the potassium at 4-5 mmol/L.
3. If serum potassium is >5 mmol/L, do not administer potassium in fluids until <5 mmol/L.
4. Consider phosphate replacement with potassium phosphate if serum levels are low (<1 mg/dL, 0.32 mmol/L) or severe symptoms are present.

Abbreviations: DKA, diabetic ketoacidosis; HHS, hyperglycemic hyperosmolar state

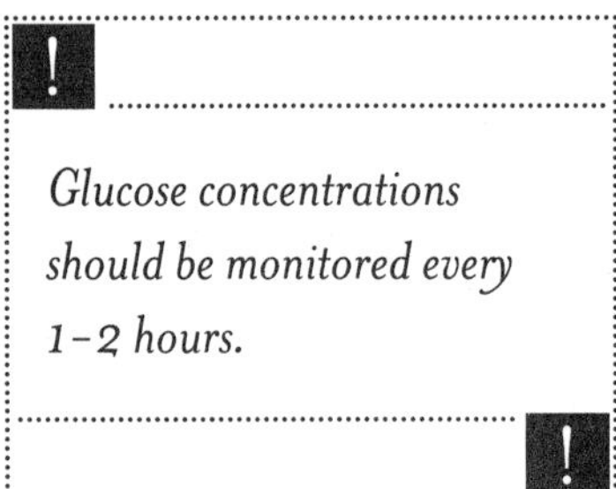

The intravenous route for insulin administration is the most reliable and easiest to titrate. Because of the short half-life of intravenous insulin, a continuous infusion is necessary with serial monitoring of the glucose and electrolyte concentrations. Smaller doses of insulin may be adequate in HHS.

Glucose-containing fluids may be started earlier than recommended if blood glucose cannot be monitored frequently. When glucose and/or serum osmolality are controlled, acidosis has cleared, and the patient is stable, subcutaneous insulin may be administered; an insulin sliding scale of regular and longer-acting preparations can be started and should overlap for 1 to 2 hours with discontinuation of the insulin infusion.

Insulin and correction of acidosis shifts potassium intracellularly and may lead to precipitous drops in serum potassium levels. Oral potassium replacement can be considered if nausea and vomiting are not present. Potassium and other electrolyte levels should be monitored frequently (especially in the first 6 hours) until levels stabilize and acidosis is resolved.

Acidosis is well tolerated by patients with DKA, and bicarbonate therapy is controversial. No benefit has been found when bicarbonate is administered to DKA patients with pH of 6.9 to 7.1, and fluid and insulin therapy result in rapid improvement in pH. Bicarbonate administration may be considered if the arterial pH is <6.9 (give 100 mmol bicarbonate over 1 hour to increase pH >7). Do not attempt to normalize blood pH with bicarbonate, because acidosis resolves as ketones are metabolized.

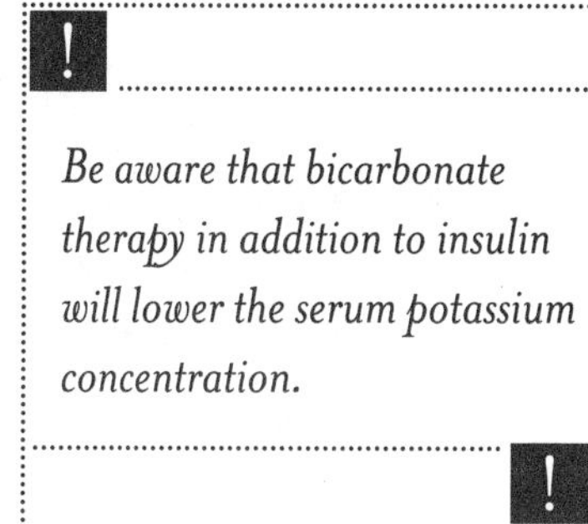

2. Hyperglycemia in Critical Illness

Hyperglycemia is common in diabetic and nondiabetic patients with critical illness and may be due to stress hormones, inflammatory mediators, glucocorticoid therapy, excessive nutritional calories, decreased activity, and other mechanisms. Significant hyperglycemia is associated with poor wound healing, impaired immune function, increased inflammation, endothelial dysfunction, and other adverse effects leading to increased illness and death. Early studies of tight glucose control (80-110 mg/dL, 4.4-6.1 mmol/L) suggested benefit in a surgical population, but this target has been difficult to achieve in subsequent studies without increasing the risk for severe hypoglycemia. In addition, in multiple subsequent trials, no consistent reduction in mortality was observed with intensive control of glucose levels. Some recent studies of tight glycemic control have actually demonstrated increased mortality associated with higher rates of hypoglycemia.

In critically ill patients, insulin therapy should be initiated for persistent hyperglycemia, starting at a threshold of no greater than 180 mg/dL (10 mmol/L). Once therapy has been initiated, a glucose range of 140-180 mg/dL (7.8-10 mmol/L) is recommended. Intravenous insulin infusions are the preferred method to achieve and maintain control. During intravenous insulin therapy, frequent monitoring of blood glucose is essential to minimize the risk of hypoglycemia and achieve optimal control.

The ability to provide adequate nursing support and monitoring may affect the blood glucose goals chosen. Different types of blood sampling and glucose measurement methods may also yield different results. The institution protocol for blood sampling, insulin infusion, and glucose management targets should be followed to achieve consistency and minimize the risk of hypoglycemia.

!

Patients with renal dysfunction require lower rates of insulin infusions.

!

Key Points

Management of Life-Threatening Electrolyte and Metabolic Disturbances

- In the presence of life-threatening arrhythmias or paralysis associated with hypokalemia, give potassium chloride, 20 mmol/h, through a central venous catheter.
- If hyperkalemia-associated ECG abnormalities are present, administer calcium chloride or calcium gluconate intravenously over 5 to 10 minutes, then consider shifting potassium intracellularly with 50% dextrose and regular insulin intravenously, inhaled β-agonists, and/or sodium bicarbonate.
- In symptomatic euvolemic hyponatremia, limit the increase in serum sodium to 8 to 12 mmol/L in the first 24 hours. Too-rapid correction of serum sodium may result in CNS injury.
- Patients with hypernatremia and hemodynamic instability should have normal saline administered until intravascular volume is corrected. Subsequently, replace water with 5% dextrose in water, 0.45% NaCl, or 0.2% NaCl with 5% dextrose.
- Emergent treatment with a glucocorticoid is indicated in critically ill patients with possible adrenal insufficiency, even if the diagnosis is not established.
- The goals of treatment in hyperglycemic syndromes are to restore the fluid and electrolyte balance, provide insulin, and identify precipitating factors.
- In diabetic ketoacidosis, insulin infusion should be continued until the ketosis and acidosis have resolved. Glucose-containing fluids should be administered to prevent hypoglycemia during insulin infusion.
- Maintain the glucose between 250 and 300 mg/dL (13.9-16.7 mmol/L) in hyperglycemic hyperosmolar syndrome until the plasma osmolality is <315 mOsm/kg and the patient is alert.
- Potassium should be added to the fluid therapy for hyperglycemic syndromes as soon as serum potassium is recognized to be <5 mmol/L and urine output is adequate.
- A protocol of blood sampling, insulin infusion, and target glucose level should be followed to avoid hyperglycemia and minimize hypoglycemia in critically ill patients.

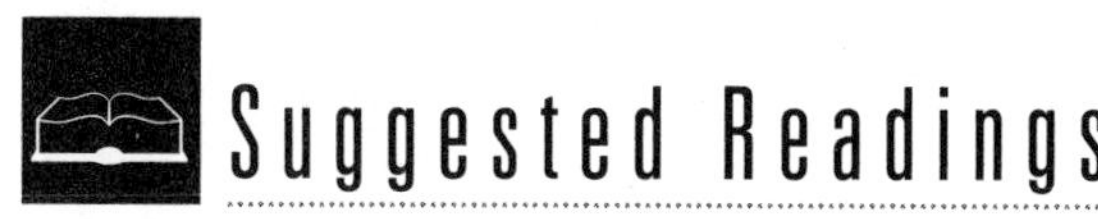

Suggested Readings

1. Adrogué HJ, Madias NE. Hypernatremia. *N Engl J Med.* 2000;342:1493-1499.

2. Adrogué HJ, Madias NE. Hyponatremia. *N Engl J Med.* 2000;342:1581-1599.

3. Brown GR, Greenwood JK. Drug- and nutrition-induced hypophosphatemia: mechanisms and relevance in the critically ill. *Ann Pharmacother.* 1994;28:626-632.

4. Charron T, Bernard F, Skrobik Y, et al. Intravenous phosphate in the intensive care unit: more aggressive repletion regimens for moderate and severe hypophosphatemia. *Intensive Care Med.* 2003;29:1273-1278.

5. Gennari FJ. Disorders of potassium homeostasis: hypokalemia and hyperkalemia. *Crit Care Clin.* 2002;18:273-288.

6. Kamel KS, Wei C. Controversial issues in the treatment of hyperkalaemia. *Nephrol Dial Transplant.* 2003;18:2215-2218.

7. Kitchabi AE, Umpierrez GE, American Diabetes Association, et al. Hyperglycemic crises in diabetes. *Diabetes Care.* 2004;27(suppl 1):S94-S102.

8. Marik PE. Critical illness-related corticosteroid insufficiency. *Chest.* 2009; 135:181-193.

9. Marik PE, Pastores SM, Annane D, et al. Recommendations for the diagnosis and management of corticosteroid insufficiency in critically ill adult patients. Consensus statements from an international task force by the American College of Critical Care Medicine. *Crit Care Med.* 2008;36:1937-1949.

10. Moghissi ES, Korytkowski MT, DiNardo M, et al. American Association of Clinical Endocrinologists and American Diabetes Association consensus statement on inpatient glycemic control. *Diabetes Care.* 2009;32:1119-1131.

11. Noronha JL, Matuschak GM. Magnesium in critical illness: metabolism, assessment, and treatment. *Intensive Care Med.* 2002;28:667-679.

12. Verbalis JG, Goldsmith SR, Greenberg A, et al. Hyponatremia treatment guidelines 2007: Expert panel recommendations. *Am J Med.* 2007;120:S1-S21.

Chapter 13

SPECIAL CONSIDERATIONS

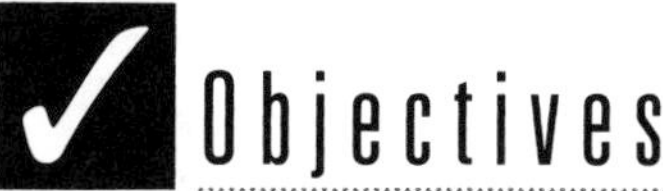

Objectives

- Outline the diagnosis and management of pulmonary embolism.
- Describe appropriate prophylactic therapy for venous thromboembolism.
- List general management principles of severe gastrointestinal hemorrhage.
- Describe appropriate prophylactic therapy for the prevention of stress-related gastritis.
- Summarize principles of poisoning management.
- Review the management of hypertensive crises.
- Outline the diagnosis and management of intra-abdominal hypertension and abdominal compartment syndrome.

Case Study

An obese woman with chronic tobacco abuse and congestive heart failure arrives at the emergency department complaining of shortness of breath and right pleuritic chest pain for the past 2 days. She has a heart rate of 110/min with clear lung fields and mild bilateral pretibial edema. When she arrived, her Spo_2 on room air was 89%; that has increased to 94% on oxygen, 3 L/min by nasal cannula. A chest radiograph did not show any infiltrates. As her primary care physician, you are called for assistance in her management.

- What risk factors and clinical findings suggest a differential diagnosis?
- What tests are indicated?

I. INTRODUCTION

In addition to the medical conditions discussed in previous chapters, the clinician may be called on to care for patients with other severe and/or life-threatening problems. The management and prevention of some of these commonly encountered conditions are reviewed in this chapter.

II. PULMONARY EMBOLISM

A. Diagnosis

A patient's history and clinical findings may be unreliable for diagnosis of a pulmonary embolism (PE). Risk factors for PE and other venous thromboembolic disease (**Table 13-1**) often contribute to a high index of suspicion. Predisposing factors include any condition that may cause venous stasis, injury to the vascular endothelium, or hypercoagulability (Virchow triad).

Table 13-1 Risk Factors for Pulmonary Embolism/Venous Thromboebolism

Family history	Central venous catheterization
Advanced age	Recent surgery
Obesity (body mass index >30)	Immobility, paralysis
Prior history of deep vein thrombosis/PE	Stroke with partial or full paralysis
Venous insufficiency	Trauma
Venous injury or repair	Malignancy (past or current)
Inherited hypercoagulable disorders	Cancer therapy
(protein C or S deficiency, lupus anticoagulant, etc)	Selective estrogen receptor modulators
Acute medical illness, ICU admission	Pregnancy and postpartum period
Heart or respiratory failure	Estrogen therapy
Nephrotic syndrome	Smoking

The classic combination of dyspnea, pleuritic chest pain, and hemoptysis occurs in a minority of patients with PE. Routine blood studies are not diagnostic. Chest radiographs are frequently unremarkable but may show nonspecific findings of atelectasis, pleural effusion, elevated hemidiaphragm, and/or infiltrates. Chest radiographs may be useful in ruling out other life-threatening problems, such as pneumothorax. The electrocardiogram (ECG) may show nonspecific ST-T wave changes, QR pattern in lead V_1, an $S_1Q_3T_3$ pattern, or right bundle-branch block, but a pattern of acute cor pulmonale is generally not present.

Sinus tachycardia and premature atrial contractions are the most frequently encountered arrhythmias. Often the most relevant information provided by the ECG is the exclusion of other potential sources of chest pain, such as acute ischemia or pericarditis. Hypoxemia, a nonspecific finding in cardiopulmonary disease, is commonly present, but a normal Pa_{O_2} value or normal alveolar-arterial oxygen partial pressure difference $[P(A - a)_{O_2}]$ does not rule out PE. Signs and symptoms of PE are shown in **Table 13-2**.

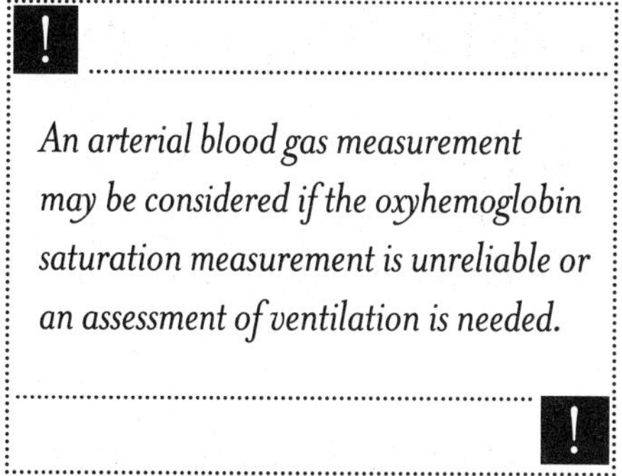

An arterial blood gas measurement may be considered if the oxyhemoglobin saturation measurement is unreliable or an assessment of ventilation is needed.

Table 13-2 Clinical Manifestations of Pulmonary Embolism

Dyspnea	Fever (usually low-grade)
Chest pain	Hypoxemia
Cough	Cyanosis
Tachypnea	Apprehension
Tachycardia	Syncope
Diaphoresis	Previously noted leg swelling
Hemoptysis	

A correct diagnosis of PE is essential because early initiation of appropriate therapy decreases mortality. The current diagnostic strategy recommends that the clinician formulate a clinical likelihood of low, moderate, or high clinical suspicion of PE (**Figure 13-1**). One scoring system used to determine pretest probability is presented in **Table 13-3.** D-dimer assays with high sensitivity and high negative predictive value are frequently used as an initial step in algorithms for the diagnosis of PE in outpatients. A negative D-dimer result in a patient with low clinical probability of PE may reliably exclude the diagnosis. Patients with a positive D-dimer result or with a moderate or high clinical probability assessment require further diagnostic evaluation. D-dimer measurements have limited utility for the evaluation of PE in hospitalized patients because of the high proportion of positive results.

Multidetector computed tomography (CT) angiography demonstrating thrombus up to the segmental-level pulmonary arteries is diagnostic for PE, whereas a negative scan can be safely used to exclude it. In patients with allergy to contrast, compression venous ultrasonography of lower limbs can be used. A positive leg study establishes the diagnosis of thromboembolism, and further diagnostic testing is not needed as therapy is similar for PE. A normal $\dot{V}/\dot{Q}$ scan can exclude PE in patients with low clinical suspicion. Similarly, a high probability $\dot{V}/\dot{Q}$ scan establishes the diagnosis of PE in patients with high clinical suspicion. In all other combinations of $\dot{V}/\dot{Q}$ scan and clinical suspicion, further tests are performed. Bedside echocardiography can be used for establishing the diagnosis in appropriate clinical circumstances and assessing right ventricular function.

Figure 13-1. A Diagnostic Approach to Pulmonary Embolism

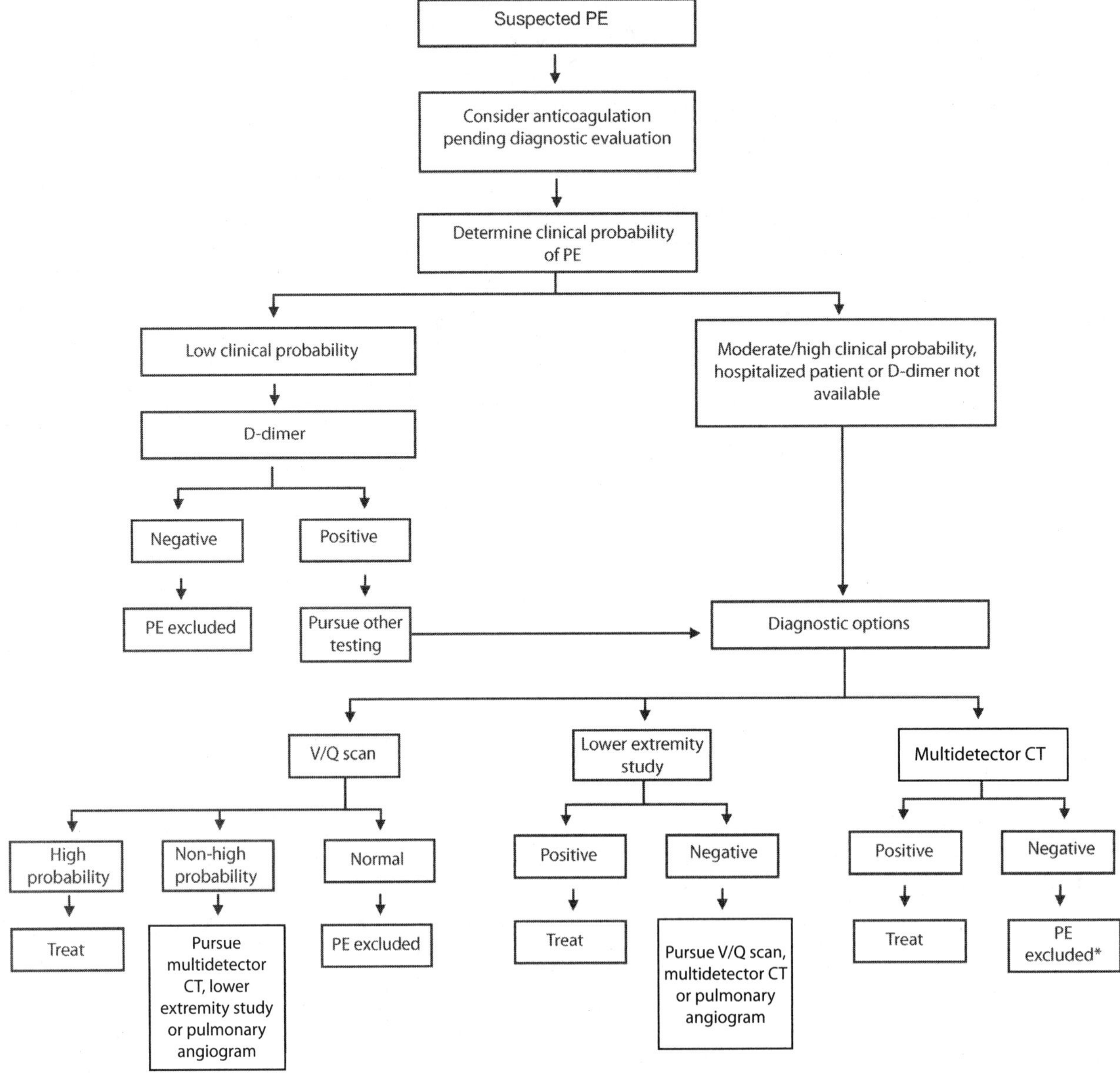

*Consider pulmonary angiogram if clinical suspicion is high; negative predictive value is increased by a negative lower extremity study

Table 13-3 Clinical Probability Assessment for Pulmonary Embolism

Clinical signs and symptoms of DVT (objective leg swelling and pain with palpation)	3
PE as likely, or more likely, than an alternative diagnosis	3
Immobilization (bed rest, except to access bathroom, for ≥3 consecutive days or surgery in previous 4 weeks)	1.5
Previous objective diagnosis of DVT or PE	1.5
Heart rate >100 beats/min	1.5
Previous objective diagnosis of DVT or PE	1.5
Heart rate >100 beats/min	1.5
Hemoptysis	1
Active cancer (treatment ongoing or within previous 6 months or palliative treatment)	1

0-1: Low probability
2-6: Moderate probability
≥7: High probability

Abbreviations: DVT, deep venous thrombosis; PE, pulmonary embolism

B. Therapy

The treatment of PE can usually be limited to anticoagulation starting with initial administration of a parenteral agent (low-molecular-weight heparin [LMWH], unfractionated heparin, fondaparinux). (See **Appendix 11** for recommended intravenous unfractionated heparin therapy for full anticoagulation.) LMWH and fondaparinux can be effective in treating PE and are preferred over unfractionated heparin due to convenient dosing, absence of need for laboratory monitoring, and low incidence of heparin-induced thrombocytopenia. Both agents are dosed based on weight and require dosage adjustment with renal impairment. Unfractionated heparin is preferred in patients with severe renal dysfunction, those at high risk of bleeding, and when thrombolytic therapy is being considered. In patients with suspected PE and no contraindications to anticoagulation, baseline-activated partial thromboplastin time, prothrombin time, and complete blood cell count should be obtained, and heparin or fondaparinux therapy should be initiated while waiting for test results unless there is a high risk of bleeding. Contraindications to heparin therapy include recent major trauma with hemorrhage, recent central nervous system hemorrhage or infarction, active gastrointestinal (GI) bleeding, and heparin-induced thrombocytopenia. When unfractionated heparin is used, the activated partial thromboplastin time should be monitored to achieve a value 1.5 to 2.5 times the mean normal value or anti-factor Xa levels can be monitored.

Oral warfarin therapy is started on day 1 and adjusted to achieve an international normalized ratio of 2 to 3. Heparin or fondaparinux therapy can be discontinued after 5 days if the international normalized ratio is 2 or above for at least 24 hours with warfarin. Oral anticoagulation should continue for at least 3 months, but some patients (those with unprovoked first PE/deep venous thrombosis or recurrent unprovoked PE/deep venous thrombosis) may have indications for longer therapy unless there is a high risk of bleeding. For patients with underlying malignancy, extended therapy with LMWH is suggested over warfarin, but the choice of agent may be influenced by costs, tolerance of injections, and need for monitoring. In patients who receive long-term anticoagulant treatment, the risk/benefit ratio of continuing such treatment should be reassessed at regular intervals.

Systemic thrombolysis for PE may improve pulmonary arterial hemodynamics, lung perfusion, and right ventricular function, but the quality of evidence suggesting improved mortality is low. The use of thrombolytic agents in the treatment of PE should take into account the patient's hemodynamic status, right ventricular function, and risk of bleeding. Systemic thrombolytic therapy is currently suggested for patients with acute PE with hypotension who are at low risk of bleeding. Thrombolysis is not recommended for most hemodynamically stable patients with PE. Although thrombolysis is suggested for a subgroup of patients with a high risk of developing hypotension, there are no validated clinical findings that can be used to identify such patients. Multiple clinical signs such as tachycardia, decrease in blood pressure, hypoxemia, evidence of hypoperfusion, and right ventricular dysfunction can be considered in decision-making. Tissue plasminogen activator is preferred at a dose of 100 mg infused over a 2-hour period. Streptokinase has also been used with a loading dose of 250,000 international units, followed by 100,000 international units each hour for 24 hours. Short administration times are preferred over prolonged infusion times. Local administration of a thrombolytic agent via a catheter is not recommended. Surgical embolectomy or extraction/fragmentation of the embolus via transvenous catheters requires specialized expertise not commonly available, but it can be considered when thrombolysis is absolutely contraindicated or has failed and when shock is likely to cause death before thrombolytics can affect clot dissolution.

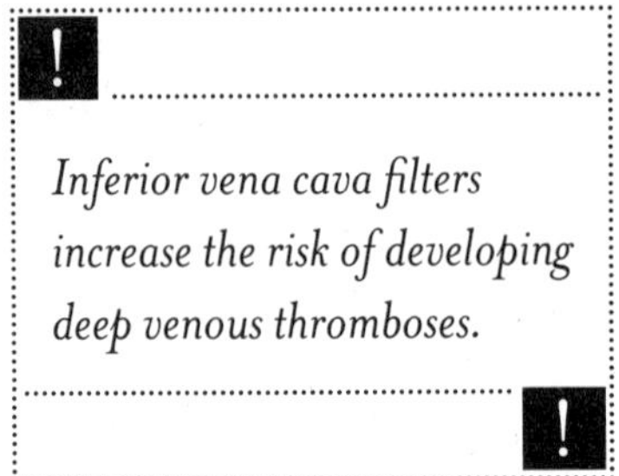

An inferior vena cava filter should be considered in patients with pulmonary embolism when:

- There is a strong contraindication to anticoagulation
- Emboli recur during anticoagulation
- Bleeding occurs during anticoagulation

Retrievable filters may be an option in some centers. If possible, anticoagulation for treatment of the embolus should be resumed as soon as possible after insertion of a filter.

C. Prevention of Venous Thromboembolism

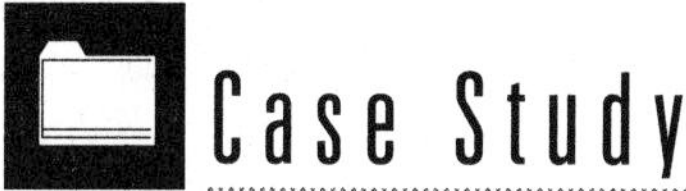

Case Study

A middle-aged man presents with an acute ischemic stroke and right hemiparesis. He received tissue plasminogen activator and experienced improvement in the neurologic deficits.

- Should this patient receive prophylaxis for venous thromboembolism?
- What type of venous thromboembolism prophylaxis would be appropriate for this patient if the decision were made to treat?

Many critically ill or injured patients are at risk of developing venous thromboembolism, either PE or deep venous thrombosis. The development of thrombosis can lead to longer hospital stays, increased resource utilization, venous abnormalities, and death. Thromboprophylaxis is cost-effective and highly efficacious in preventing venous thromboembolism. Both pharmacologic (heparins, direct thrombin inhibitors such as fondaparinux and dabigatran [not approved for this indication in U.S.], factor Xa inhibitors such as rivaroxaban and warfarin) and mechanical interventions (intermittent pneumatic compression device, graduated compression stockings) may be used for prophylaxis in hospitalized patients (**Appendix 12**). Mechanical methods for prophylaxis are generally less effective but are acceptable options for patients at high risk of bleeding and when combined with anticoagulants.

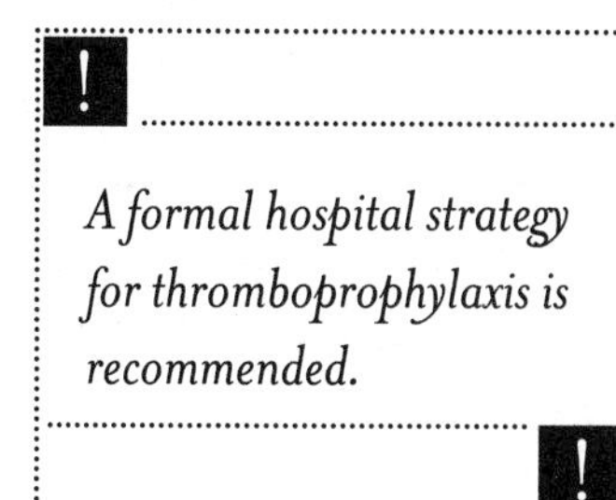

A formal hospital strategy for thromboprophylaxis is recommended.

Recommendations are based on specific patient groups (nonsurgical, nonorthopedic surgical, orthopedic surgical), level of risk for venous thromboembolism, and risk of bleeding. Clinicians should follow manufacturers' instructions for dosing of LMWH, especially in the setting of renal failure and obesity. Caution must be used when instituting anticoagulant therapy in patients with recent or ongoing hemorrhage, renal failure, or concomitant use of antiplatelet therapy.

III. SEVERE GASTROINTESTINAL HEMORRHAGE

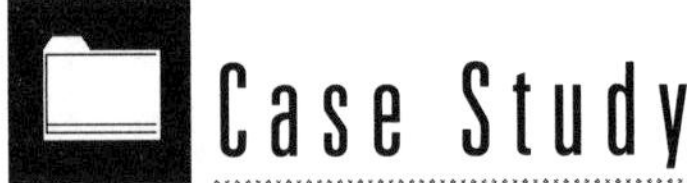

Case Study

A 64-year-old man with arthritic pain had been taking ibuprofen four times daily for months without significant relief. He starts to complain of fatigue and progressive weakness. Today he developed nausea and started vomiting bright red blood. He called an ambulance and was brought to the emergency department. He is pale, tachycardic, and dizzy with a blood pressure of 95/60 mm Hg and hematocrit of 28%.

- What additional clinical and laboratory assessments are indicated?
- How would you prioritize interventions?

A. General Management Principles

Medications for ulcer prophylaxis and treatment have reduced the incidence of stress gastritis and severe upper GI bleeding. However, when present, such bleeding can be life threatening and requires early surgical consultation as well as rapid assessment, diagnosis, and intervention. The distinction between upper and lower GI sources of hemorrhage is important in determining the appropriate diagnostic/therapeutic approach. The ligament of Treitz is the anatomic marker that separates the upper GI tract from the lower GI tract when discussing hemorrhage.

Typically, patients with life-threatening GI hemorrhage are older and have other chronic organ system disease(s). Therefore, the critical consequences of hemorrhage, hypotension, and anemia may be poorly tolerated and may lead to other systemic manifestations of poor oxygen delivery, such as myocardial ischemia. Prompt assessment, resuscitation, early diagnosis (even during resuscitation), and intervention are needed to prevent these secondary consequences.

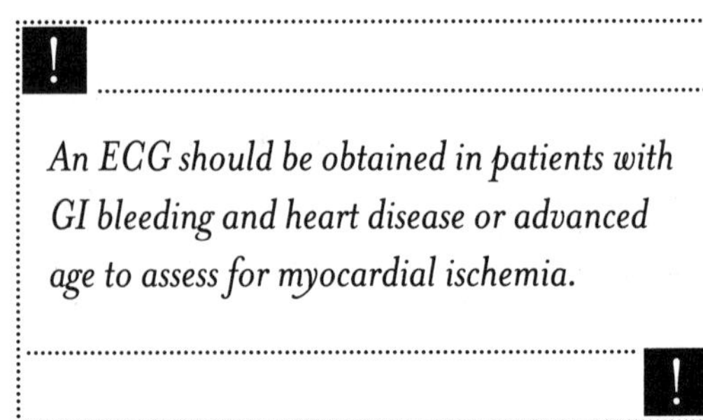

An ECG should be obtained in patients with GI bleeding and heart disease or advanced age to assess for myocardial ischemia.

A general approach to managing GI bleeding is outlined in **Table 13-4**. Obtain blood for typing and cross matching as soon as possible. An appropriate hemoglobin level should be maintained based on patient condition and coexisting disease. Two large-bore peripheral catheters or a large-bore central venous catheter should be maintained at all times. Gastroenterology and surgery consultations (in case of severe bleeding) should be requested. If a reserve of blood products (eg, 4 units packed red cells) is not immediately available, early patient transfer should be planned.

Table 13-4 Management of Gastrointestinal Bleeding

Assessment	Airway
	    Protective reflexes
	    Level of consciousness
	Volume status
	    Vital signs, orthostatic changes
	    Central venous pressure
	    Urine output
	Severity of condition
	    Visible blood loss
	    Hemoglobin, hematocrit, platelet count
	    Coagulation status (APTT, PT)
	    Hypoperfusion abnormalities (ie, cardiac ischemia)
	Nasogastric or orogastric tube
	    Confirm or rule out upper-GI source
	    Lavage stomach for upper endoscopy

Resuscitation	Consider intubation
	    Altered mental status
	    Inability to protect airway
	    Copious hematemesis
	    Need for sedation/endoscopy
	IV access
	    Large-bore (≥16 gauge) peripheral catheter(s) or
	    large central venous catheter (9F-12F)
	Fluid administration
	    Normal saline or lactated Ringer's solution
	Transfusion of red blood cells

Diagnostic/Therapeutic Interventions	Endoscopy with directed therapy
	Surgical assessment/intervention
	Correct coagulopathy
	    Fresh frozen plasma for factor deficiency
	    Platelet transfusion if $<50{,}000/mm^3$
	Pharmacologic therapy for variceal bleeding
	IV proton pump inhibitors
	Transfer to facility with diagnostic and/or therapeutic capability

Continuing Care	Monitored environment
	Adequate blood bank resources
	Frequent assessment
	    Volume status
	    Hypoperfusion abnormalities
	    Laboratory parameters

Abbreviations: APTT, activated partial thromboplastin time; PT, prothrombin time; GI, gastrointestinal

B. Severe Upper Gastrointestinal Hemorrhage

Severe upper GI hemorrhage is diagnosed by hematemesis or the presence of blood in the gastric aspirate, although 10% to 15% of patients with duodenal ulcer may have little or no blood in the gastric aspirate due to bleeding below the level of the pylorus. When obtaining a patient's history and physical examination, it is important to note previous upper GI bleeding, the presence of ulcer disease, alcohol consumption, stigmata of cirrhosis, coagulation disorders, and use of aspirin and other antiplatelet medications, nonsteroidal anti-inflammatory agents, or anticoagulants. Upper GI hemorrhage is categorized as variceal (VUGIH) and non-variceal hemorrhage (NVUGIH) because of differing prognosis and management. Common causes of NVUGIH include duodenal and gastric ulcers, Mallory-Weiss tear, malignancy, and gastritis.

Endoscopy is needed to establish the diagnosis and control hemorrhage. If this procedure is not quickly available, consider transfer to a facility with endoscopic capabilities. In patients on anticoagulants, correction of coagulopathy is recommended but should not delay early endoscopy.

When uncontrolled variceal bleeding is suspected before endoscopic diagnosis, the following splanchnic vasoconstrictors may be considered:

- Somatostatin, 250-μg bolus, followed by 250 μg/h
- Octreotide, 25- to 100-μg bolus, followed by 25 to 50 μg/h
- Vasopressin, 20 units over 20 minutes, followed by 0.1 to 0.4 units/min
- Terlipressin 1 to 2 mg every 4 hours (not available in the United States)

Somatostatin or a somatostatin analogue, such as octreotide, is the agent of choice because of the favorable side-effect profile. Nausea and abdominal pain are sometimes associated with bolus doses, but significant adverse effects are uncommon. Maintenance infusions are usually continued for 3 to 5 days and may be effective in stopping acute variceal bleeding and preventing early rebleeding from varices. Vasopressin is an alternative choice but may cause coronary artery vasospasm, angina, or hypertension. Concomitant nitroglycerin may prevent the deleterious effects of vasopressin on the coronary circulation. Terlipressin is a synthetic vasopressin analogue with fewer side effects and a longer half-life. None of the above agents are recommended in the routine management of NVUGIH. Antibiotics – usually a third-generation cephalosporin, should be administered in cirrhotic patients with VUGIH. If hemorrhage cannot be controlled, balloon tamponade can be considered as a temporizing measure (maximum 24 hours) if expertise in placement is available until more definitive therapy can be instituted.

Following endoscopy, an intravenous bolus of a proton pump inhibitor, followed by continuous infusion for 72 hours, is effective in decreasing NVUGIH repeat bleeding and mortality due to peptic ulcer disease. Preendoscopic administration of a proton pump inhibitor may reduce the need for endoscopic therapeutic interventions, particularly if endoscopy is delayed. If endoscopy is unsuccessful in controlling the bleeding, surgical intervention or angiographic embolization may be needed for control.

C. Severe Lower Gastrointestinal Hemorrhage

Frequent causes of lower GI hemorrhage are diverticular disease, angiodysplasia, large hemorrhoids, colonic polyps, inflammatory bowel disease, rectal ulcer/tear, upper GI source, and malignancy. Evaluation should include special attention to a history of diverticular disease, inflammatory bowel disease, previous abdominal aortic aneurysm repair (may suggest life-threatening aortoenteric fistula), or the presence of a coagulation disorder. Physical examination must include inspection and a careful rectal examination to identify hemorrhoids or rectal carcinoma.

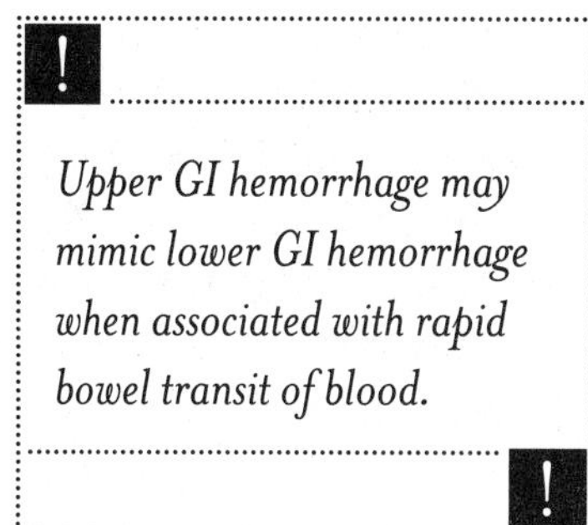

Gastric aspiration should be performed to eliminate an upper GI source of hemorrhage. A nasogastric aspirate that is negative for occult blood and contains bile makes an upper GI bleeding source unlikely. Upper GI endoscopy may be considered based on assessment of the most likely bleeding source. Lower GI endoscopy is important for diagnosis, treatment, anticipation of rebleeding, and planning other diagnostic interventions or surgery. If endoscopy is unavailable, transfer to another facility or direct surgical intervention is dictated by the patient's condition. Angiography with embolization therapy may be considered for unstable patients or those who are poor surgical risks.

D. Prevention of Stress-Related Gastritis

Identification and treatment of patients at risk for stress-related gastritis will reduce complications, length of stay, and costs. To minimize the potential complications of pharmacologic prophylaxis for stress ulceration (ie, nosocomial pneumonia), routine use of such therapy should be limited to patients with known risk factors for stress gastritis. The risk of stress ulceration and GI bleeding depends on a patient's underlying illness, its severity, and related comorbidities. Significant risk factors include mechanical ventilation for longer than 48 hours, coagulopathy, severe infection, hypotension, severe head trauma (Glasgow Coma Scale score <10), severe burns or trauma, renal or hepatic failure, major surgery, and prolonged ICU stay. Appropriate therapeutic agents include histamine receptor-blocking agents (H_2-receptor antagonists) and proton pump inhibitors.

IV. POISONING AND DRUG TOXICITY

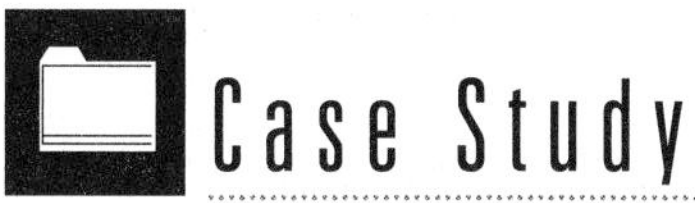

Case Study

A young woman was found on the bathroom floor by her parents the morning after a party. She was difficult to arouse and, when she was stimulated, she became agitated and violent. Her parents transported her to the emergency department.

- What are the immediate priorities and interventions in caring for this patient?
- What are the likely toxins, based on the patient's history and clinical presentation?

Patients who have ingested prescription, over-the-counter, or recreational drugs present with a variety of clinical manifestations. General categories of patient presentation and possible responsible agents are listed in **Table 13-5**. Reliable information about the substance(s), amount(s) ingested, and time of ingestion is often not available. Similarly, although qualitative urine toxicology screens and quantitative blood tests may be available, they cannot identify all agents that could have been ingested. Quantitative drug levels should be obtained if the patient's medication or medical history suggests ingestion of a specific drug, or if the signs and symptoms are compatible with toxicity from that drug. Acetaminophen levels should be checked in all cases. The anion gap should be calculated in cases of unknown toxins.

Table 13-5 Clinical Characteristics That Aid in Diagnosis of Poisoning/Overdose

Clinical Examination	Possible Agents
Agitation, confusion, bizarre behavior	Cocaine, amphetamines, antidepressants, phencyclidine, hallucinogens, SSRIs
Bradycardia/hypotension	β-Blockers, barbiturates, calcium-channel blockers, clonidine, digoxin, sedatives/hypnotics
Coma, lethargy	Alcohols, antidepressants, barbiturates, benzodiazepines, gamma hydroxybutyrate, lithium, opiates, salicylates, SSRIs
Hyperadrenergic, hyperthermia	Amphetamines, anticholinergics, cocaine, theophylline
Hypotension	Antidepressants, antihypertensives, opiates, organophosphates/carbamates, sedatives/hypnotics
Hypothermia	Ethanol, hypoglycemic agents, opiates, sedatives/hypnotics
Miosis	Cholinergic drugs, opiates, organophosphates, phencyclidine
Mydriasis	Antihistamines, atropine, tricyclic antidepressants, ethanol, sympathomimetic drugs
Nausea/vomiting	Acetaminophen, alcohols, iron, salicylates, theophylline
Nystagmus	Alcohols, carbamazepine, phenytoin, phencyclidine, sedative/hypnotics
Seizures	Amphetamines, antidepressants, cocaine, cyanide, isoniazid, lithium, organophosphates/carbamates, salicylates, SSRIs, theophylline
Tachyarrhythmias	Amphetamines, antidepressants, caffeine, cocaine, digoxin, theophylline
Ventilatory compromise (respiratory acidosis)	Opiates, alcohols, antidepressants, barbiturates, benzodiazepines, gamma hydroxybutyrate
Laboratory Tests	**Possible Agents**
Increased osmolar gap	Ethanol, methanol, ethylene glycol, acetone, isopropyl alcohol, propylene glycol
Increased oxygen saturation gap	Methemoglobinemia, carbon monoxide
Metabolic acidosis	Acetaminophen, salicylates, methanol/ethylene glycol, iron, isoniazid, carbon monoxide, cyanide, propylene glycol, propofol

Abbreviation: SSRI, selective serotonin reuptake inhibitor

These patients often require a symptom-based initial evaluation and treatment. Specific antidotes, treatments, and/or precautions based upon historical or laboratory evidence of particular ingestants can be utilized when applicable. In some countries, specialized resource centers are available to assist in the treatment of poisoning. The overall mortality from acute poisoning is low, but the treating clinician must quickly evaluate critical issues and attempt to identify patients at highest risk.

A. General Management

1. Initiate airway support as required. Assessing the patient to ensure adequate ventilation, oxygenation, and protective airway reflexes is critical.

> **!** *Respiratory failure is a common cause of death in overdose and poisoning.* **!**

2. Initiate management of cardiovascular compromise as indicated. Obtain adequate venous access and establish monitoring (eg, pulse oximeter, ECG, automated blood pressure device). Address initial concerns in monitored variables (eg, isotonic fluid administration, supplemental oxygen, seizure control, cooling or warming the patient, vasopressors, or inotropes).

3. Consider the following interventions for a patient with altered mental status:

   a. 50% dextrose (50 g), 50 mL intravenously, preferably after a blood glucose test.

   b. Naloxone, 0.2 to 2 mg, intravenously, intramuscularly, or via an endotracheal tube. Larger doses (6 to 10 mg), repeat dosing, or an infusion may be required, especially when synthetic and long-acting opiates are involved.

   c. Thiamine, 100 mg, slow intravenous administration. Administer before concentrated dextrose solutions to reduce the risk of Wernicke encephalopathy.

4. Develop a patient database with further information from the history, physical examination, laboratory studies, and other testing (eg, chest radiograph, ECG).

5. Little evidence exists for use of gastric-emptying procedures. Ipecac is not used in poisoned patients, and gastric lavage may be considered only in life-threatening overdoses within 1 hour of ingestion. Contraindications include an unprotected airway and ingestion of substances with high potential for aspiration injury, including hydrocarbons and acid or alkali ingestions.

6. Administer activated charcoal to patients with significant toxic ingestions within 1 to 2 hours of ingestion at an initial dose of 1 g/kg. The effectiveness of activated charcoal decreases with time from ingestion, so early administration is indicated. Caution is required with decreased level of consciousness and an unprotected airway.

7. Be aware that although cathartics have been used in overdoses, there is no evidence of efficacy. Caution is warranted in the very young and elderly (because of potential fluid losses) and those with potential for obstruction.

8. Recognize that hemodialysis, rather than continuous renal replacement therapy, is the preferred intervention in patients with life-threatening overdoses of dialyzable substances. Common dialyzable drugs include carbamazepine, valproic acid, lithium, toxic alcohols, salicylates, and metformin.

B. Specific Management

> *Do not overlook the possibility of acetaminophen ingestion in patients with drug overdoses.*

After the patient is stabilized, more specific therapy may be warranted. Specific antidotes and/or interventions that may be considered are listed in **Table 13-6**. The use of more advanced interventions, such as hemodialysis or hemoperfusion, should be individualized to each patient and may require consultation or transfer.

Table 13-6 Antidotes and Interventions for Specific Toxins

Toxin	Antidote or Intervention
Acetaminophen	N-acetylcysteine
Alcohols (methanol, ethylene glycol)	Ethanol, fomepizole, hemodialysis, thiamine and pyridoxine (vitamin B_6) for ethylene glycol, folic acid for methanol
Amphetamines	Benzodiazepines
Benzodiazepines	Flumazenil[a]
ß-Blockers	Glucagon, calcium chloride, pacing, catecholamines, insulin and dextrose
Calcium-channel blockers	Calcium chloride, glucagon, insulin and dextrose, pacing, catecholamines
Carbon monoxide	100% oxygen, hyperbaric oxygen
Cocaine	Benzodiazepines
Cyanide	Nitrites and thiosulfate, hydroxocobalamin
Cyclic antidepressants	Benzodiazepines (for seizures), blood alkalinization/sodium loading (pH 7.5-7.55), hypertonic saline, magnesium, alpha-agonist for hypotension (norepinephrine)
Digoxin	Digoxin-specific Fab fragments, atropine, lidocaine, pacing
Heparin	Protamine sulfate
Hypoglycemic agents	50% dextrose, somatostatin or octreotide
Iron	Deferoxamine
Isoniazid	Pyridoxine (vitamin B_6)
Lithium	Hemodialysis
Nitrites	Methylene blue
Opiates	Naloxone, intubation/ventilation
Organophosphates, carbamates, nerve gases	Atropine, pralidoxime or obidoxime
Salicylates	Urine alkalinization, hemodialysis
Theophylline	Multiple-dose charcoal, hemoperfusion
Warfarins	Vitamin K_1

[a]Flumazenil should not be administered to patients who chronically ingest benzodiazepines or have overdosed on cyclic antidepressants.

V. HYPERTENSIVE CRISES

A. Clinical Presentation

Acute hypertension or severe elevation in blood pressure (BP) may occur as a primary or secondary condition in seriously ill patients. Frequently, patients have an underlying diagnosis of chronic hypertension. New or progressive end-organ injury secondary to elevation in BP constitutes a *hypertensive emergency*, while severely elevated BP without evidence of organ injury is defined as *hypertensive urgency*. Although the BP is often >180/120 mm Hg, no specific BP defines a hypertensive emergency. The rate of blood pressure increase may be more important than the absolute value. The organs most severely affected by elevations of BP are the brain, heart, and kidney, and injury can manifest as encephalopathy, stroke, intracranial hemorrhage, unstable angina or myocardial infarction, acute left ventricular dysfunction (with pulmonary edema), acute aortic dissection, deteriorating renal function, and hypertensive disorders associated with pregnancy (see **Chapter 14**).

Symptoms related to an elevated BP at presentation reflect the organ affected and consequent injury but may be nonspecific. The patient's history of use of monoamine oxidase inhibitors, recreational drugs (including cocaine and amphetamines), over-the-counter medications, and antihypertensive agents as well as medication compliance should be ascertained. Physical examination and laboratory investigation should be directed to determine the presence of end-organ injury. Initial workup usually includes complete blood count, renal function, urinalysis with microscopy, ECG to assess for cardiac ischemia, and chest radiography to evaluate for pulmonary edema or widened mediastinum. Patients with altered mental status or focal neurological deficits warrant imaging of the brain.

A complication of uncontrolled hypertension is acute aortic dissection. Symptoms are often severe and can include unrelenting chest pain, frequently associated with back or epigastric pain, and neurological deficits such as altered mental status, focal deficits, hemiplegia, and paraplegia. A patient with severe hypertension, severe chest pain, and a wide mediastinum on chest radiograph should be evaluated for possible aortic dissection. Aortic dissection is frequently misdiagnosed as acute myocardial infarction, PE, stroke, esophagitis, pancreatitis, peptic ulcer disease, biliary colic, and ureteral colic. Physical examination should include careful auscultation for a new murmur of aortic insufficiency, assessment for asymmetric blood pressure or pulses in upper extremities, and careful palpation of pulses in all extremities for significant asymmetry. The diagnostic standard has been contrast angiography, but computed tomography angiography is more commonly used. Magnetic resonance imaging and transesophageal echocardiography may also be useful for diagnosis.

Acute hypertension secondary to increased sympathetic drive and catecholamine surge is also a frequent manifestation of common disease processes in seriously ill patients, such as respiratory failure, acute pain, alcohol or drug withdrawal syndromes, agitated delirium, and increased intracranial pressure (Cushing reflex). Initial therapy in such circumstances should be targeted to treating the underlying problem and not lowering of elevated BP.

B. Therapy

Hypertensive urgency can be managed with oral or intravenous agents, and gradual blood pressure control over 24 to 48 hours. The goal is to reduce the pressure over hours to days to a safer, but not necessarily normal, level of BP. Hypertensive emergencies require continuous monitoring of BP, neurological status, urine output, and other parameters in a monitored environment. Parenteral and titratable antihypertensive agents should be administered to lower the BP within minutes to hours. The initial goal of therapy should be to reduce mean arterial pressure by no more than 20-25% in first few hours. If the BP is lowered too rapidly, it may result in hypoperfusion of major arterial beds, resulting in cerebral infarction, myocardial infarction, and blindness secondary to changes in auto-regulation of organ blood flow.

Table 13-7 Parenteral Antihypertensive Agents Used in the Management of Hypertensive Emergencies

Primary Condition	Therapy
Acute aortic dissection	Labetalol Esmolol Nicardipine
Hypertensive encephalopathy	Labetalol Nicardipine Clevidipine Fenoldopam Nitroprusside
Acute myocardial ischemia	Nitroglycerin Labetalol Fenoldopam
Systolic heart failure	Nicardipine Nitroglycerin Loop diuretic
Eclampsia/severe preeclampsia	Hydralazine Labetalol Nicardipine
Pheochromocytoma	Phentolamine Labetalol
Diastolic dysfunction with pulmonary edema	Nicardipine Labetalol Fenoldopam Nitroglycerin Nitroprusside
Acute ischemic stroke/ intracerebral bleed	Nicardipine Labetalol Fenoldopam Clevidipine
Acute renal failure	Nicardipine Labetalol Fenoldopam
Perioperative hypertension	Nicardipine Nitroglycerin Clevidipine Labetalol Esmolol

Rapid-acting antihypertensives are preferred, including labetalol, esmolol, nitroprusside, nicardipine, nitroglycerin, and fenoldopam. Agents that can be considered in some specific situations are given in **Table 13-7**. Oral antihypertensives appropriate for the patient can usually be initiated within 6 to 12 hours of presentation and parenteral agents weaned.

Specific Situations:

1. In patients with acute aortic dissection, a rapid reduction of systolic BP to 100 to 120 mm Hg with a heart rate 60 to 80 beats per minute should be achieved within 5 to 10 minutes. Beta blockers or an agent with combined α and β blockade such as labetalol are preferentially used in this condition to decrease the shear forces on the aorta and hopefully limit the extent of dissection. Additionally, opiate analgesics may be needed for pain control.

2. In patients with normal renal function and signs of volume depletion (due to pressure natriuresis), gentle volume expansion with normal saline will help suppress renin secretion and prevent significant hypotension from vasodilating medications.

VI. INTRA-ABDOMINAL HYPERTENSION AND ABDOMINAL COMPARTMENT SYNDROME

Increased intra-abdominal pressure (IAP), the pressure within the abdominal cavity typically measured as bladder pressure, has been increasingly recognized as both the cause and consequence of many complications in critically ill patients. The perfusion pressure to the abdomen, termed abdominal perfusion pressure (APP), is the mean arterial pressure minus the IAP. Similar to cerebral perfusion pressure, APP is the critical determinant of perfusion to the abdominal visceral organs.

Intra-abdominal hypertension (IAH) is defined as a sustained pathological increase of IAP to >12 mm Hg, while abdominal compartment syndrome is defined as IAP >20 mm Hg or new onset of organ failure at a lower IAP.

While normal IAP is in the range of 5 to 7 mm Hg, it can reach 9 to 14 mm Hg in obese individuals. Hence, physiologic state must be taken into account when interpreting IAP measurements. Increases can come from increased abdominal volume, decreased abdominal compliance, or more commonly a combination of the two. Some conditions leading to IAH/abdominal compartment syndrome are listed in **Table 13-8**. Abdominal compartment syndrome is classified as primary, secondary, or recurrent. Primary abdominal compartment syndrome is a condition associated with injury or disease in the abdominopelvic region that frequently requires early surgical or radiological intervention, whereas secondary abdominal compartment syndrome develops from conditions that do not originate primarily from the abdominopelvic region (eg, sepsis, capillary leak, burns). Abdominal compartment syndrome can progress and recur even after initial therapy is successful.

Table 13-8 Conditions Associated with Intra-abdominal Hypertension/Abdominal Compartment Syndrome[a]

Increased Intra-abdominal Volume	Decreased Abdominal Wall Compliance	Combination
Gastrointestinal tract dilatation • Gastroparesis • Gastric distention • Ileus • Volvulus • Colonic pseudo-obstruction Intra-abdominal or retroperitoneal masses • Abdominal tumor Ascites or hemoperitoneum Pneumoperitoneum (eg, during laparoscopy)	Abdominal surgery, especially with tight abdominal closures Abdominal wall bleeding or rectus sheath hematomas Surgical correction of large abdominal hernias, gastroschisis, or omphalocele	Obesity Sepsis, severe sepsis, and septic shock Severe acute pancreatitis Massive fluid resuscitation Major burns (with or without abdominal eschars) Complicated intra-abdominal infection

[a]Classified partly using Malbrain ML, Cheatham ML, Kirkpatrick A, et al. Results from the International Conference of Experts on Intra-abdominal Hypertension and Abdominal Compartment Syndrome. I. Definitions. *Intensive Care Med.* 2006;32:1722-1732.[7]

IAH has deleterious effects on both intra- and extra-abdominal organ systems. Most of these effects are either from decreased abdominal perfusion causing ischemia of intra-abdominal organs or from reduced thoracoabdominal compliance leading to reduced cardiac output and respiratory compromise. Specifically:

1. Decreases in APP can cause acute kidney injury, splanchnic hypoperfusion, and gut ischemia. These effects may occur in the absence of decreased cardiac output.
2. Intrathoracic pressure increases secondary to reduced thoracoabdominal compliance and cephalad displacement of the diaphragm (20% to 80% transmission of abdominal pressure). This has negative effects on the cardiovascular, respiratory, and central nervous systems:
    a. Cardiovascular
        i. Decreased venous return leading to diminished preload and end-diastolic volume
        ii. Increased systemic afterload
    b. Respiratory
        i. Decreased total compliance
        ii. Increased inspiratory pressures or decreased tidal volumes depending on the mode of mechanical ventilation

c. Intracranial

i. Increased intracranial pressures secondary to elevated thoracic pressures and diminished cerebral venous return

Significant IAH will lead to increased measured filling pressures, such as central venous pressure, secondary to reduced chest wall compliance; however, venous return is significantly reduced, and the transmural pressures are actually low. Thus, these values will have different interpretations with IAH, and higher physiological targets may be appropriate for resuscitation.

IAP measurements are made at end-expiration with the patient in the supine position, after ensuring that abdominal muscle contractions are absent and with the transducer zeroed at the level of the mid-axillary line. The reference standard for intermittent IAP measurement is via the bladder with a maximal instillation volume of 25 mL of sterile saline.

A. Management

The cornerstones of management of IAH/abdominal compartment syndrome are early recognition by serial monitoring of IAP (every 4 to 6 hours), maintenance of abdominal (APP >60 mm Hg) and systemic perfusion, prompt institution of medical therapies to reduce IAP and prevent adverse consequences on organ function, and early surgical decompression for refractory IAH.

Medical Therapies

1. Evacuate intraluminal contents by nasogastric or colonic decompression, use of prokinetic agents, and administration of enemas.

2. Evacuate intra-abdominal space-occupying lesions (eg, drainage of large volume ascites).

3. Optimize fluid administration and avoid both hypo- and hypervolemia. Consider diuretics and renal replacement therapy in cases of hypervolemia.

4. Improve thoracoabdominal compliance by ensuring adequate sedation and analgesia, and drainage of pleural effusions and ascites. Avoid constrictive bandages, and consider neuromuscular blockade.

5. Ensure abdominal and systemic perfusion by keeping APP >60 mm Hg.

Surgical Therapies

1. Prophylactic open abdomen in patients with high risk of developing IAH/abdominal compartment syndrome, especially in trauma patients.

2. Decompressive laparotomies

3. Ultrasound-guided percutaneous drainage of excessive free intra-abdominal fluid may be an option in selected patients.

Key Points

Special Considerations

- A negative result with a high-sensitivity D-dimer assay in outpatients with low clinical probability of pulmonary embolism can exclude the diagnosis, whereas those with moderate or high clinical probability of pulmonary embolism and hospitalized patients require further diagnostic testing.
- In patients with suspected pulmonary embolism and no contraindications to anticoagulation, unfractionated or low-molecular-weight heparin or fondaparinux therapy should be initiated while diagnostic tests are being obtained.
- Patients at risk for venous thromboembolism should receive appropriate pharmacologic and/or mechanical prophylaxis.
- In facilities that are unable to maintain 4 units of blood in reserve for potential transfusion, consideration should be given to transferring patients with serious GI bleeding to a facility with a higher level of care.
- Endoscopy is needed to establish the etiology of upper gastrointestinal hemorrhage and to institute potentially definitive therapy.
- Lower gastrointestinal endoscopy is important for diagnosing, treating, and planning interventions for patients with severe lower gastrointestinal hemorrhage.
- Patients at risk for stress-related gastritis should be started on an H_2-receptor antagonist or proton pump inhibitor.
- In the treatment of patients with known or suspected poisoning/overdose, maintaining airway patency and circulatory stabilization are initial priorities.
- Control of blood pressure and heart rate is critical in the management of patients with aortic dissection.
- Intra-abdominal pressure should be monitored frequently in patients at risk for developing intra-abdominal hypertension and abdominal compartment syndrome.
- Therapy for control of intra-abdominal pressure and maintenance of abdominal and systemic perfusion should be initiated promptly.

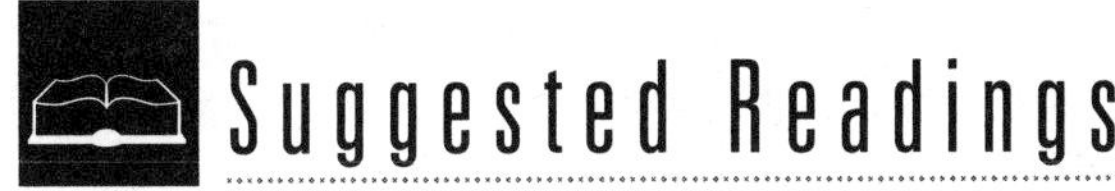

Suggested Readings

1. Alapat PM, Zimmerman JL. Toxicology in the critical care unit. *Chest.* 2008;133: 1006-1013.

2. Anderson FA Jr., Spencer FA. Risk factors for venous thromboembolism. *Circulation.* 2003(suppl);107:I-9–I-16.

3. Barkun AN, Bardou M, Kuipers EJ, et al. International consensus recommendations on the management of patients with nonvariceal upper gastrointestinal bleeding. *Ann Intern Med.* 2010;152:101-113.

4. Braverman AC. Aortic dissection: prompt diagnosis and emergency treatment are critical. *Cleve Clin J Med.* 2011;10:685-696.

5. Cheatham ML. Abdominal compartment syndrome. *Curr Opin Crit Care.* 2009;15: 154-162.

6. Cheatham ML, Safcsak K. Percutaneous catheter decompression in the treatment of elevated intra-abdominal pressure. *Chest.* 2011;140:1428-1435.

7. Falck-Ytter Y, Francis CW, Johanson NA, et al. Prevention of VTE in orthopedic surgery patients: Antithrombotic Therapy and Prevention of Thrombosis, 9th ed: American College of Chest Physicians Evidence-Based Clinical Practice Guidelines. *Chest.* 2012;141:e278S-e325S.

8. Garcia-Tsao G, Sanyal AJ, Grace ND, et al. Prevention and management of gastroesophageal varices and variceal hemorrhage in cirrhosis. *Hepatology.* 2007; 46:922-938.

9. Gould MK, Garcia DA, Wren SM, et al. Prevention of VTE in nonorthopedic surgical patients: Antithrombotic Therapy and Prevention of Thrombosis, 9th ed: American College of Chest Physicians Evidence-Based Clinical Practice Guidelines. *Chest.* 2012;141:e227S-e277S.

10. Kahn IA, Nair CK. Clinical, diagnostic, and management perspectives of aortic dissection. *Chest.* 2002;122:311-328.

11. Kahn SR, Lim W, Dunn AS, et al. Prevention of VTE in nonsurgical patients: Antithrombotic Therapy and Prevention of Thrombosis, 9th ed: American College of Chest Physicians Evidence-Based Clinical Practice Guidelines. *Chest.* 2012; 141:e195S-e226S.

12. Kearon C, Akl EA, Comerota AJ, et al. Antithrombotic therapy for VTE disease: Antithrombotic Therapy and Prevention of Thrombosis, 9th ed: American College of Chest Physicians Evidence-Based Clinical Practice Guidelines. *Chest.* 2012; 141:e419S-e494S.

13. Konstantinides S. Clinical practice. Acute pulmonary embolism. *N Engl J Med.* 2008;359:2804-2813.

14. Malbrain ML, Cheatham ML, Kirkpatrick A, et al. Results from the International Conference of Experts on Intra-abdominal Hypertension and Abdominal Compartment Syndrome. I. Definitions. *Intensive Care Med.* 2006;32:1722-1732.

15. Marik PE, Varon J. Hypertensive crises: challenges and management. *Chest.* 2007;131:1949-1962.

16. Papadopoulos DP, Mourouzis I, Thomopoulos C, et al. Hypertension crisis. *Blood Press.* 2010;19:328-336.

17. Torbicki A, Perrier A, Konstantinides S, et al. Guidelines on the diagnosis and management of acute pulmonary embolism: the Task Force for the Diagnosis and Management of Acute Pulmonary Embolism of the European Society of Cardiology (ESC). *Eur Heart J.* 2008;29:2276-2315.

18. Wells PS, Anderson DR, Rodger M, et al. Excluding pulmonary embolism at the bedside without diagnostic imaging: management of patients with suspected pulmonary embolism presenting to the emergency department by using a simple clinical model and D-dimer. *Ann Intern Med.* 2001;135:98-107.

19. Zimmerman JL, Rudis M. Poisonings. In: Parrillo JE, Dellinger RP, eds. *Critical Care Medicine.* 3rd ed. Philadelphia, PA: Mosby Elsevier; 2008:1453.

Web Sites

1. Institute for Clinical Systems Improvement. http://www.icsi.org. *This Web site contains guidelines and order sets for venous thromboembolism management and prophylaxis.*

2. World Society of Abdominal Compartment Syndrome. http://www.wsacs.org. *This Web site contains guidelines for the diagnosis and management of abdominal compartment syndrome.*

Chapter 14

Critical Care in Pregnancy

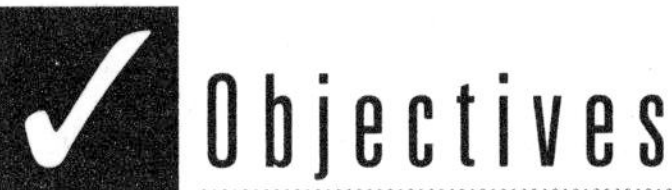

Objectives

- Describe the physiologic and metabolic alterations unique to pregnancy.
- Discuss the diagnosis and management of hypertensive disorders of pregnancy.
- Identify clinical manifestations and treatment of the HELLP syndrome.
- Outline the approaches to managing peripartum cardiomyopathy, thromboembolic disease, and other conditions in pregnancy.
- List priorities for managing the traumatized pregnant patient.

Case Study

You are called to assess a 25-year-old primigravid woman in labor at 34 weeks' gestation who has an increased blood pressure (BP) of 180/110 mm Hg, heart rate 120/min, oxygen saturation (Spo$_2$) 88% while receiving room air, and severe respiratory distress. A chest radiograph shows pulmonary edema.

- What are possible diagnoses?
- What immediate interventions are needed?
- What additional evaluations are indicated?

I. INTRODUCTION

A pregnant woman may present for critical care support either with a disease state that is unique to pregnancy or with a critical illness that is not unique to pregnancy. Diseases specific to pregnancy include preeclampsia, eclampsia, HELLP syndrome (hemolysis, elevated liver enzymes, and low platelet count), and amniotic fluid embolism syndrome, all of which usually require immediate therapy that may be lifesaving. Some critical illnesses not unique to pregnancy—such as preexisting maternal hypertension, thromboembolic disease, cardiac and respiratory diseases, and trauma—can be unmasked, precipitated, or aggravated by pregnancy. The normal physiologic, metabolic, and hormonal changes of pregnancy may alter the presentation of disease processes and add a level of complexity to diagnosis and treatment. Understanding the normal physiologic changes during pregnancy, delivery, and the postpartum period is the key to managing critically ill obstetric patients with underlying medical diseases and pregnancy-related complications. The most common critical illnesses in obstetric patients are hypertensive disorders and hemorrhage.

II. PHYSIOLOGIC ALTERATIONS

A. Cardiovascular Alterations

Alterations in blood volume and cardiovascular status are among the most dramatic changes that occur in pregnancy. These are adaptive mechanisms that accommodate the increased metabolic needs of both the mother and the fetus during pregnancy, labor, and delivery. Blood volume increases in each trimester, reaching 40% to 50% above prepartum values by the end of gestation. Cardiac output also increases up to 50% above prepartum values by the 24th week of gestation and then plateaus until labor and delivery; this is primarily a result of increased stroke volume during the first and second trimesters and a heart rate raised 15 to 20 beats/min during the third trimester until term. Improved myocardial contractility may account in part for the increase in cardiac output. A significant decrease of 25% to 30% in this output may occur during the third trimester if the patient is placed in the supine position; this causes the gravid uterus to compress the aorta and inferior vena cava, increasing afterload and restricting venous return to the heart. The left lateral decubitus position is the preferred position for pregnant women with serious illness, particularly as gestation progresses and the gravid uterus increases in size. The decrease in cardiac output is exaggerated in women with poorly developed venous collaterals who exhibit significant hypotension and bradycardia in the supine position, known as the supine hypotensive syndrome of pregnancy. Filling pressures, such as the central venous and pulmonary artery pressures, typically do not change during pregnancy. A decrease in BP is seen in the second trimester as a result of diminished systemic vascular resistance secondary to the vasodilating effects of progesterone. Peak reduction in BP occurs at 24 weeks; systolic pressures are reduced by 5 to 10 mm Hg and diastolic pressures by 10 to 15 mm Hg. By term, the BP should return to prepartum values.

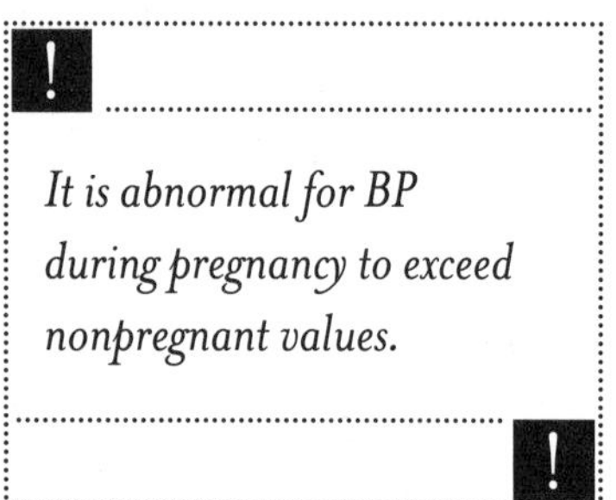

Another normal cardiovascular change of pregnancy that may cause or exacerbate illness is remodeling of the heart with enlargement of all four chambers. In particular, left atrial enlargement may precipitate supraventricular and atrial arrhythmias. Systolic ejection murmurs and a third heart sound are commonly detected during pregnancy, but diastolic, pansystolic, and late systolic murmurs suggest a more serious underlying cardiac disorder.

In addition to chamber enlargement, the heart is rotated upward and to the left as the uterus enlarges and the diaphragm elevates. Because of this displacement, cardiomegaly and increased vascular markings may be seen on the chest radiograph. These changes have no clinical significance if the patient has no other evidence of cardiac disease.

Healthy pregnant women tolerate the cardiovascular and hemodynamic effects associated with pregnancy, as do patients with mild to moderate cardiac disease, although the incidence of heart failure and arrhythmias is higher in patients with cardiac disease. Concurrent hemodynamic and fetal monitoring is often necessary for pregnant patients with New York Heart Association (NYHA) functional class III or class IV heart disease.

B. Pulmonary Alterations

The pregnant woman is considered to have a "difficult airway" complicated by edema of the upper respiratory tract as a result of increased blood volume and hormone-induced mucosal edema and hypervascularity. Pulmonary changes in pregnancy include an increase in tidal volume of approximately 40%, a decrease in functional residual capacity of 25%, and an increase in oxygen consumption as a result of the rising metabolic needs of the mother and the fetus. During pregnancy, metabolic demands can be elevated up to 32% above nonpregnant values by term. The increases in metabolic demands are due to the expanding uterine mass and the size of the fetus, but only 4% is attributed to maternal metabolic demands. The combination of decreased functional residual capacity and increased oxygen consumption during pregnancy diminishes maternal oxygen reserves and subsequently increases the hypoxic risk to both the mother and the fetus in the event of maternal hypoventilation or apnea.

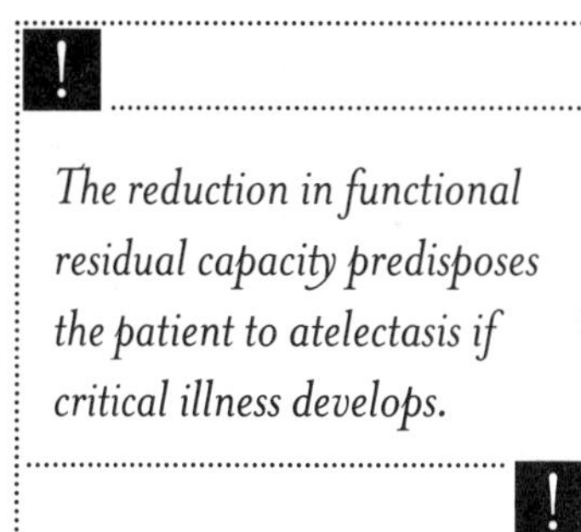
The reduction in functional residual capacity predisposes the patient to atelectasis if critical illness develops.

Oxygen requirements rise by approximately 30 to 40 mL/min in pregnancy and are met by an increase in minute ventilation, primarily as a result of an expanded tidal volume. The increase in minute ventilation results in a mild compensated respiratory alkalosis with a decline in the $Paco_2$ to 27 to 34 mm Hg (3.6 to 4.5 kPa). The pH does not change due to renal compensation, which results in a decrease in serum bicarbonate concentration. Pregnant women who present with a "normal" $Paco_2$ level of 35 to 40 mm Hg (4.7 to 5.3 kPa) should prompt the clinician to look for a cause of impending ventilatory failure.

C. Gastrointestinal Alterations

Hormonal and anatomic changes in pregnancy affect the gastrointestinal tract. Starting at the end of the first trimester, a reduction in lower esophageal sphincter tone caused by high progesterone levels contributes to an increased risk for aspiration. Gastroesophageal reflux and decreased gastric emptying are also present during pregnancy. Alterations in gastric motor function may cause nausea, vomiting, and dyspepsia.

D. Hematologic Alterations

The 40% to 60% increase in plasma volume that occurs by the third trimester is associated with a gain in red cell mass of only 25% at term. The disproportionate rise in plasma volume results in dilutional anemia (physiologic anemia of pregnancy); hemoglobin concentration is ~11 g/dL (110 g/L) at 24 weeks, when it stabilizes; however, it may increase slightly later in the pregnancy, when there is less discrepancy between the increases in blood volume and red cell mass. The white blood cell count climbs to 10,000 cells/µL (10.0 x 109/L) at term, with a slight reduction in platelet count. Plasma concentrations of all clotting factors except XI, XIII, and antithrombin III increase in pregnancy. Fibrinogen levels may be as high as 600 mg/dL (6.0 g/L) at term. Fibrinogen levels <150 mg/dL (<1.5 g/L) are considered abnormal. Although coagulation test results and bleeding times do not change, these compositional changes result in a hypercoagulable state that, in association with venous stasis and vessel wall trauma, raises the risk for thromboembolic disease. Increased coagulation factors, fibrin generation, inhibited fibrinolysis, and venous stasis contribute to the hypercoagulable state of pregnancy.

E. Metabolic Alterations

Creatinine levels are lower in pregnancy as a result of a rise in the glomerular filtration rate due to increased blood flow to the kidneys. Corticotropin and cortisol levels are increased during pregnancy, with an enlargement of the pituitary gland resulting in a greater risk of postpartum infarction (Sheehan syndrome) if significant blood loss occurs. Occult adrenal insufficiency can result in adrenal crisis from the stress of labor and delivery.

III. HYPERTENSIVE DISORDERS

De novo hypertensive disorders associated with pregnancy are not uncommon, but pregnancy can precipitate or unmask underlying maternal essential hypertension. Women with a preexisting history of diabetes mellitus, renal disease, or vascular disease, or with a family history of hypertension are more predisposed to developing hypertension during pregnancy.

A. Diagnosis of Hypertensive Disorders

1. Pregnancy-Induced Hypertension

Pregnancy-induced hypertension is defined as gestational hypertension without the presence of proteinuria. It usually manifests as diastolic hypertension that resolves 1 to 2 months after delivery, although many women will later develop chronic hypertension. A relatively high rate of recurrence of diastolic hypertension occurs with subsequent pregnancies.

2. Essential Hypertension

Essential hypertension, which accounts for approximately one-third of all causes high BP during pregnancy, may present at any time during gestation. If it occurs in the last trimester, it is differentiated from preeclampsia by the lack of proteinuria, and it should be considered in older multiparous women who present with hypertension. Echocardiography can reveal left ventricular hypertrophy, which suggests chronic disease. Other causes of hypertension that are not related to pregnancy, such as renal artery stenosis, pheochromocytoma, and Cushing syndrome, may need to be considered. If BP is well controlled, there is no significant increase in maternal or fetal complications such as placenta previa, abruption, or preeclampsia.

3. Preeclampsia

Preeclampsia, a multisystem disease that occurs during pregnancy, is defined by the development of hypertension with proteinuria, usually presenting after the 20th week of gestation but possible up to 1 week after delivery. Generalized peripheral edema may develop, but it is no longer considered a hallmark of the disease.

Preeclampsia is classified as severe with end-organ involvement if at least one of the following signs is present:

- Resting BP ≥160 mm Hg systolic or 110 mm Hg diastolic at any time, or 140 mm Hg systolic or 90 mm Hg diastolic associated with any of the complications listed below. Diastolic hypertension, rather than isolated systolic hypertension, is more commonly observed.

- Proteinuria ≥5 g/24 h or 3+/4+ on urine dipstick.

- Oliguria (urine output <30 mL/h for 3 consecutive hours).

- A wide spectrum of systemic symptoms including, but not limited to, acute renal failure, pulmonary edema, right upper quadrant pain, impaired liver function, headache, visual changes, and thrombocytopenia.

4. Eclampsia

Eclampsia is defined as severe preeclampsia with generalized tonic-clonic seizures. In some cases, it may present initially with eclamptic seizures. Although seizures are its most dramatic manifestation, other intracranial catastrophes, such as hemorrhage, stroke, or intracranial hypertension, are more likely to cause death.

Eclampsia usually occurs after 20 weeks' gestation or within 48 hours after delivery, but it should be considered in the differential diagnosis of seizures occurring up to 14 days after delivery. Eclampsia that occurs >48 hours after delivery is likely to be misdiagnosed

Benzodiazepines are appropriate as initial therapy for seizures in eclampsia.

B. Management of Hypertensive Disorders

1. General Guidelines

Patients with eclampsia or severe preeclampsia require hospital admission. Administration of magnesium sulfate for the prevention of seizures, judicious control of BP, and maternal and fetal monitoring should be initiated early. Issues such as intensive care unit admission, management, and delivery of the fetus should be discussed with an obstetrician and the critical care physician as soon as possible. Preventing maternal injury, ensuring maternal and fetal oxygenation, and initiating seizure prophylaxis are the most important aspects of therapy. The treatment of choice in severe preeclampsia is delivery, but fetal maturity must be considered. In most cases of severe preeclampsia that occur after 32 weeks' gestation, delivery is indicated. Consultation with a maternal-fetal medicine specialist is recommended.

2. Seizure Prophylaxis

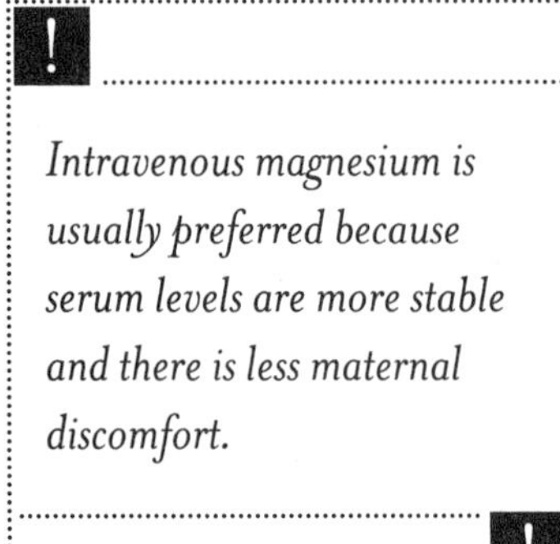
Intravenous magnesium is usually preferred because serum levels are more stable and there is less maternal discomfort.

Magnesium sulfate (20% solution) is used prophylactically in preeclampsia to avoid progression to eclampsia and to prevent recurrent eclamptic seizures. This drug is not thought to jeopardize the fetus. Therapy is usually initiated when the diastolic BP is >100 mm Hg and signs of impending seizure, such as visual blurring, scotomata, hyperreflexia, or signs of severe preeclampsia are present.

Magnesium can be administered intravenously or intramuscularly. A loading dose of 4 to 6 g in 200 to 250 mL normal saline over 10 to 15 minutes is followed by an intravenous infusion of 1 to 2 g/h. Magnesium levels are checked 2 to 4 hours later and should in the range of 2.0 to 3.5 mmol/L (4-7 mEq/L). Maternal respiratory rate, deep tendon reflexes, level of consciousness, and urine output are monitored regularly and correlate well with serum levels. Respiratory depression, somnolence, or loss of patellar reflexes suggests magnesium levels in excess of the therapeutic range (>3.5 mmol/L or 7 mEq/L). Because magnesium is excreted renally, the infusion rate should be decreased if urine output drops. The maintenance infusion should be decreased or withheld on the basis of the serum creatinine level. The antidote for magnesium toxicity is 1 g calcium chloride (10 mL of 10% solution) given intravenously over several minutes.

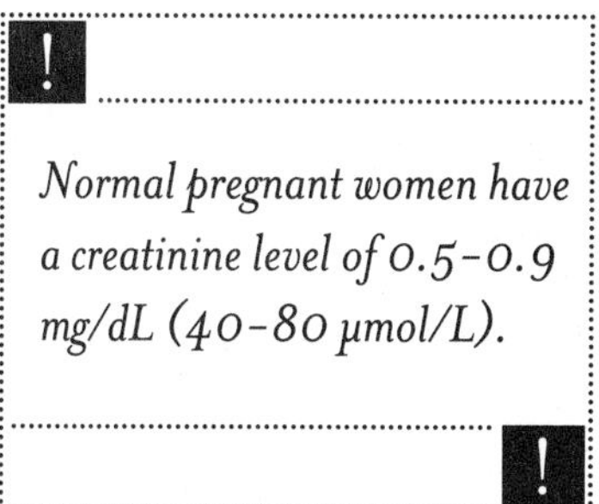

Normal pregnant women have a creatinine level of 0.5-0.9 mg/dL (40-80 μmol/L).

3. Blood Pressure Control

The goal of antihypertensive therapy is prevention of maternal complications such as stroke, intracranial hemorrhage, and acute heart failure. There are no convincing data to determine the optimal BP with antihypertensive medications. The BP need not be lowered to normal levels, although the diastolic pressure should be reduced gradually to 90 to 100 mm Hg. In patients with extremely elevated BP, the mean arterial pressure should be lowered gradually in increments of 10% to 15%. Aggressive antihypertensive therapy that results in precipitous drops could further compromise an already stressed fetus by shunting blood away from the placental circulation. Therapy is necessary if the systolic BP is >160 mm Hg or the diastolic BP is >110 mm Hg, or if the systolic BP is >30 mm Hg or the diastolic BP is >15 mm Hg above the patient's baseline pressure. Lower levels may need to be treated if they are associated with evidence of end-organ damage. Admission to the hospital for acute antihypertensive therapy is recommended for marked elevations in BP or if the patient has end-organ involvement. Treatment in these instances includes immediate delivery of the fetus and antihypertensive management. Intravenous therapy is the standard method of delivering antihypertensive agents for life-threatening conditions.

Drugs that are generally used to treat hypertension associated with severe preeclampsia are parenteral hydralazine (2.5-5.0 mg administered as a slow intravenous push every 15-20 minutes) and labetalol (20 mg intravenously initially, and titrated every 10-15 minutes). If the initial 20-mg dose of labetalol is not effective, 40 mg should be given. If the 40-mg dose does not lower the BP to the desired level, it should be followed by an 80-mg dose. Precipitous drops in BP can occur with hydralazine therapy, particularly in the volume-depleted preeclamptic patient, and labetalol use can result in fetal bradycardia. Diuretics should usually be avoided because most preeclamptic patients have a significantly decreased plasma volume. Nitroprusside also has been used, despite reports of cyanide toxicity in animal models. Nitroglycerin, a venodilator, may be effective when used to treat pulmonary edema associated with severe preeclampsia but is less effective in preeclamptic hypertension. Intravenous calcium channel blockers, such as diltiazem and nicardipine, also may be useful for treating severe hypertension. Although not used in the United States, oral nifedipine therapy for hypertension in preeclampsia has been effective.

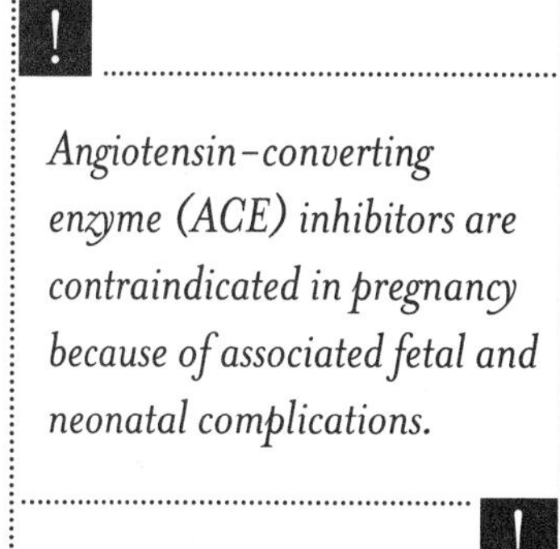

Angiotensin-converting enzyme (ACE) inhibitors are contraindicated in pregnancy because of associated fetal and neonatal complications.

4. Supportive Measures

Cardiogenic and noncardiogenic pulmonary edema often occurs during severe preeclampsia. Treatment includes supplemental oxygen to maintain maternal Pa_{O_2} >70 mm Hg (>9.3 kPa) with Sp_{O_2} ≥94% to prevent fetal hypoxia and acidosis. The indications for tracheal intubation and mechanical ventilation are the same as those for the nonpregnant patient. Because of increased maternal oxygen consumption and a decrease in the functional lung surface area, the mother is at greater risk for hypoventilation and apnea. Intubation should be approached cautiously in the pregnant woman due to the potential for hypoxemia during induction, the increased risk of aspiration, and the possibility of oropharyngeal edema. Usually, smaller endotracheal tubes (6.5 or 7.0 mm) are necessary. A pregnant woman who requires intubation should be approached as a full-stomach intubation. Ventilation with a bag-mask device and intubation should proceed with cricoid pressure throughout the procedure due to the increased risk of aspiration. Because preeclamptic and eclamptic patients frequently have intravascular volume depletion, invasive hemodynamic monitoring may be required to optimize management of pulmonary edema. Central venous pressure values have not been shown to correlate with pulmonary artery filling pressures during pregnancy but may guide volume resuscitation. Noninvasive techniques such as echocardiography may be used to assess cardiac output, volume status, and ejection fraction. Vasoconstriction of the renal vasculature in severe preeclampsia frequently leads to oliguria. Intravenous fluid challenges should be instituted cautiously. The empiric use of diuretics without invasive hemodynamic monitoring of intravascular volume is discouraged. Most preeclamptic women with oliguria will respond to 1 to 2 L of crystalloid without the need for invasive monitoring. Failure of the patient to respond to repeated fluid challenges, or the presence of cardiac or respiratory failure, should prompt consideration of hemodynamic monitoring and critical care consultation. Vasodilator therapy may be beneficial if intravascular volume is adequate.

5. Monitoring

All patients should have the BP monitored regularly, and those who are hypertensive require more frequent assessment. When magnesium sulfate is used, monitoring includes checking patellar reflexes, respiratory rate, and periodic magnesium levels. Invasive hemodynamic monitoring of preeclamptic patients is infrequently required, although it is recommended for those with significant cardiac, respiratory, or renal abnormalities.

IV. HELLP SYNDROME

The HELLP syndrome is a life-threatening condition that can occur during pregnancy or in the immediate postpartum period. Seen in 4% to 12% of preeclamptic patients, the syndrome is characterized by the following:

- Hemolysis: hemolytic microangiopathic anemia with an abnormal result on peripheral smear, a total bilirubin level >1.2 mg/dL (21 μmol/L), or serum lactate dehydrogenase level >600 U/L
- Elevated liver enzymes: aspartate aminotransferase value >70 U/L or lactate dehydrogenase level >600 U/L
- Low platelet count: <150,000/μL

Variations of the syndrome do not necessarily include all of these manifestations. Patients can present with a variety of nonspecific clinical signs and symptoms, including epigastric or right upper quadrant pain, bleeding gums or nose, petechiae, malaise, nausea, and vomiting. Most HELLP syndrome cases occur at a gestational age of 27 to 36 weeks. Postpartum presentations occur in 20% of cases, usually within 1 to 2 days after delivery. One-third of patients with the HELLP syndrome have no evidence of preeclampsia with either proteinuria or hypertension during the pregnancy.

The HELLP syndrome can be confused with acute fatty liver of pregnancy, thrombotic thrombocytopenic purpura, or adult hemolytic-uremic syndrome, and it may mimic or mask severe sepsis. Laboratory tests that are helpful in differentiating acute fatty liver and the HELLP syndrome are listed in **Table 14-1**. The HELLP syndrome almost always indicates a need for urgent delivery because of significantly increased fetal and maternal morbidity and mortality rates.

Table 14-1 Laboratory Findings in Acute Fatty Liver, HELLP Syndrome, and Eclampsia/Preeclampsia

Test	Acute Fatty Liver	HELLP	Eclampsia/Preeclampsia
Fibrinogen	↓	Normal or ↑	Normal or ↑
Glucose	↓	Normal	Normal
Ammonia	↑	Normal	Normal
ALT (usual range)	300 U/L	150 U/L	60 U/L
Bilirubin	↑	Normal, mild ↑	Normal, mild ↑
DIC	75%	20%–40%	Rare

Abbreviations: ALT, alanine aminotransferase; DIC, dissemintated intravascular coagulation

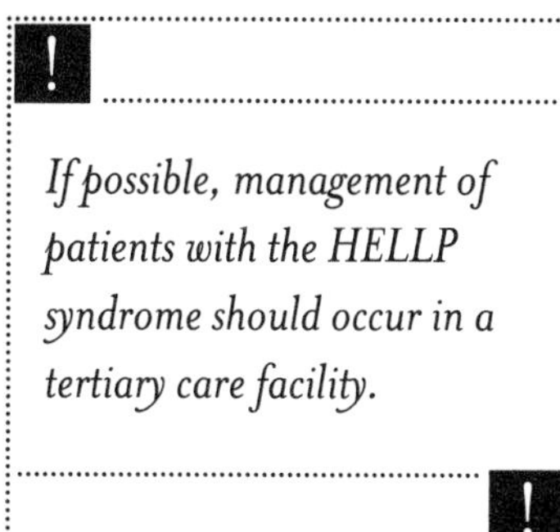

Treatment of the HELLP syndrome includes supportive care, intravenous magnesium sulfate, and antihypertensive therapy (see section, "Hypertensive Disorders"). Dexamethasone for postpartum-onset HELLP syndrome (10-12 mg every 12 hours) may improve some maternal outcomes, although it has no beneficial effect on maternal mortality rates. Early plasmapheresis has also been performed when symptomatic and severe thrombocytopenia continues after aggressive platelet replacement, especially when the possibility of thrombotic thrombocytopenic purpura is being considered. Patients complaining of persistent, severe, or worsening epigastric or right upper quadrant pain should be carefully examined for spontaneous fracture or rupture of the liver. Computed tomography or magnetic resonance imaging can be useful in diagnosing intrahepatic bleeding. Other complications of the HELLP syndrome may include intracerebral hemorrhage, acute renal failure, and fulminant hepatic failure.

V. POSTPARTUM HEMORRHAGE

Primary postpartum hemorrhage is defined as excessive bleeding within 24 hours of a vaginal or cesarean delivery. It is the leading cause of postpartum death worldwide. The usual signs of tachycardia and hypotension associated with severe bleeding may occur late because of the hypervolemia associated with pregnancy. Concealed pelvic hematomas with ongoing blood loss may be masked initially. The most frequent cause of primary postpartum hemorrhage is uterine atony, which occurs in 5% of deliveries; risk factors for this include overdistension of the uterus, retained placental products, uterine muscle fatigue, and the use of halogenated anesthetic agents. The diagnosis is made clinically by palpation of a large and boggy uterus. The second most frequent cause of primary postpartum hemorrhage is lacerations of the lower genital tract that occur spontaneously or as a result of traumatic labor. Disseminated intravascular coagulation resulting from placental abnormalities, HELLP syndrome, and amniotic fluid embolism syndrome may also cause hemodynamically significant postpartum hemorrhage.

General treatment measures include aggressive and early fluid resuscitation and attempts to locate the source of the bleeding. Maternal mortality rates increase when treatment is delayed and blood loss is underestimated. Patients with ongoing blood loss, any amount of blood loss resulting in hemodynamic instability, or a total loss exceeding 2,000 mL require packed red blood cell transfusions in addition to fluid administration. Depending upon the amount of blood loss and the presence of coagulopathy, additional blood products may be needed. Angiographic embolization and surgical therapy, including hysterectomy, may be required for severe uterine hemorrhage unresponsive to uterotonic drug therapy.

VI. THROMBOEMBOLIC DISEASE

The incidence of thromboembolic disease in pregnant women during the immediate postpartum period is five times that in nonpregnant women. Risk rises with increased parity, cesarean delivery, operative vaginal delivery, previous deep venous thrombosis, and increased maternal age.

Although manifestations of pulmonary embolism in pregnant women are similar to those in nonpregnant women (**Chapter 13**), the physiologic changes of pregnancy complicate evaluation. Lower-extremity edema, leg pain, and dyspnea are common in pregnancy and create a diagnostic dilemma for the clinician. If a chest radiograph is obtained to rule out other pulmonary problems, such as pneumonia, the fetus must be shielded. After 16 weeks' gestation, D-dimer values are elevated above the usual normal range and are of little diagnostic utility. Doppler scanning of the lower extremities (compression ultrasound), when available, is usually the first diagnostic test for deep vein thrombosis in pregnancy, but it is less accurate for calf and isolated iliac vein thrombosis. For diagnosing pulmonary embolism, ventilation/perfusion scanning is reliable in a pregnant woman, and it may be beneficial to perform perfusion scanning alone initially. If there are no perfusion defects, the scan can be considered negative. Spiral computed tomography is an alternative method and is more sensitive for emboli in the central arteries and less sensitive for subsegmental emboli. The teratogenic and oncogenic risks to the fetus from these diagnostic tests are not significant, and the potential for maternal death from undiagnosed thromboembolic disease outweighs the risk of radiation exposure. An appropriate diagnostic evaluation should always be performed when indicated. Heparin therapy should be initiated immediately when the diagnosis of pulmonary embolism is suspected and should be continued if the diagnosis is confirmed.

!

Patients receiving heparin are at risk for heparin-induced thrombocytopenia and osteoporosis.

!

The treatment of stable pulmonary embolism in the pregnant patient parallels that in the nonpregnant patient, except that warfarin is relatively contraindicated in pregnancy and absolutely contraindicated during the first trimester, when the risk of teratogenicity is greatest. Instead, unfractionated heparin can be administered intravenously by a weight-adjusted dose regimen to achieve an activated partial thromboplastin time of 1.5 to 2.5 times control. Treatment is then converted to subcutaneous administration, starting at 5,000 IU of unfractionated heparin every 12 hours and aiming for the same activated partial thromboplastin time measured 6 hours after administration. Low-molecular-weight heparins are safe for the fetus and can be used for the treatment of thromboembolic disease. Due to the decreased half-life of this agent in pregnancy, twice-daily dosing is preferred; the dose must be adjusted proportionately for weight change or antifactor Xa levels must be monitored weekly.

After delivery, warfarin can be substituted for 3 to 6 months of total therapy, depending upon risk factors. Intrapartum management requires that unfractionated heparin be discontinued at least 4 to 6 hours before delivery and that low-molecular-weight heparin be discontinued 24 hours before elective delivery. Heparin usually can be resumed 6 to 24 hours after delivery. The risks with intrapartum use include a significantly increased likelihood of hemorrhage with cesarean delivery, bleeding and hematoma formation if a regional or epidural anesthetic is used, and increased bleeding if an episiotomy or operative vaginal delivery is performed. Patients with massive pulmonary embolism and/or hemodynamic instability should be managed much like nonpregnant patients, with careful consideration of risks (**Chapter 13**).

VII. PERIPARTUM CARDIOMYOPATHY

A. Clinical Manifestations

Peripartum cardiomyopathy is defined as systolic heart failure that occurs during the last month of pregnancy or in the first 5 months postpartum. Clinical symptoms include severe progressive dyspnea, progressive orthopnea, paroxysmal nocturnal dyspnea, or syncope with exertion. Signs include evidence of right and left heart failure, generalized or chamber-specific cardiomegaly seen on a chest radiograph, evidence of pulmonary hypertension, murmurs, prominent jugular vein distension, cyanosis, clubbing, or dysrhythmias. Most patients present with dramatic symptoms soon after delivery. Peripartum cardiomyopathy is associated with maternal age >30 years, first pregnancy, twin pregnancies, gestational hypertension, and pregnant women who receive tocolytic agents. The course tends to be more severe in older patients of higher parity with later onset of symptoms after delivery.

B. Management

Initial evaluation of the patient with possible peripartum cardiomyopathy includes a chest radiograph, electrocardiogram, and echocardiogram. Initial therapy includes bed rest, sodium restriction, diuretics, and possibly vasodilators. Patients who present with pulmonary edema and cardiac decompensation often require invasive hemodynamic monitoring for careful and judicious fluid management, intravenous inotropic support, and afterload reduction. Useful drugs include digoxin, dobutamine, and milrinone as inotropic agents and angiotensin-converting enzyme inhibitors for afterload reduction, although the latter are contraindicated before delivery. Loop diuretics can help with symptomatic relief of systemic and pulmonary congestion, but should be used cautiously in the last month of gestation due to their effect on uteroplacental perfusion. If symptoms develop in the antepartum period, consultation with the obstetrician, critical care physician, and anesthesiologist can guide decisions regarding early delivery. Early delivery is not usually recommended because many patients experience worsening of symptoms postpartum. Urgent delivery may be considered in pregnant women with advanced heart failure or hemodynamic instability. Critically ill patients who require inotropic and mechanical support should undergo cesarean delivery. Anticoagulation should be considered in peripartum cardiomyopathy, enlarged cardiac chambers, ejection fraction <35%, and atrial fibrillation as systemic and pulmonary emboli are significantly more common than in other cardiomyopathies. Cardiac function returns to normal in approximately 50% of patients. Those who continue to have symptoms have a mean survival of ≤5 years. Right and left ventricular-assist devices may serve as a bridge for patients who may eventually recover or who require cardiac transplantation as the definitive treatment because of failure of pharmacologic therapy. Subsequent pregnancies are discouraged in women who have no resolution of the signs and symptoms of heart failure 6 months after delivery.

VIII. SEVERE ASTHMA

Patients with severe asthma who require intubation and mechanical ventilation should have the minute ventilation adjusted to avoid hyperventilation and respiratory alkalosis. An alkalotic pH may lead to reduction of uteroplacental blood flow, impairing fetal oxygenation. Occasionally, life-threatening asthma can be refractory despite mechanical ventilation and intensive medical therapy; in such cases, cesarean delivery is an option.

IX. AMNIOTIC FLUID EMBOLISM

Amniotic fluid embolism, a catastrophic event with significant morbidity and mortality rates, may be associated with miscarriages, abortions, and amniocentesis. It occurs most often during labor and delivery or immediately postpartum. The presentation includes typical findings of hypoxia, shock, altered mental status, and disseminated intravascular coagulation; seizure activity, agitation, fetal distress, fever, chills, nausea, and vomiting may also be present. The diagnosis of amniotic fluid embolism is clinical and a diagnosis of exclusion. It should be considered in pregnant or postpartum women who abruptly and dramatically present with profound shock and cardiovascular collapse associated with severe respiratory distress. Occasionally, disseminated intravascular coagulation is the first presenting sign. Other life-threatening conditions, such as pulmonary embolism, sepsis, air embolism, eclampsia, and myocardial infarction, should be excluded. Radiographic evidence of pulmonary edema with bilateral interstitial and alveolar infiltrates is possible. Management is supportive and focuses on rapid maternal cardiopulmonary stabilization (as mentioned previously) and prevention of subsequent end-organ damage.

X. TRAUMA IN PREGNANCY

Treatment priorities for the pregnant patient with traumatic injury are the same as those for nonpregnant patients (**Chapter 9**). There are, however, unique changes that should be taken into account during clinical assessment. The gravid uterus complicates the initial abdominal assessment. The height of the uterus is roughly at the symphysis pubis at 12 weeks and the umbilicus at 20 weeks; thereafter, the height increases by 1 cm each week up to 36 to 40 weeks, when the uterus encompasses almost the entire abdomen. Late in pregnancy, a widened symphysis pubis and widened sacroiliac joints are possible. All pregnant patients with major traumatic injuries should be admitted to a facility with surgical obstetric capabilities. When evaluating the patient's mental status, be aware that neurologic symptoms of eclampsia may mimic head injury. Aortocaval compression in the supine position can contribute to hypotension by restricting the return of blood to the heart. Whenever possible, the patient should be placed in the left lateral decubitus position; at a minimum, the right hip can be raised by 4 to 8 cm to displace the uterus off the inferior vena cava. If any question of spinal injury exists, spinal alignment is maintained and the patient is logrolled.

The pregnant patient can lose up to 35% of blood volume before significant tachycardia, hypotension, and other signs of hypovolemia are seen. Therefore, the fetus may actually be in a state of hypoperfusion while the mother's condition seems stable. An assessment of the fetal heart rate is an essential part of the initial survey and can be accomplished easily with a fetoscope or a Doppler fetoscope. A conventional stethoscope can be used to auscultate the fetal heart rate in the third trimester, although it may be difficult to differentiate between maternal and fetal heart tones if the mother is tachycardic. If available, ultrasonography is effective for documenting fetal cardiac activity and function. Late or persistent decelerations of the fetal heart rate are an ominous sign. If the fetus cannot be examined adequately at the facility, the patient should be stabilized and transported as soon as possible. A minimum of 4 hours of fetal monitoring is necessary after trauma.

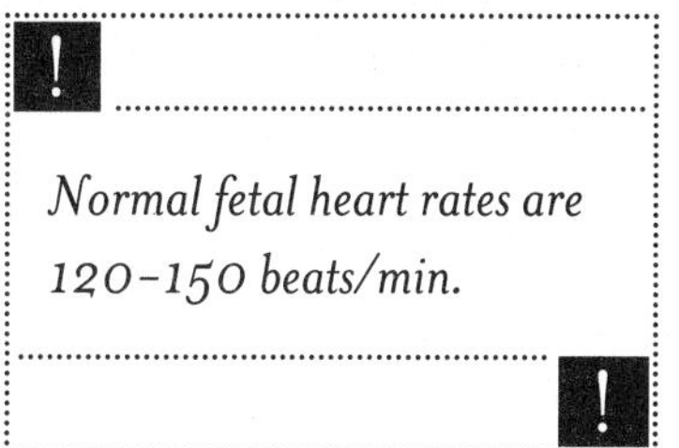

Secondary assessment should evaluate uterine irritability (spasms of the uterus), fetal heart rate, and fetal movement. A pelvic examination should be performed if necessary. If there is any question of blood from the vagina, a qualified, experienced caregiver should do a sterile speculum examination, preferably following a sonographic examination to exclude placenta previa. A manual vaginal examination is contraindicated if placenta previa is possible.

Definitive care of the pregnant trauma patient includes adequate hemodynamic and respiratory resuscitation, stabilization of the mother, continued fetal monitoring, and radiographic studies as necessary, in addition to obstetric care, critical care, and surgical consultation. If the mother is Rh-negative, Rh_0(D) immune globulin (RhoGAM®, Ortho Clinical Diagnostics, Raritan, NJ) should be given within 72 hours of injury, even when trauma is minimal. An assessment of the amount of fetal red blood cells in the maternal circulation by means of a Kleihauer-Betke stain is advised. Obstetrical consultation for appropriate dosage of Rh_0(D) immune globulin is recommended.

XI. SEPTIC PELVIC THROMBOPHLEBITIS

Septic pelvic thrombophlebitis, characterized by infected clot(s) in the pelvic veins, can occur in the peripartum period after vaginal and cesarean deliveries as well as after both spontaneous and therapeutic abortions. Physical findings are nonspecific. Fever that fails to respond to empiric antibiotics in a postpartum patient should prompt consideration of septic pelvic thrombophlebitis. Evidence of systemic septic emboli from sepsis, metastatic abscesses, and septic pulmonary emboli may be present. Ultrasonography or computed tomography studies are not diagnostic but occasionally may show evidence of a clot. Because this is a diagnosis of exclusion, patients are typically treated on the basis of clinical suspicion. Heparin, as outlined previously, is administered in addition to antibiotics. A reduction in fever usually occurs within 24 hours. Anticoagulant therapy is continued for 3 to 6 months postpartum.

XII. MECHANICAL VENTILATION DURING PREGNANCY

The indications for intubation and mechanical ventilation in pregnant patients are the same as those for nonpregnant patients. The maternal oxygen reserve is decreased and significant arterial desaturation occurs if the patient is hypoventilating or apneic for even a short time. Such episodes increase the hypoxic risk to the fetus as well. Mechanical ventilator parameters should be adjusted to maintain the $PaCO_2$ in the range of 30 to 32 mm Hg (4.0-4.3 kPa). Availability of data about permissive hypercapnic ventilation in the pregnant patient is limited, although chronic elevations of maternal PCO_2 up to 60 mm Hg (8.0 kPa) in those with congenital heart diseases have not been shown to be detrimental to the fetus. Caution should be used when considering noninvasive ventilation due to the increased risk of aspiration during pregnancy.

Expeditious delivery in the patient requiring mechanical ventilation during pregnancy is indicated only with evidence of placental disruption, disseminated intravascular coagulation, chorioamnionitis, or severe preeclampsia. It may also be indicated for patients with stiff, noncompliant lungs requiring high peak airway pressures or pressure control ventilation. Delivery while the mother is receiving mechanical ventilation may improve diaphragmatic excursion and decrease elevated airway pressures. Successful spontaneous delivery is possible during mechanical ventilation.

XIII. ADVANCED LIFE SUPPORT IN PREGNANCY

When cardiac arrest occurs in a pregnant woman, standard advanced life support resuscitative methods can and should be undertaken. With advanced gestation or a large uterus, a wedge should be placed under the right flank to displace the uterine contents to the left, improving venous return to the heart. Alternatively, the uterus can be displaced manually to the left. Chest compressions are performed slightly above the center of the sternum to account for elevation of the diaphragm. If initial attempts with standard advanced cardiac life support resuscitative measures are unsuccessful and the gestational age and size are estimated to be ≥24 weeks, then a decision to perform a perimortem cesarean delivery should be made rapidly so that it is accomplished within 4 to 5 minutes of arrest. This option is applicable only when the uterus is deemed large enough to impede life support efforts by significant aortocaval compression, which further worsens maternal hemodynamics. The principal reason for performing a perimortem delivery is to improve cardiac output by augmenting venous return to the heart with effective cardiac compressions. Standard medications for cardiopulmonary resuscitation should be used. Obstetric and neonatology assistance should be sought if at all possible.

XIV. PHARMACOTHERAPY

Choice of medications for the pregnant woman must take into account the potential for adverse effects on the fetus (**Table 14-2** and **Table 14-3**). Certain medications, such as warfarin, angiotensin-converting enzyme inhibitors, diazepam, and phenytoin, have known or potential adverse effects and should be avoided when acceptable alternatives are available. In general, the selection of any new medication for a critically ill or injured pregnant patient should include a review of its indications and pharmacology as well as alternative approaches to management. A clinical pharmacist should be consulted to obtain information about fetal risk associated with drug therapy.

Table 14-2 US Food and Drug Administration Categories of Fetal Drug Toxicities

Category	Description
A	Controlled studies in pregnant women have not demonstrated any risk to the fetus in the first trimester. These drugs are considered to be relatively safe for use during pregnancy.
B	No known specific risks are associated with the use of the drug in pregnancy, but controlled human studies are lacking. If adverse effects were shown in animal reproduction studies, they were not confirmed in controlled human trials.
C	Studies in women and animals are not available or studies in animals have revealed adverse effects on the fetus. Most new drugs fall into this category. These drugs should be given only if the potential benefit justifies the potential fetal risk.
D	These drugs have shown a definite fetal risk in controlled human trials. However, their use may be necessary during pregnancy, and a risk-benefit assessment needs to be performed before they are used.
X	These drugs have shown a definite risk to the fetus and their use is contraindicated because the potential risks outweigh the potential benefits.

Table 14-3 Toxicity Categories for Selected Drugs During Pregnancy[a]

Drug	Category
Antiarrhythmics	
Amiodarone	D
Lidocaine	B
Procainamide	C
Antibiotics	
Acyclovir	B
Aminoglycosides	
Ophthalmic gentamicin	C
Injectable gentamicin	D
Ophthalmic tobramycin	B
Injectable tobramycin	D
Amikacin	D
Azithromycin	B
Cefotetan (avoid)	B
Ceftriaxone (avoid)	B
Cephalosporins	B
Clindamycin	B
Metronidazole	B[b]
Penicillins	B
Quinolones	C
Sulfonamides	B
Trimethoprim	C
Vancomycin	
PO	B
IV	C
Anticonvulsants	
Carbamazepine	D
Magnesium sulfate	B
Phenobarbital	D
Phenytoin	D
Antihypertensives	
ACE inhibitors	
1st Trimester	C
2nd and 3rd Trimesters	D
β-Blockers	
Metoprolol	C
Atenolol	D
Carvedilol	C
Labetalol	C
Clonidine	C
Hydralazine	C
Labetalol	C
Cardiovascular Medications	
Amrinone/milrinone	C
Aspirin	D
Atropine	C
Digoxin	C
Dobutamine	B
Dopamine	C
Epinephrine	C
Nitroglycerin	C
Nitroprusside	C
Norepinephrine	C
Thrombolytics	C
Vasopressin	C
Verapamil	C
Diuretics	
Furosemide	C
Spironolactone	C
Neuromuscular Blockers	
Cisatracurium	B
Rocuronium	C
Succinylcholine	C
Vecuronium	C
Sedatives/Analgesics/Anxiolytics	
Benzodiazepines	D
Codeine	C
Haloperidol	C
Morphine	C
Propofol	B
Steroids	
Dexamethasone	C
Hydrocortisone	C
Prednisolone	C
Other	
Aminophylline	C
H_2 blockers	B
Heparin	C
Insulin	B
Mannitol	C
Warfarins	X

Abbreviations: ACE, angiotensin-converting enzyme; PO, by mouth

[a]Data from Lexi-Comp's Drug Information Handbook, 2011-2012. Hudson, OH: Lexicomp, Inc.; 2011.[20]

[b]Contraindicated in 1st trimester

Key Points

Critical Care in Pregnancy

- A significant decrease in cardiac output may occur with advanced gestation or a large uterus when the patient is placed in the supine position because the gravid uterus restricts venous return and aortic blood flow.
- The diagnosis of preeclampsia is based on the development of pregnancy-induced hypertension with proteinuria after 20 weeks' gestation.
- Eclampsia is defined as preeclampsia with generalized tonic-clonic seizures.
- Magnesium sulfate (20% solution), used as seizure prophylaxis in preeclampsia and as treatment for eclamptic seizures, requires close monitoring.
- Lowering BP to normal levels is not necessary in the hypertensive states associated with pregnancy.
- Anticoagulation with heparin (unfractionated or low-molecular-weight) is used to treat pulmonary embolism in pregnancy. Warfarin is contraindicated, particularly in the first trimester.
- Early and aggressive treatment with fluid and blood products is necessary in primary postpartum hemorrhage.
- Priorities for the resuscitation of the pregnant trauma patient are the same as those for nonpregnant patients.
- The pregnant woman can lose up to 35% of her blood volume before tachycardia, hypotension, and other signs of hypovolemia are seen. This can mask significant fetal compromise as well as ongoing maternal blood loss.
- If the mother is Rh-negative, Rh_0(D) immune globulin (RhoGAM®) should be given, even after minimal trauma.
- Indications for intubation and ventilation are the same for pregnant patients as for nonpregnant patients. Adjust mechanical ventilator settings to maintain the P_{CO_2} level in the range of 30 to 32 mm Hg (4.0-4.3 kPa).
- If initial resuscitative measures are ineffective, a perimortem cesarean delivery should be considered within 4 to 5 minutes to improve maternal hemodynamics.
- When choosing medications for the pregnant woman, it is important to take into account their potential adverse effects on the fetus.

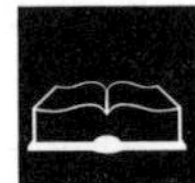

Suggested Readings

1. ACOG Committee on Obstetric Practice. ACOG practice bulletin. Diagnosis and management of preeclampsia and eclampsia. *Int J Gynaecol Obstet.* 2002;77:67-75.

2. Ahonen J, Stefanovic V, Lassila R. Management of post-partum haemorrhage. *Acta Anaesthesiol Scand.* 2010;54:1164-1178.

3. Bates SM, Greer IA, Pabinger I, et al. Venous thromboembolism, thrombophilia, antithrombotic therapy, and pregnancy: American College of Chest Physicians evidence-based clinical practice guidelines. *Chest.* 2008;133(suppl):844S-886S.

4. Chesnutt AN. Physiology of normal pregnancy. *Crit Care Clin.* 2004;20:609-615.

5. Clark SL. Amniotic fluid embolism. *Clin Obstet Gynecol.* 2010;53:322-328.

6. Cruz MO, Briller J, Hibbard JU. Update on peripartum cardiomyopathy. *Obstet Gynecol Clin North Am.* 2010;37:283-303.

7. Guntupalli SR, Steingrub J. Hepatic disease in pregnancy: an overview of diagnosis and management. *Crit Care Med.* 2005;33(suppl):S332-S339.

8. Hardy-Fairbanks AJ, Baker ER. Asthma in pregnancy: pathophysiology, diagnosis and management. *Obstet Gynecol Clin North Am.* 2010;37:159-172.

9. Leung AN, Bull TM, Jaeschke R, et al. An official American Thoracic Society/Society of Thoracic Radiology Clinical Practice Guideline: Evaluation of suspected pulmonary embolism in pregnancy. *Am J Respir Crit Care Med.* 2011;184:1200-1208.

10. Mallampalli A, Guy E. Cardiac arrest in pregnancy and somatic support after brain death. *Crit Care Med.* 2005;33(suppl):S325-S331.

11. Marik PE. Venous thromboembolism in pregnancy. *Clin Chest Med.* 2010;31:731-740.

12. Miller MA, Chalhoub M, Bourjeily G. Peripartum pulmonary embolism. *Clin Chest Med.* 2011;32:147-164.

13. Montan S. Drugs used in hypertensive diseases in pregnancy. *Curr Opin Obstet Gynecol.* 2004;16:111-115.

14. Munnur U, Suresh MS. Airway problems in pregnancy. *Crit Care Clin.* 2004;20:617-642.

15. Oxford CM, Ludmir J. Trauma in pregnancy. *Clin Obstet Gynecol.* 2009;52:611-629.

16. Pearson GD, Veille JC, Rahimtoola S, et al. Peripartum cardiomyopathy: National Heart, Lung, and Blood Institute and Office of Rare Diseases (National Institutes of Health) workshop recommendations and review. *JAMA.* 2000;283:1183-1188.

17. Tan M, Huisman MV. The diagnostic management of acute venous thromboembolism during pregnancy: recent advancements and unresolved issues. *Thromb Res.* 2011; 127(Suppl 3):S13-S16.

18. Whitty JE. Maternal cardiac arrest during pregnancy. *Clin Obstet Gynecol.* 2002; 45:377-392.

19. Yeomans ER, Gilstrap LC 3rd. Physiologic changes in pregnancy and their impact on critical care. *Crit Care Med.* 2005;33(suppl):S256-S258.

20. Lexi-Comp's Drug Information Handbook, 2011-2012. Hudson, OH: Lexicomp, Inc.; 2011.

Chapter 15

ETHICS IN CRITICAL CARE MEDICINE

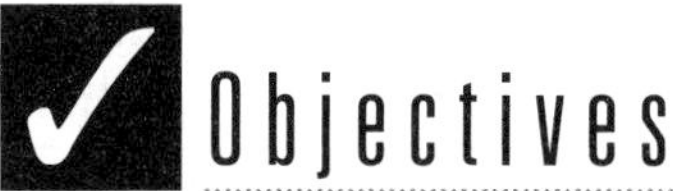

Objectives

- Review ethical principles.
- Discuss ethical dilemmas that involve withdrawal of life support in critically ill patients, do-not-attempt-resuscitation orders, medical futility, and triage.
- Define types of advance directives used to guide care.
- Discuss examples that outline the decision-making process used in medical ethics.

Case Study

A 68-year-old man collapsed at home and sustained a cardiac arrest. Cardiopulmonary resuscitation was not initiated until paramedics arrived 6 minutes later. The man was found in ventricular fibrillation, but he responded to intubation, defibrillation, and epinephrine. In the emergency department 30 minutes later, he is unresponsive to painful stimuli, pupils are dilated and fixed, and corneal reflexes are absent. He is breathing spontaneously and is hemodynamically stable. He is transferred to the ICU, but 3 days later he remains in a deep coma.

- Who should make decisions regarding the patient's medical care, and on what basis?
- What are the goals of care for this patient?
- Should further therapy be limited or withdrawn?
- What process should be utilized to address these issues?
- What potential dilemmas might arise in discussions with the patient's family?

I. INTRODUCTION

Ethics is one of the foundations of laws, statutes, and regulations that govern the practice of medicine in many countries. Application of ethical principles may vary in different regions and nations. Ethics is not identical to existing laws; often ethics is in critical tension with laws leading to statutory change. Ethics is closely related to mortality, culturally accepted norms regarding right and wrong, but is not reducible to prevailing or conventional values. At its best, ethics may lead to substantive moral reform.

Ethics is the critical, reflective consideration of moral practices in light of basic principles of conduct and value. When applied to medicine, this involves critical reflection on practices such as clinical research, resource allocation criteria, relationships between patients and their healthcare providers, and healthcare policy formulation. Medical ethics is at the heart of the patient-clinician relationship, which is grounded in trust. Healthcare professionals have an obligation to act in their patients' best interests, recognizing an inequality of knowledge, information, and experience. Clinicians possess medical expertise but are limited in their knowledge of patients' goals and values. Shared decision-making is one way of productively engaging these differences to produce what is in the best interest of the patient while preserving the clinician's professional integrity.

Focusing on the critical care context, three sets of circumstances typically bring patients at risk of dying in the hospital to the emergency department: (1) an acute event in an otherwise healthy person (such as trauma, stroke, myocardial infarction, or pneumonia); (2) a recurrent or relapsing decompensation in a patient with a chronic and progressive disease (such as respiratory failure in chronic lung disease, pneumonia complicating dementia, heart failure in cardiomyopathy); or (3) the patient's arrival at a critical point in a progressive, unrelenting decline (such as cancer or dementia). Many of these at-risk patients may be admitted to an ICU. Such patients may be unable to participate in decisions about their medical care and depend upon advance directives or surrogate decision makers to guide the healthcare team regarding treatment decisions.

The critical care team is involved in end-of-life care decision-making in three key situations: (1) limitation of therapy and/or resuscitation attempts, (2) withdrawal of life support, and (3) triage. Therefore, the critical care team must be able to effectively communicate with patients and their families about prognosis and futility, reasonable goals of therapy, healthcare advance directives, and options for limitation of resuscitation efforts or removal of life support. Without formal discussions, patients' preferences are difficult to predict; assumptions based upon quality of life, age, or functional status may be inaccurate; and physicians' choices may reflect their own preferences rather than those of their patients.

Healthcare providers must be both cognitively and emotionally prepared to communicate among themselves and with patients and families regarding: (1) realistic goals, (2) expectations for treatments and alternatives, (3) patients' expressed and implied desires regarding medical interventions and the implications of those desires, and (4) acceptable therapeutic options. Meaningful discussions of these issues are grounded in a thorough understanding of medical ethics, individual and collective cultural values, and pertinent legal principles. The competency of providers as communicators correlates directly with patients' and families' satisfaction with the medical care provided and also enhances the professional integrity of the providers.

II. THE GUIDING ETHICAL PRINCIPLES OF HEALTHCARE

In healthcare, ethical principles protect patient interests and inform professional integrity. The guiding ethical principles of healthcare are a conceptual framework for providing patient-centered care (care that is appropriately respectful of patients), and for grounding the healthcare professional standards of practice that define excellence. These principles are also helpful in identifying, analyzing, and contributing to the resolution of ethical problems that occur in the practice of medicine. The four commonly accepted ethical principles of healthcare are:

- Autonomy: Respect the right of an individual to be self-directing and to make decisions freely and independently; this recognizes the patient's sovereignty over his or her own body.

- Beneficence: Act in the best interest of patients and promote their well-being. Different value systems can lead to different concepts of what is best for an individual patient.

- Nonmaleficence: *Primum non nocere*, the Latin tenet which translates as "above all else, do no harm." *Harm* can be defined as the intentional or careless infliction of physical, psychological, or emotional distress through either actions or omissions.

- Justice: Treat all persons fairly and equitably; treat similar cases in the same manner and different cases differently.

III. ETHICAL DILEMMAS IN CRITICAL CARE

Many, if not all, ethical dilemmas can be handled professionally with utmost respect for patient needs and professional integrity when decisions involve consideration of the treatment situation, truthful exchange of information, thorough discussion of the patient's wishes and expectations, understanding of pertinent ethical principles, and coordination among members of the healthcare team. Uncertainty and ambiguity on the part of the physician, critical care team, patient, or family make meaningful discussion and decisions difficult. The team leaders are responsible for ensuring that the healthcare environment is characterized by open communication, caring, and support. In rare situations where some members of the team have conflicting deeply held beliefs, serious emotional conflicts, or conflicts of interest that preclude open and objective communication and decision-making, they may request to be excused and transfer patient care responsibilities to a colleague. Patients and families can sense uncertainty and ambiguity, and are likely to react with suspicion and confusion. A consensus on the goals of care and treatment plan also facilitates consistent communication and documentation and minimizes liability risks. In institutions where ethics consultation teams are available, their involvement has been regarded favorably by most participants.

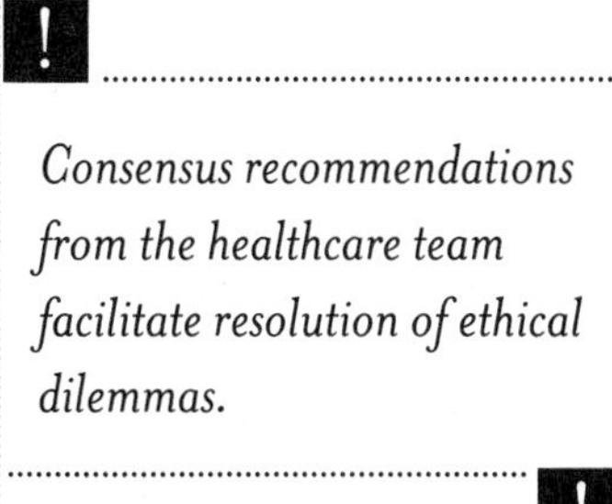

A. Advance Directives

To make binding decisions such as refusal of recommended medical care or limitation of resuscitation, a person must be legally able to do so. *Incompetency* is determined by a court and is a judgment that a person lacks the abilities required to give or withhold informed consent. While competent patients are legally empowered to make decisions, unemancipated minors or mentally impaired individuals may not be competent for decision-making purposes. Distinct from legal competence, the capacity to make decisions refers to the ability to make informed, voluntary decisions in a specific circumstance; because of medications, injuries, or metabolic derangements that impair judgment, a patient may lack capacity. Patients must have both competence and capacity to consent, to refuse, or to limit medical care, as well as to establish advance directives regarding medical care. Their agreement must be obtained without fraud, duress, or coercion after full, reasonable disclosure. The basis, process, and outcome of all discussions leading to such decisions should be carefully documented to supplement any required forms and clinician orders. Unlike consent to treatment, limitation or refusal of treatment is never implied.

An *advance directive* is an instructional statement that takes effect at some time in the future when specific conditions are met. A capable, competent person can often leave verbal or written instructions directly for healthcare professionals and/or select a surrogate to guide medical decisions. If patients have left unambiguous and detailed instructions regarding their preferences for life-sustaining therapy in the event they become incapacitated, such instructions are usually binding and carried out. However, most patients' instructions are neither sufficiently detailed nor unambiguous for the circumstances of their future illness. The role of the surrogate decision-maker is to inform the healthcare team of what the patient's wishes and values would be under the circumstances; the wishes and values, therefore, are not those of the surrogate but of the patient. The surrogate makes a substituted judgment based on explicit instructions or direct and indirect communication of the patient's preferences and expectations. The following tools may be used to convey a patient's preferences:

- Advanced healthcare directive: This document contains specific, substantive statements of the patient's values and wishes regarding medical care. It may also specify procedures that the patient wants to receive or forgo in specific circumstances. In most cases, this document also enables the patient to name a healthcare agent who will make decisions for the patient when incapacitated.

- Durable power of attorney for healthcare: A durable power of attorney is a proxy directive that assigns one person authority to perform specified actions on behalf of the signer. The power is "durable" because, unlike the usual power of attorney, it continues to be in effect if the signer becomes incompetent.

- Healthcare proxy: A proxy is a person appointed by the patient specifically for the purpose of making healthcare decisions on the patient's behalf.

- Next of kin: Under some circumstances, in some countries or states, the next of kin are authorized by law to speak on behalf of an incapacitated patient. Surrogacy hierarchies that must be considered in healthcare decision-making are usually defined by law.

Ethically, the person who knows the patient best is the appropriate surrogate decision-maker. This person may not be the legally identified next of kin.

- The healthcare provider should be certain that the conditions for invoking an advance directive as intended by the patient have occurred before acting upon the directive. Similarly, acquiescing to requests made by surrogates occurs only after consideration of proper medical and ethical decision-making principles. If an incapacitated patient's specific wishes and values are unknown, a surrogate is usually expected to act in the best interests of the patient.

B. End-of-Life Care and Termination of Life Support

The goal of end-of-life care is to allow patients to die with dignity and respect and to exercise an element of control over their death. It is paramount that in all communications it is made clear that *care is not being withdrawn;* rather, it is life support or unwanted medical interventions that are withdrawn after the goals of treatment have changed. In many cases, the intensity of care may actually escalate following termination of life support as comfort needs are addressed. "Do not attempt resuscitation" never means "do not treat." Before the removal of life support, a proper do-not-attempt-resuscitation (DNAR) order should be in effect based on local and institutional regulations. A plan for comfort measures should be developed by the healthcare team and must address anxiolysis and analgesia. Though they may have this effect, comfort care interventions are not intended to directly hasten death; this distinguishes comfort care from euthanasia and physician-assisted suicide.

C. Do-Not-Attempt Resuscitation Orders

DNAR orders, also known as do-not-resuscitate (DNR) orders, are explicit physician orders restricting specific medical interventions in the event of a cardiopulmonary arrest. Because resuscitation efforts are not always successful, it is more accurate to refer to these as limitations on attempts to resuscitate. Such orders are usually based on a patient's expressed or written wishes or on such wishes as they are known to a proxy or surrogate decision-maker. DNAR orders may include categorical specifications that limit blood transfusions, intubation and mechanical ventilation, defibrillation, cardiopulmonary resuscitation in an already mechanically ventilated patient, or an escalation of existing ICU treatment. If such orders are agreed upon, it is usually advisable to review all other treatment modalities to determine if they continue to be compatible with the changed goals of care (eg, dialysis, medically provided fluids and nutrition, antibiotics). Factors that suggest a discriminatory intent must never form the basis for initiating DNAR discussions; these factors include gender, age, race, and economic or social status. Suicidal ideation and treatable depression must be excluded as reasons for a patient's wishes to limit resuscitation or terminate life support.

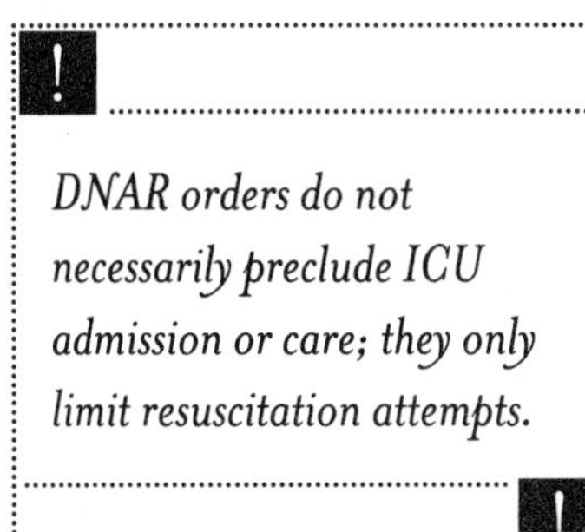

D. Medical Futility

Medical futility generally refers to medical interventions that are highly unlikely to contribute to a beneficial outcome. The key problem associated with futility judgments is that they are based on particular situations. Interventions perceived as futile in one institution by some providers at a certain point in time may not be perceived as such by others at a different time. Futility is also based on the anticipated outcome in terms of probability of survival, values regarding minimally acceptable quality of life, and prognosis or time frame for possible recovery. Thus, a determination of medical futility should take into account the predicted outcome, available medical evidence or experience, and patient expectations and wishes. Futility differs from cost-effective and cost-benefit analyses, which are based on principles of utility and distributive justice rather than strict assessment of the probability of benefits derived from aggressive medical interventions. There is considerable ethical debate about whose views should prevail in decisions regarding discontinuation or limitation of medical interventions when providers and families disagree about the futility of an intervention. Depending on the circumstances, a determination of medical futility may be made by a team of clinicians, an ethics team, or a legal process. Local conditions and policies will prescribe the course to follow to implement a judgment that a medical intervention is futile.

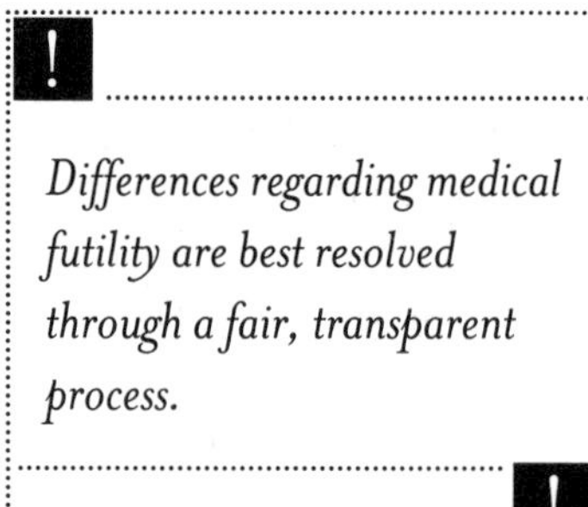
Differences regarding medical futility are best resolved through a fair, transparent process.

E. Triage

The ICU is characterized by resource-intensive medical care. Because the technology, physician presence, and staffing that characterize the ICU are costly and limited, triage decisions regarding the allocation of these physical and personnel resources are frequently necessary. Triage is most often necessary when demand for critical care beds exceeds their supply. Thus, patients may either be denied admission based on resource constraints; transferred from the ICU to another level of care based on severity of illness, prognosis, or wishes; or transferred to another institution. The minimum severity of illness required to meet ICU admission criteria is likely to fluctuate within an institution (such as during influenza season or disaster situations). Increasingly, however, patients who do not meet some minimum objective criteria for ICU admission are cared for on the wards regardless of the preference of patients, attending physicians, or staff. Critically ill patients who are not admitted to ICUs may have significantly greater morbidity and mortality rates. Therefore, triage choices represent life-and-death decisions that must be based upon criteria that are as objective as possible and applied uniformly. The ethical principle of beneficence is applied at the group or social level in such cases (maximize the benefit to the most) and is restrained by the principle of justice (treat all similar cases the same and different cases differently).

F. Organ Donation

After discussions regarding the extent of medical treatments have been completed and a decision to withdraw life support has been made, organ-procurement representatives should be allowed to evaluate the patient and conduct discussions with the patient's family or surrogate decision maker about the potential for organ donation. Options include both conventional organ recovery after declaration of neurological death and potential organ donation after cardiac death. See **Appendix 9** for more information on brain death and organ donation.

IV. ETHICS AT THE BEDSIDE

When faced with an ethical dilemma, clinicians should incorporate one or more of the guiding principles of healthcare into a framework for resolution. As each principle is systematically addressed, specific components of conflict can be identified and their analysis can often be simplified. The clinician should always start with the medical facts of the patient's case and then proceed to related topics. Specific issues may include:

- Which persons it is appropriate to involve in the discussion
- Whether time constraints apply
- Whether the chronology of events or decisions is important
- What additional medical, legal, or social information is needed to facilitate decision-making
- What communication pathways will work best to resolve possible conflict
- What values or rules are important to the patient, the family, and the institution
- What areas of consensus already exist among the participants

Any unsettled matters often can be organized into a series of steps within the process of resolution. Depending on the nature of the dilemma, other experts may be called upon for specific input. An ethics consultant is often able to clarify the ethical issues involved and to work toward a successful resolution of any differences. Some issues may need repeated examination to determine how to provide the highest level of medical and moral good for the patient. Some important elements of ethical decision-making are summarized in **Table 15-1**.

Each patient's situation is unique and requires continual, caring communication and reassessment of needs and goals. Clinical judgment, practical wisdom, common sense, compassion, and empathy are the key attributes required by clinicians involved in any ethically complex problem.

Table 15-1 Key Elements of Ethical Decision-Making

- Whenever possible, initiate discussions with patients regarding their preferences for life support before a medical crisis occurs and they lose capacity to make informed decisions.
- Utilize hospital and/or unit end-of-life care protocols. If such protocols are not in place, healthcare providers should work with appropriate legal and ethical advisers to develop them.
- Direct discussions with patients and families to set appropriate goals of care, based on patient values, wishes, and preferences, taking into account best diagnostic and prognostic judgments.
- Ensure that all decisions related to consent, refusal to consent, limitation of resuscitation attempts, or termination of life support are clearly determined and documented according to policy and regulation.
- Make certain that all end-of-life care decisions are made with full disclosure of alternatives, implications, and potential conflicts of interest; are free of duress and coercion; and are made by persons who are competent and have decision-making capacity.
- Ensure adherence to ethical principles and professional and legal standards of medical conduct.
- Communicate clearly and document extensively.
- Develop consensus and a plan with the care team and, when indicated, involve support services such as clergy, an ethics committee or consultant, social services, palliative care services, or hospital counsel.

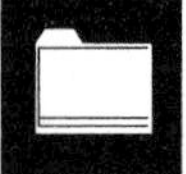

V. CASE STUDIES

A. Case 1: Advanced Directives and Treatment Limitations

A 68-year-old man, Mr. Hill, collapsed at home and sustained a cardiac arrest. Cardiopulmonary resuscitation was not initiated until paramedics arrived 6 minutes later. He was found in ventricular fibrillation, but he responded to intubation, defibrillation, and epinephrine. In the emergency department 30 minutes later, he is unresponsive to painful stimuli, pupils are dilated and fixed, and corneal reflexes are absent. He is breathing spontaneously and is hemodynamically stable. He is transferred to the ICU, but 3 days later he remains in a deep coma.

Analysis

This scenario is frequent in critical care and often involves issues of limitation or withdrawal of treatments. The principles of autonomy, beneficence, nonmaleficence, and justice are presumed to apply in all clinical situations, though the role of each in a specific case may be more or less important. Whenever possible, the members of the healthcare team should reach a consensus regarding their prognosis and recommendations before discussions are initiated with the family. However, early in the course of ICU care, there needs to be a determination of whether the patient had defined his wishes in advance, and/or who is authorized to speak and make decisions on the patient's behalf. The patient's preferences and attitudes regarding acceptable minimum quality of life are essential here. The ICU team should work closely with the patient's primary care physician, with whom the family is likely to have a close rapport. The early involvement of clergy and members of the ethics team may be beneficial in establishing the values and goals of care that the patient would find acceptable.

The care team needs to convey a realistic attitude, using evidence-based data, accepted prognosis models, case studies, and anecdotal experience whenever possible, while acknowledging that all prognostication has a subjective component and everyone knows of someone who has survived as a "miracle." Communication of medical information is important, especially regarding reflexes and responses that the family witnesses and may place great hope in for eventual recovery. Further diagnostic data that may be more determinative should be considered if it may guide the surrogate decision-maker. For example, if the cause of the initial event was a massive cerebrovascular accident, computed tomographic scan data is likely to result in a stronger prognostic stance. The help of a neurologist may be indicated to underscore estimates of recovery from anoxic brain injury.

Melding the patient's values, wishes, and directives with the diagnostic and prognostic information should lead to establishing the appropriate goals of continued medical care. In light of these goals, the issues of tracheostomy, the medical provision of fluids and nutrition, and further resuscitation attempts in the event of another cardiac arrest must be explored. It is appropriate to discuss both possible ramifications of discontinuing life support and long-term care issues. Documentation is important, and the elements of each conversation and the bases for prognosis should be clear.

Finally, if the patient has left no advance directives and the surrogate cannot decide on the goals of care or the appropriateness of specific medical treatments, providers cannot coerce a decision based on their personal values, the guilt of the surrogate, or resource constraints. Continued support and guidance are always warranted; a decision may be forthcoming at a later date. However, when the patient is no longer critically ill and unstable, transfer to another unit is acceptable. The critical care team may then choose to continue in an advisory role, if appropriate.

B. Case 2: Triage

Six months pass and Mr. Hill develops urosepsis and becomes hemodynamically unstable on a long-term ventilator unit. He has not been weaned from mechanical ventilatory support despite continued attempts. In addition, he has experienced repeated episodes of aspiration pneumonia (for which he was successfully treated), has developed multiple decubitus ulcers, and is moderately malnourished. There has been no interval change in his mental status examination since ICU discharge. You receive a call from the pulmonary service requesting a transfer to the ICU. The unit is presently full and there are no truly good candidates for discharge; you reasonably believe that all ICU patients have the potential to survive to discharge. The best potential candidate for transfer is a 35-year-old man with a closed head injury who was admitted 8 hours ago, is hemodynamically stable, and is not currently ventilated. He is in danger of developing worsening cerebral edema and may or may not require intubation for airway protection.

Analysis

This is a triage/resource-allocation dilemma. The demand for ICU beds at the institution exceeds the supply, which requires a caring application of distributive justice. To be fair, defined hospital and ICU policies and protocols must be adhered to, if they exist. The attending intensivist, as the leader of the critical care team, is responsible for determining how those resources will be allocated. The patient with the closed head injury is at high risk for acute decompensation outside the monitored setting of the ICU, and his long-term prognosis may not be better than that of Mr. Hill; however, his clinical course is indeterminate at this time. On the other hand, the course of events since Mr. Hill's cardiac arrest suggests medical futility—beneficial outcomes may not be possible despite continued aggressive care. It is assumed that the family has continued to hope for recovery and has chosen not to limit resuscitation attempts. It is appropriate to revisit the topic of limiting resuscitation attempts, calmly and dispassionately; however, to avoid coercing the surrogate into a decision based on feelings of guilt, the triage considerations should not be a focus of the resumed discussion. The triage decision is made on the basis of criteria that take into account the good of all patients, not just that of Mr. Hill. This is a medical staff decision, not an individual patient care decision. There are three feasible alternatives: transfer Mr. Hill to the ICU in place of the patient with closed head injury; transfer Mr. Hill to another institution with available ICU beds, if possible; or deny Mr. Hill ICU admission at the present time.

Based on the immediate clinical situation, denial of ICU admission may be the most reasonable option. Though patient autonomy must be respected, it is not the preeminent ethical principle in situations of triage. Promoting the well-being of the patient with closed head injury (beneficence) must be weighed against possible harm to the older patient with anoxic injury (nonmaleficence). If justice requires maximizing the good to be produced by the allocation of scarce resources, and this is achieved by refusing to admit Mr. Hill to the ICU, it is the ethically correct decision. Supportive measures for Mr. Hill should continue to the extent possible on the ward. The family should be notified that he has taken a turn for the worse and that best available care is being provided. If there is continued deterioration without a response to therapy and an ICU bed remains unavailable, discussions with Mr. Hill's family regarding the medical futility of life support may be appropriate. Careful documentation must accompany all treatment decisions and discussions. Clergy and the ethics committee may be notified if appropriate. Administrative notifications or advice of hospital counsel may also be needed.

C. Case 3: Advance Directive

Robert is a 17-year-old male patient with cystic fibrosis. He has written an advance directive. After much deliberation, Robert's parents and pediatrician have agreed to his wishes in writing. Robert has been getting progressively worse over the last 3 months, and in the last 24 hours he has had increasing respiratory distress. Robert developed respiratory failure at home while his parents were away, so a temporary caretaker called paramedics, who intubated him and placed him on mechanical ventilation, unaware of his advance directives. When Robert's parents arrive in the emergency department, they demand that he be extubated, that life support be withdrawn, and that he be made comfortable. Robert, who has been medicated with sedatives, is unable to participate in the discussions.

Analysis

Assume that Robert has a clear and unambiguous advance directive, and that he evidenced sufficient maturity to make such momentous decisions. If we cannot make such an assumption, it is important to take a reasonable length of time to validate this assumption. Although he is legally a minor, his wishes have been endorsed by his parents. An advance directive written by a 17-year-old may not have binding legal status, but it is of ethical value as a document that expresses the wishes of an autonomous individual. The physician, when confronted with an advance directive, should always pursue, if possible, the true intent of the document and its validity. The paramedics, unaware of Robert's directive, appropriately initiated life support under the principle of beneficence and made a reasonable presumption of implied consent under the circumstances. However, given the information and documentation now available, it is important to consider discontinuation of life support to adhere to Robert's clearly stated wishes. Appropriate sedation and pain relief are indicated, and the ICU care team or palliative care services should be available to provide comfort care. It must be noted, however, that in some countries or institutions, laws and regulations may limit the ability of the care team to follow Robert's directive. What may be ethically warranted may not receive legal sanction.

Key Points

Ethics in Critical Care Medicine

- Healthcare professionals have an obligation to act in their patients' best interests based upon the ethical principles of autonomy, beneficence, nonmaleficence, and justice.
- When faced with an ethical dilemma, consensus from the healthcare team on the diagnosis, prognosis, and recommended treatment plan facilitates consistent communication and documentation and minimizes liability risks.
- Specific components of conflict within an ethical dilemma can be identified and the analysis can often be simplified when each ethical principle is addressed systematically.
- Life support may be withdrawn at the end of life, but care is never withdrawn.

Suggested Readings

1. Beauchamp TL, Childress JF. *Principles of Biomedical Ethics.* 4th ed. New York, NY: Oxford University Press; 2008.

2. Cassell J, Buchman TG, Streat S, et al. Surgeons, intensivists, and the covenant of care: Administrative models and values affecting care at the end of life. *Crit Care Med.* 2003; 31:1263-1270.

3. Consensus statement of the Society of Critical Care Medicine's Ethics Committee regarding futile and other possibly inadvisable treatments. *Crit Care Med.* 1997; 25:887-891.

4. Davidson JE, Powers K, Hedayat KM, et al. Clinical practice guidelines for support of the family in the patient-centered intensive care unit: American College of Critical Care Medicine Task Force 2004-2005. *Crit Care Med.* 2007;35:605-622.

5. Giacomini M, Cook D, DeJean D, et al. Decision tools for life support: A review and policy analysis. *Crit Care Med.* 2006;34:864-870.

6. Kummer HB, Thompson DR, eds. *Critical Care Ethics: A Practice Guide.* 2nd ed. Mount Prospect, IL: Society of Critical Care Medicine; 2009.

7. Luce JM. A history of resolving conflicts over end-of-life care in intensive care units in the United States. *Crit Care Med.* 2010;38:1623-1629.

8. Prendergast TJ, Puntillo KA. Withdrawal of life support: Intensive caring at the end of life. *JAMA.* 2002;288:2732-2740.

9. Siegel MD. Alone at life's end: Trying to protect the autonomy of patients without surrogates or decision-making capacity. *Crit Care Med.* 2006;34:2238-2239.

10. Szalados JE. Do-not-resuscitate and end-of-life care issues: Clinical, ethical, and legal principles. *Curr Rev Clin Anesth.* 2003;24:47.

11. Truog RD, Cist AF, Brackett SE, et al. Recommendations for end-of-life care in the intensive care unit: the Ethics Committee of the Society of Critical Care Medicine. *Crit Care Med.* 2001;29:2332-2348.

12. West Yorkshire Critical Care Network. End of Life Care Bundle. http://www.wyccn.nhs.uk/Pages/Care%20Bundles.aspx.

13. White DB, Curtis JR, Lo B, et al. Decisions to limit life-sustaining treatment for critically ill patients who lack both decision-making capacity and surrogate decision-makers. *Crit Care Med.* 2006;34:2053-2059.

14. Wueste DE. A philosophical yet user-friendly framework for ethical decision making in critical care nursing. *Dimens Crit Care Nurs.* 2005;24:70-79.

Chapter 16

Critical Care in Infants and Children: The Basics

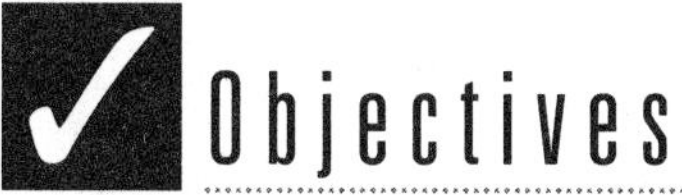

Objectives

- Review physiologic differences between pediatric and adult critical illnesses.
- Evaluate the differences in the incidence of conditions, consequences, and complications between adults and children.
- Identify modifications to adult therapies needed to support children appropriately.

Case Study

A 3-month-old infant with a history of prematurity was brought to the emergency department by her father, who reported that she had nasal congestion, cough, wheezing, post-tussive emesis, tachypnea, and fever for the past week. On arrival, the infant's vital signs revealed a heart rate of 182/min, respiratory rate 72/min, Spo_2 87%, and temperature 101.7°F (38.7°C). She was tachypneic, grunting, retracting intercostal muscles, and cyanotic. The staff administered nebulized albuterol with 100% oxygen. You have been asked to assist in her management.

- What is the most important initial intervention?
- What are the most immediate treatment strategies?

I. INTRODUCTION

The preceding chapters in the FCCS program have emphasized principles of critical care and specific management of a variety of conditions in adult patients. This chapter focuses on the basic management of certain pediatric conditions only. An in-depth review of this subject can be found in the Pediatric Fundamental Critical Care Support (PFCCS) program. This chapter will introduce a key PFCCS learning and management concept that can be summarized with the DIRECT acronym: **D**etection, **I**ntervention, **R**eassessment, **E**ffective **C**ommunication, and **T**eamwork. Each section is preceded by a case study that will illustrate this notion further.

Due to issues related to maturation, habitus, anatomy, and physiology, the manifestations of critical illness in infants and children may differ from those in adults and may lead to different interventions.

II. GENERAL EXAMINATION

Because young children are unable to verbalize specific complaints, evaluation by the healthcare provider depends upon general and specific features of examination in addition to information obtained from a parent or guardian. Although many of the early signs of distress are subtle, their recognition can increase the likelihood that interventions will be successful and prevent more serious progression. If healthcare providers miss these elusive signs of illness, they sometimes assume that a child's condition has suddenly deteriorated when in fact the seemingly abrupt change reflects an advanced point along a continuum of physiologic compromise. Important factors to be considered in the general examination of a pediatric patient are listed in **Table 16-1**. **Tables 16-2** and **16-3** provide age-appropriate normal values for vital signs and blood volume.

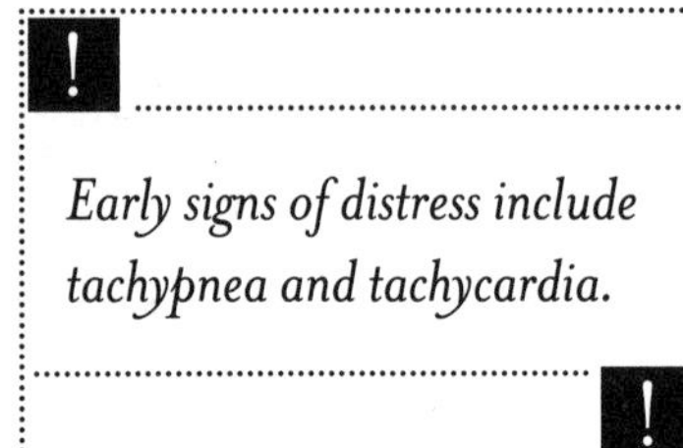

Table 16-1 Important Aspects of the Physical Examination

Skin perfusion: Check for loss of normal pink mucosa and nail beds, mottling that has replaced the usually uniform skin color over the trunk and extremities, skin that has lost its warmth, and the slowing of capillary refill. To prevent an erroneous assessment, capillary refill should be determined with the extremity above the level of the patient's heart.

Degree of hydration: A dehydrated infant may have a sunken fontanelle in addition to signs that may be seen in older children, such as absent tears, sunken eyes, skin tenting, and dry mucous membranes.

Level of spontaneous reactivity and responsiveness: Ill children may have increased irritability initially, often followed by decreased responsiveness and increasing flaccidity. In most infants, alertness can be evaluated by observing their ability to fixate on objects, particularly a parent's face. Infants should turn toward sound and should follow an object horizontally and, within 1 month of age, vertically. Older children should exhibit stranger anxiety and show clear recognition of parents.

Position spontaneously assumed for comfort: Illness may be marked by the inability to find a position of comfort or to find more than a single position of comfort. Patients should not be forced to assume another position, as this could potentially compromise a tenuous airway.

Tachypnea: Very rapid breathing is an important sign of illness in infants and young children. Etiologies include respiratory disease, hypovolemia, hyperviscosity syndromes, hyperglycemia, heart failure, adverse drug effect, metabolic acidosis, fever, pain, and anxiety.

Bradypnea: This ominous sign may be due to hypothermia, central nervous system injury, drug-induced depression, neuromuscular disease, severe shock, or some metabolic disorders.

Grunting during exhalation: Such grunting is ominous and occurs as part of respiratory distress, pain, or intra-abdominal disorders.

Nasal pathway: The nasal pathway is the primary route for normal breathing in an infant. Total airway resistance and the potential for compromised breathing are increased significantly in infants with nasal congestion or increased secretions, or by the presence of a nasogastric tube. Nasal flaring is a sensitive indicator of respiratory distress in the infant.

Early hypovolemic shock: The most reliable indicators of early, but compensated, hypovolemic shock in children are persistent tachycardia, cutaneous vasoconstriction, and diminution of the pulse pressure. The best clinical evidence of decreased tissue perfusion is the combination of skin mottling, prolonged capillary refill, and cool extremities. Systemic arterial blood pressure is frequently normal at this stage because of a compensatory increase in systemic vascular resistance. The neurologic status is normal or only minimally impaired. It remains important to measure blood pressure, as an abnormally low value suggests a decompensated state and requires immediate intervention.

Seizures: In infants seizures may be characterized by decreased alertness (the infant does not regard parents or track an object across the visual field), autonomic changes (tachycardia, elevated blood pressure, and dilated pupils), apnea, and subcortical muscle activity (bicycling movements of the legs, swimming movements of the arms, sucking, or tongue-thrusting movements). Tonic-clonic muscle motion may not occur in infants because neurons and their connections have not fully developed.

Infection: Fever should always suggest the possibility of serious bacterial disease. In the neonate, infections usually involve the bloodstream, although respiratory distress, temperature instability (including hypothermia), and gastrointestinal signs are frequent clinical findings of sepsis.

Table 16-2 Vital Signs in Children

Age Group	Heart Beat (beats/min)	Respiratory Rate (breaths/min)	Systolic Blood Pressure (mm Hg)	Diastolic Blood Pressure (mm Hg)
Newborn	100-180	30-60	50-70	25-50
Infant	80-180	30-40	85-100	50-60
2-4 years	70-140	20-30	87-105	53-66
4-7 years	60-110	20-30	95-105	53-66
7-12 years	60-100	16-20	97-112	57-71
≥13 years	50-90	12-16	112-128	66-80

Table 16-3 Blood Volume in Children

Age Group	Weight (kg)	Blood Volume (mL/kg)	Total Volume (mL)
Newborn	2.5-4.0	90	290
Infant	4-12	75	600
2-4 years	10-20	75	1200
4-7 years	15-30	75	2000
7-12 years	20-50	75	2500
≥13 years	≥40	70	3,000-5,000

III. EVALUATION BY ORGAN SYSTEM

Healthcare providers attending to seriously ill pediatric patients must be able to promptly recognize respiratory, cardiovascular, metabolic, immunologic, and neurologic problems that affect children. Important differences between children and adults and basic treatment strategies are summarized below.

A. Respiratory System/Airway

Airway management is challenging due to the anatomic differences that exist between small children and adults as well as among children of different ages. Recognition and interruption of the progression from respiratory compromise to respiratory failure is fundamental to pediatric airway management. The ability to recognize airway compromise and to establish and maintain a patent airway is essential.

1. Anatomic and Physiologic Considerations

The airway of a child changes continuously from birth until approximately 8 years of age, when it becomes anatomically similar to an adult's airway. In addition to airway disorders related to small size and normal anatomic development, congenital abnormalities can affect the airway. After children reach age 8, their upper airway problems become similar to those found in adults. **Table 16-4** in the Airway Management section highlights some differences between infant and adult airways.

In addition to normal maturational differences between the pediatric and adult airways, there are other important thoracic and pulmonary differences. The thorax is more cartilaginous in infants and young children and is, therefore, more compliant. Increased intrathoracic pressure during respiratory distress is less efficient in augmenting tidal volume because the chest retracts inward, reducing tidal ventilation and indirectly increasing the work of breathing. Soft-tissue retractions similarly reduce thoracic volume during vigorous respiratory efforts. In addition, the infant's ribs are aligned in a more horizontal plane and decrease the inspiratory displacement of the thorax in the anteroposterior plane, further decreasing the efficiency of the bellows effect.

The points of muscular insertion of the diaphragm on the thorax are more horizontal in the infant, as they are in the adult with obstructive lung disease and a flattened diaphragm. Therefore, the lower thorax may be drawn inward during inspiration, causing reduced inspiratory volume. Immature intercostal muscles cannot assist active ventilation for several years after birth; thus, more dependency is placed upon diaphragmatic function and excursion. Compromise of diaphragmatic excursion by gastric distention, abdominal distension, and surgery may quickly compromise respiratory function.

Alveolar size and number, as well as lung compliance, increase substantially during childhood. Tidal volume remains fairly constant through childhood at 6 to 7 mL/kg body weight, but the fact that this small volume must also be available quickly indicates a need for high intrinsic or externally supplied airflow rates. Smaller anatomic conducting airways may produce high resistance if further narrowed by inflammation, edema, mucus, bronchospasm, and bronchiolitis. Such high peripheral airway resistance may also alter exhalation and induce dynamic closure of the airways and auto-positive end-expiratory pressure.

2. Airway Management

The first consideration in airway management is head position. A child who is obtunded or otherwise unable to maintain a position of comfort should be placed in the sniffing position to minimize upper airway obstruction from soft tissues. The sniffing position is accomplished by placing the child on a hard surface and rotating the head back so that the child's face is directed upward. A roll beneath the shoulders can work well to maintain the head position of an infant. In the child older than 2 years, the sniffing position may be accomplished by placing a folded towel or sheet under the child's occiput. It must again be emphasized that, if able, children should be allowed to choose a position of comfort. After trauma involving a possible cervical spine injury, gentle in-line stabilization in the neutral position is used, and further manipulation is restricted to the jaw-thrust maneuver or insertion of an oropharyngeal or endotracheal airway.

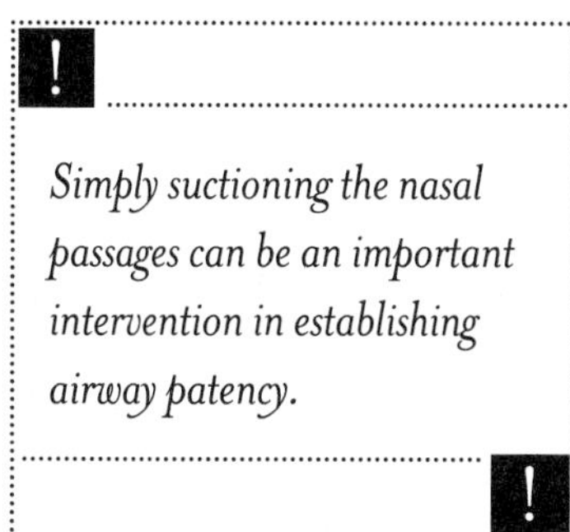

Oxygen consumption by an infant is two to three times that of an adult. Residual oxygen reserves in the lung are rapidly depleted if oxygen availability is compromised, and this situation quickly leads to hypoxemia and its consequences. Because children have lower hemoglobin levels than adults and because cyanosis occurs only when a critical level of unsaturated hemoglobin is present, blood oxygen content must fall to very low levels before cyanosis is evident. Therefore, 100% oxygen should be administered to all dyspneic children or those in whom respiratory compromise is suspected. Pulse oximetry is accurate and should be used to titrate the fraction of inspired oxygen. The mask used for oxygen supplementation may cause agitation in children, and several devices should be available for trial. Supplemental oxygen should be warmed and humidified to avoid heat and evaporative water loss from the airway or secretion thickening. The nasopharynx in infants is large compared to the tidal volume and inspiratory flow achieved, so a nasal cannula will provide a much higher inspired oxygen concentration than in an adult. Issues relating to intubation are summarized in **Table 16-4**.

!

100% oxygen should be promptly administered to children in distress.

!

Table 16-4 Factors in Endotracheal Intubation in Children

- Positive pressure created during bag-mask ventilation may quickly cause gastric distension; a nasogastric tube may be needed. Gastric distension not only promotes vomiting and aspiration but also interferes with ventilation and leads to acceleration of hypoxemia during mask ventilation.
- Because the infant has a large occiput, the head flexes forward onto the chest when the infant is lying in supine position and the head is in the midline. In the absence of neck injury, the child's head should be placed in the sniffing position. However, extreme neck extension can obstruct the airway.
- The tongue in infants and children up to approximately 2 years of age occupies a relatively large portion of the oral cavity and may cause obstruction to spontaneous or assisted ventilation and intubation.
- The anterior and cephalad position of the larynx makes blind nasal intubation very difficult. In addition, the adenoidal tissue may be enlarged. Blind passage of a relatively rigid tube through this area can cause uncontrollable bleeding. This route is discouraged.
- The epiglottis often obscures the glottic opening because of its angle of attachment to the larynx and its relative lack of cartilage.
- Cricoid pressure may improve exposure of the glottis and reduce the risk of gastric distension, regurgitation, and aspiration by occluding the esophagus. The maneuver is accomplished by applying gentle pressure toward the spine at the level of the cricoid cartilage without displacing the larynx in the cephalad direction. Grasping the surface of the cricoid cartilage between the thumb and forefinger and pushing straight down will cause less lateral displacement than is sometimes seen when the tips of one or two fingers are used to push down on the trachea.
- The upper airway is narrowest at the cricoid ring. An oversized endotracheal tube may cause permanent injury to this area. In general, a properly sized tube is about the diameter of the child's small finger. In children older than 2 years, the following formula is used to determine the appropriate endotracheal tube size: [16 + (age in years)] /4.The use of cuffed endotracheal tubes is safe for infants beyond the newborn period and in children. Cuffed endotracheal tubes may be used in certain clinical conditions (poor lung compliance, large air leak, or high airway resistance) as long as the tube size and position are correct and the cuff inflation pressure is monitored.
- A straight blade is most often used for children weighing <20 kg and should be long enough to reach the epiglottis.
- The trachea is short enough that special care must be taken to avoid bronchial placement of the endotracheal tube.

3. Respiratory Failure

The anatomical and developmental factors described earlier combine to produce low respiratory reserve in the pediatric patient. Therefore, the etiology of cardiopulmonary arrest in pediatric patients is most commonly a primary respiratory disorder. The majority of deaths in children (especially those younger than 1 year) involve respiratory disorders resulting from infection, poisonings, trauma, submersion or suffocation, and sudden infant death syndrome. Airway obstruction, aspiration, and apnea are also among the major hazards to respiratory function. Thus, assuring a patent airway is the important first step in care of the child with respiratory compromise. Neonates and young infants are dependent on their nasal airways (obligate nasal breathing). In young children, common causes of respiratory failure include airway obstruction, congenital disorders, infections (viral croup, bacterial tracheitis, or less commonly, epiglottitis), or ingestion of a foreign body (**Table 16-5**). Clinical examination may help identify the site of obstruction and treatment options.

Table 16-5 Causes of Respiratory Failure

Premature neonates	Apnea of prematurity Infant respiratory distress syndrome (surfactant deficiency and ineffective chest bellows)
Term neonates	Bacterial pneumonia Sepsis Meconium aspiration Congenital airway abnormalities
Infants, toddlers	Pneumonia Bronchiolitis Asthma Foreign-body aspiration Upper-airway obstruction due to infection

- Airway obstruction above the thoracic inlet tends to cause stridor (inspiratory noise), whereas intrathoracic obstruction tends to cause wheezing (expiratory noise).

- Upper airway infection (viral croup) and other conditions (eg, laryngeal edema) may be relieved by racemic epinephrine nebulization (0.05 mg/kg, maximum of 0.5 mg in 3 mL normal saline) and intravenous steroids (dexamethasone 0.3 mg/kg q 6 h).

- Lower airway infections of viral origin (respiratory syncytial virus) are frequent in small children and can produce significant wheezing that may respond to bronchodilators.

- The causes of respiratory failure in older children are similar to those found in adults.

- Children with asthma should receive supplemental oxygen, inhaled β-agonist, and corticosteroids (methylprednisolone). β-Agonists may be administered intermittently or as continuous nebulization therapy. The suggested initial dosage for methylprednisolone is 1 mg/kg intravenously every 6 hours. Anticholinergic therapy such as ipratropium bromide maybe beneficial.

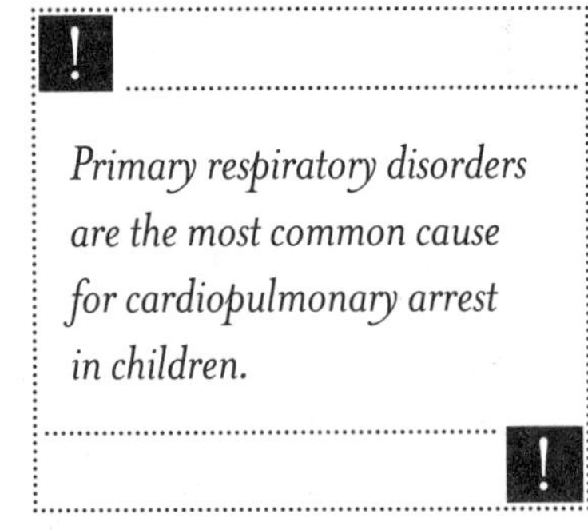

- Patients with upper or lower conditions, including bronchiolitis or asthma requiring low oxygen concentrations, may benefit from an oxygen-helium mixture (30% oxygen, 70% helium).

4. Mechanical Ventilation

The principal concepts of mechanical ventilation are similar in pediatric patients, but specific settings and adjustments may vary. The suggested initial mechanical ventilation settings for infants who weigh <5 kg are presented in **Table 16-6**.

Table 16-6 Initial Mechanical Ventilator Settings: Infants Weighing <5 kg

Mode	Time-cycled, pressure-limited ventilation
Peak inspiratory pressure	Start at 18-20 cm H_2O and titrate to a pressure that provides adequate chest movement and tidal volume not to exceed 10 mL/kg
Tidal volume	Approximately 8 mL/kg
Respiratory rate	30-40 breaths/min, adjust to maintain acceptable $Paco_2$ levels
Positive end-expiratory pressure	3-5 cm H_2O

Remember that tidal volumes measured at the ventilator also incorporate breathing circuit expansion and gas compression volumes, which can constitute a substantial portion of the total volume. Loss of ventilation can occur because the ventilator tubing is distended lengthwise and circumferentially by increases in peak airway pressure that create a back pressure. The amount of gas from the tidal inhalation that is trapped in the ventilator tubing is a function of the airway pressure and the distensibility (compliance) of the tubing. Soft plastic used in ventilator tubing distends more than hard plastic, increasing the compliance volume. As much as 3 to 4 mL of gas per centimeter H_2O airway pressure may be trapped in the tubing at end inspiration. This volume of gas remains in the tubing at peak inhalation without entering the lung and then exits the circuit through the exhalation valve as exhalation begins. This loss of alveolar ventilation is of less consequence in an adult with a tidal volume of 500 mL than it is in a child with a tidal volume of 150 mL.

Increased airway pressure is most often due to increased resistance or decreased compliance in the lung or ventilatory path.

Suggested initial ventilator settings for pediatric patients >5 kg are summarized in **Table 16-7**. If volume-controlled ventilation is used, attention to the peak inflation pressure (keep <30 cm H_2O) is required to prevent barotrauma. If pressure-controlled ventilation is used, attention to tidal volume is necessary to prevent hypoventilation or volutrauma. Always observe the chest rise at initiation of mechanical ventilation and when tidal volume is adjusted. Sedation may be useful with increased respiratory rates and/or increased tidal volume.

Table 16-7 Initial Mechanical Ventilator Settings: Infants Weighing >5 kg

Mode	Time-cycled, synchronized intermittent mandatory ventilation (volume- or pressure-limited)
Tidal volume (SIMV volume-limited)	8-10 mL/kg for normal lungs or 6 mL/kg for acute lung injury/acute respiratory distress syndrome (do not exceed 10 mL/kg)
Peak inspiratory pressure (pressure-limited SIMV)	Start at 18-20 cm H_2O and titrate to a pressure that provides adequate chest movement and tidal volume not to exceed 10 mL/kg
Inspiratory time	Babies 0.5-0.6 sec Toddlers 0.6-0.8 sec School-age children/teens 0.8-1.2 sec
Respiratory rate	Rates vary according to age: toddlers 25-35/min, preschool 20-30/min, school age 15-25/min, teens 10-20/min; adjust to maintain acceptable $Paco_2$ levels
Pressure support	5-10 cm H_2O to overcome resistance of endotracheal tube
Positive end-expiratory pressure	5 cm H_2O; higher levels in acute lung injury for alveolar recruitment

Abbreviation: SIMV, synchronized intermittent mandatory ventilation

B. Cardiovascular System

1. Anatomic and Physiologic Considerations

The circulating blood volume is higher per kilogram in children than in adults, but the absolute volume remains low because of the small body size. Therefore, small amounts of blood loss are less tolerated by children. Blood replacement is indicated when 5% to 10% of the circulating volume has been lost.

Cardiac output is high per kilogram of weight at birth, but the absolute amount is small (~600 mL/min) and largely depends on a rapid heart rate because the small heart size results in low stroke volume. In children, cardiac output remains dependent upon changes in heart rate. Therefore, bradycardia may greatly limit systemic perfusion and is most often an ominous sign of significant hypoxemia or acidosis. Other arrhythmias usually do not produce significant changes in cardiac output unless sustained supraventricular tachycardia occurs. Ventricular arrhythmias are uncommon but, when present, may signify congenital heart disease, myocarditis, cardiomyopathy, electrolyte abnormalities, or asphyxia.

Myocardial maturation influences the heart's response to volume challenges intended to increase preload. Before the age of 8 weeks, infants may not respond to a fluid bolus by increasing cardiac output, but thereafter the response is similar to that of adults. The central venous pressure, however, does not necessarily reflect circulatory blood volume or left ventricular efficiency.

> **!** *Maintaining an optimal hemoglobin concentration for the patient's age is desirable for patients in shock (minimum 10 g/dL).* **!**

Pulmonary vascular resistance falls quickly after birth, reaching normal adult levels by 8 weeks of age. However, the pulmonary vasculature may remain very reactive to hypoxia, hypercapnia, hypothermia, or acidosis, thereby increasing afterload to the right ventricle. Myocardial anatomy changes in such a way that after birth, the larger right ventricle decreases its mass and the left ventricle increases in size and mass. Similarly, the neonatal response to catecholamines is limited until sympathetic nervous system innervation and β1-receptors increase over several weeks. Therefore, the physiologic effects of exogenous catecholamine administration may be quite variable, and careful titration to the individual child's response is essential.

2. Shock

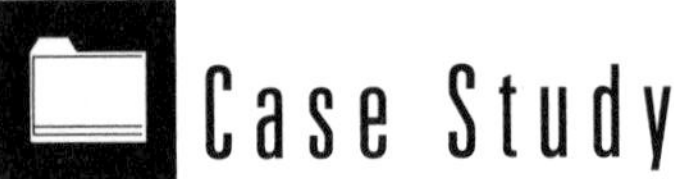

Case Study

A 4-month-old infant with non-bilious vomiting and loose stools for the past 4 days has had 14 watery stools and vomited 10 times since yesterday. He has refused anything by mouth for the past 24 hours, before which time he was only being offered water and tea by his grandmother. The patient was given 10 mL/kg of dextrose 5% in 1/4 normal saline (0.225% sodium chloride) injection intravenously. The intravenous line has subsequently infiltrated.

On arrival, the infant is found to have: heart rate 192/min, respiratory rate 60/min, Spo_2 98%, blood pressure 50/30 mm Hg, and temperature 97.7°F (36.5°C). He appears lethargic, mottled, and pale.

- What is the possible diagnosis?
- What interventions are appropriate?
- What diagnostic modalities are indicated?

Children are particularly susceptible to shock states. Shock in pediatric patients is defined and categorized as in adults (**Chapter 7**), but the etiologies may differ. Timely recognition of the shock state and aggressive intervention are essential to obtaining an optimal outcome (**Table 16-8**). As soon as the diagnosis of shock is considered, early cardiopulmonary monitoring, vascular access, and treatment must be implemented. Fluid resuscitation is the initial therapy for most forms of shock. Rapid restitution of circulating intravascular volume is critical to restore tissue oxygenation and perfusion and avoid end-organ damage. Initial volume expansion with isotonic crystalloid solutions (normal saline or Ringer's lactate solution) at 20 mL/kg is recommended, repeated up to a total of 60 mL/kg in the first 15 minutes. Smaller volumes of 5 to 10 mL/kg should be used in patients with suspected myocardial dysfunction. Although hepatomegaly can be a sign of fluid overload in the pediatric patient, it must be viewed with caution. Disease processes common to children (eg, asthma, respiratory syncytial virus, pneumonitis) can cause lung hyperinflation and displacement of the liver. Other signs of volume overload also should be considered in the evaluation of these patients. If a child with an enlarged liver fails to respond to initial fluid administration, radiologic examination of the chest may help to evaluate heart size. In children, crackles may occur late in the process of developing heart failure, and a gallop may be difficult to discern in infants due to their rapid heart rate.

Table 16-8 Management of Pediatric Shock

Detection	Evaluate and perform assessment of general appearance, airway, breathing, circulation, pertinent history, and physical exam
	Attach appropriate monitoring devices
	Recognize the type of shock (hypovolemic and categorize the severity)
Intervention	Provide 100% oxygen
	Obtain appropriate intravenous/intraosseous access (preferred)
	Administer appropriate intravenous fluids
	– 20 mL/kg bolus of isotonic crystalloids
	– Repeat fluid boluses with reassessment
	Place urinary catheter
Reassessment	Re-evaluate airway, breathing, circulation, and mental status after each intervention
	Repeat fluid at 20 mL/kg
	Monitor ongoing losses
	Check therapeutic end points in resuscitation
	End-organ function
	Heart rate, blood pressure, signs of perfusion
	Mental status
	Urinary output
	Obtain serum electrolyte measurements; monitor hypo-/hypernatremia, acidosis, blood urea nitrogen/creatinine, glucose
Effective communication	Define team member roles and responsibilities
	Communicate effectively with other caregivers
	Promote collegial interaction and knowledge sharing

a. Hypovolemic Shock

The most common cause of shock in the pediatric patient is acute hypovolemia resulting from increased fluid and electrolyte losses (gastrointestinal disorders) or blood loss resulting from severe trauma. Hypovolemia also can result from capillary leak due to intestinal ischemia caused by volvulus, intussusception, or necrotizing enterocolitis.

A detailed medical history should be obtained from the patient's caregiver and/or referring institution. A history of increased fluid losses (vomiting and diarrhea), lethargy, and decreased urine output is usually found in infants with hypovolemic shock. Blood pressure is maintained longer in hypovolemic children than in adults. Capillary refill and extremity temperature are much more reliable indicators of hypovolemia because they may become abnormal much earlier than blood pressure in the child with shock. Children with hypovolemic shock may require 40 to 60 mL/kg of isotonic fluids (normal saline or Ringer's lactate solution). Hypotonic or dextrose-containing fluids are not indicated during the initial treatment phase. A transfusion of packed red blood cells (10-15 mL/kg) should be considered in patients with hemorrhagic shock when signs of shock persist despite adequate isotonic fluid resuscitation. Inotrope/vasopressor support should be considered for patients who do not respond to isotonic fluids. Those with concurrent adrenocortical problems can be refractory to fluids and inotropes and will respond only to glucocorticoid replacement (hydrocortisone 1-2 mg/kg/day).

b. Distributive Shock

As in adults, the most common cause of distributive shock in pediatric patients is sepsis. Other etiologies are similar to those in adults with the addition of congenital adrenal hyperplasia. Septic shock is characterized by changes in mental status, fever or hypothermia, and perfusion abnormalities such as vasodilation (warm shock) or vasoconstriction (cold shock). The therapeutic goal in septic shock is to restore and maintain optimal organ perfusion and oxygenation. Acceptable goals include restoration of the patient's mental status and urine output (1 mL/kg/h). Children in septic shock are usually severely hypovolemic and will respond to aggressive fluid resuscitation. Initial rapid fluid resuscitation with isotonic fluids (20 mL/kg) is suggested. Typical fluid requirements range from 40 to 200 mL/kg during the initial phase of resuscitation. Fluid choices are crystalloids (normal saline, Ringer's lactate solution) and colloids (5% albumin, dextran, gelatin). Vasopressor support with central norepinephrine (0.05 to 0.3 µg/kg/min) is recommended as the first choice in patients with fluid-refractory vasodilated shock. Vasopressin (0.001 U/kg/min) or epinephrine (0.05-0.3 µg/kg/min) may be considered in patients unresponsive to norepinephrine. Dopamine (5-10 µg/kg/min) is recommended as the first choice in patients with fluid-refractory cold shock. Epinephrine (0.05-0.3 µg/kg/min) may be considered in patients unresponsive to dopamine. Dobutamine may be administered to patients with low cardiac output and elevated systemic vascular resistance states (vasoconstricted) after fluid resuscitation. Use of corticosteroids is indicated in patients with vasopressor-resistant shock, purpura fulminans, or suspected adrenocortical problems (chronic steroid use in immunodeficiency, malignant disease, collagen vascular disorders). The initial recommended dose is 1-2 mg/kg/day of hydrocortisone. Early transfer to a pediatric intensive care unit for inotropic support and invasive cardiopulmonary monitoring is indicated in patients not responding to fluid resuscitation. Infants with sepsis are often profoundly hypoglycemic on presentation and glucose determinations should be performed on all infants with suspected sepsis.

c. Cardiogenic Shock

Congestive heart failure is the most common presentation of congenital heart anomalies in children and often precedes cardiogenic shock. Congestive heart failure can often be the result of acute or chronic changes in the heart's preload, afterload, contractility, or heart rate and rhythm. Signs and symptoms vary depending on the type of lesion. Newborn (0-28 days) infants with ductal-dependent lesions (eg, coarctation of the aorta, transposition of the great vessels, tricuspid atresia) will typically present in profound shock with a history of poor feeding, tachypnea, lethargy, cyanosis, thready or absent femoral pulses, and poor or absent urine output (obstructive shock). These patients will require prompt initiation of prostaglandin E_1 (PGE_1) and inotropes in addition to isotonic fluids. Patients with non-ductal dependent lesions can present beyond the newborn period with a history of tachycardia, gallop rhythm, heart murmur, tachypnea, hepatomegaly, and failure to thrive. These patients will often respond to diuresis with a loop diuretic (furosemide 0.5-1 mg/kg) rather than fluid resuscitation and to inotropic support (milrinone 0.5-1 µg/kg/min or dobutamine 5-10 µg/kg/min) and/or afterload reduction. Fluid resuscitation must be titrated cautiously. Early transfer to a pediatric intensive care unit for further monitoring, inotropic support, and a complete evaluation by a pediatric cardiologist is recommended. Other common etiologies of cardiogenic shock include hypoxic-ischemic episodes after acute life-threatening events, near drowning, or strangulation.

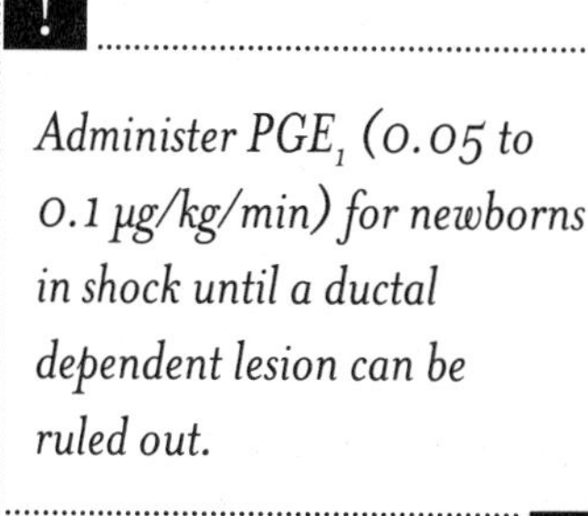

d. Obstructive Shock

Congenital lesions that interfere with outflow from the left ventricle, such as coarctation of the aorta or interrupted aortic arch, commonly cause obstructive shock in infants. They develop signs of shock when the ductus arteriosus closes, thus interfering with blood delivery to the distal aorta. A history of poor feeding, lethargy, decreased or absent urine output, decreased or absent femoral pulses, and metabolic acidosis is frequent. When treating hypotension in a child with non-hypovolemic shock, initial titrated boluses of 10 to 20 mL/kg crystalloid, up to 40 mL/kg, may not be effective. Inotropic support with dobutamine 5 to 10 µg/kg/min and a PGE_1 infusion should be initiated rapidly to reopen the ductus arteriosus and restore perfusion to the distal aorta in infants and children with suspected left heart lesions. The usual dose is PGE_1 0.05 to 0.1 µg/kg/min as a continuous infusion. The side effects of PGE_1 infusion include periodic breathing, apnea, and peripheral vasodilatation, so the clinician must be prepared to support the patient's airway, provide ventilation, and administer additional fluids. Once the ductus arteriosus has reopened, hyperventilation and hyperoxia must be avoided, because both of these conditions will lead to preferential pulmonary blood flow through the ductus and will worsen systemic shock and distal perfusion.

C. Metabolism/Temperature

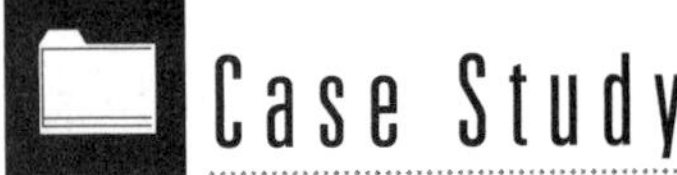

Case Study

A 6-month-old infant is brought by ambulance to the emergency department from his grandmother's house. He has been sick with diarrhea for 6 days. He refused to drink fluids except for water, rice water, and some juice. His grandmother found him unresponsive. En route to the hospital he develops tonic-clonic seizure activity and receives diazepam 5 mg by rectum. On arrival to the emergency department, the patient is unresponsive, cyanotic, and apneic.

- What is the possible diagnosis?
- What interventions are appropriate?
- What diagnostic modalities are indicated?

Pediatric patients are particularly susceptible to water and electrolyte abnormalities and experience temperature regulation problems frequently (**Table 16-9**). The more common issues that can result in critical illness are discussed.

1. Water/Temperature

Insensible water loss is higher in children than in adults because children have a higher ratio of surface area to body mass. This higher evaporative fluid loss, combined with a higher metabolic rate, emphasizes that dehydration may occur quickly. Therefore, children require a greater amount of fluid per kilogram than adults do, but this volume is still a low absolute amount because of a child's small size. Titration of these small volumes usually requires infusion pumps for precise administration and frequent adjustment of fluids to assure adequate replacement of deficits lost from all sites. Several approaches to fluid (**Table 16-10**) and electrolyte replacement help the clinician estimate the actual requirements.

The method most widely used is the Holliday-Segar method, which relates caloric expenditure to body weight for a resting healthy patient. For every 100 calories expended, 100 mL of water is lost (65% urine + 35% insensible water) plus 2 to 4 mEq sodium and potassium. Thus, a child weighing 25 kg would receive 1,600 mL water daily (1,500 mL + 100 mL), sodium 50 to 100 mmol/day, and potassium 25 to 50 mmol. Unfortunately this method underestimates electrolyte requirements in sick patients. Pediatric patients have been shown to develop hyponatremia when given hypotonic fluids within the hospital setting. The amount of dextrose required will depend on the patient's age and metabolic needs. Children who weigh <10 kg should receive a solution of 10% dextrose or higher. Children who weigh >10 kg will typically require a 5% dextrose-containing solution. Dextrose solutions should be withheld in hyperglycemic patients (glucose >180 mg/dL [9.9 mmol/L]). The recommended solution for the previously mentioned patient weighing 25 kg would then be 5% dextrose in normal saline with 20 mmol potassium chloride in each 1,000 mL (D5 0.9% sodium chloride + 20 mmol potassium chloride/L) or 5% Ringer's lactate solution to run at 66 mL/h (1,600 mL/24 h).

Table 16-9 Pediatric Management of Water and Electrolyte Abnormalities

Detection	Evaluate and perform assessment of general appearance, airway, breathing, circulation, pertinent history, and physical exam Attach appropriate monitoring devices Recognize the respiratory physiologic disorder and type of dehydration (hyponatremic), and categorize the severity
Intervention	Provide ventilation with bag-mask with 100% oxygen Obtain appropriate intravenous/intraosseous access (preferred) – Administer appropriate intravenous fluids – 20 mL/kg bolus of isotonic crystalloids – Repeat fluid boluses with reassessment – Start 3% saline 3 mL/kg over 15 min – Administer lorazepam 0.05 mg/kg Place urinary catheter Obtain serum electrolyte measurements; monitor hypo-/hypernatremia, calcium, and glucose
Reassessment	Reevaluate airway, breathing, circulation, and mental status after each intervention Repeat fluid at 20 mL/kg if needed Correct confirmed hyponatremia with 3% saline to bring sodium >120 mmol/L Monitor ongoing losses Check therapeutic end points in resuscitation – End-organ function – Heart rate, blood pressure, signs of perfusion – Mental status – Urinary output Monitor serum electrolytes, hypo-/hypernatremia, acidosis, blood urea nitrogen/creatinine, glucose at least every 4-6 h
Effective Communication	Define team member roles and responsibilities Communicate effectively with other team members and pediatric intensive care unit Promote collegial interaction and knowledge sharing

Table 16-10 Estimating Fluid Requirements

Body Weight	Fluid
<10 kg	100 mL/kg/day
11-20 kg	1000 mL + 50 mL/kg for each kg above 10 kg
>20 kg	1500 mL + 20 mL/kg for each kg above 20 kg

Under normal conditions, maintenance fluid needs are derived from normal urine, stool, and insensible water losses. Stool water losses are usually negligible in patients without gastrointestinal abnormalities. Minimally acceptable urine output is ~2 mL/kg/h for a well-hydrated infant and 1 mL/kg/h for a child.

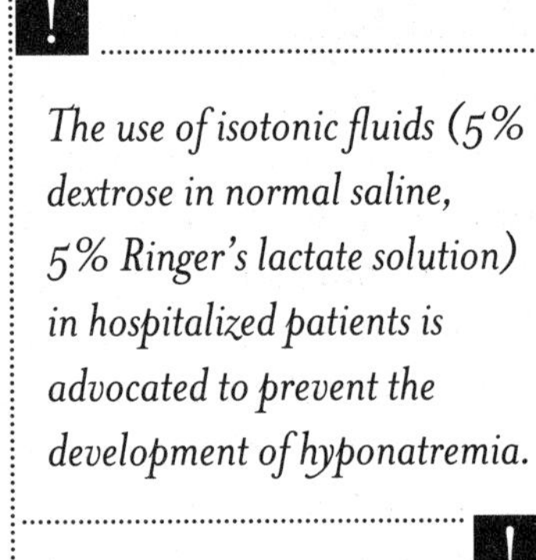

The use of isotonic fluids (5% dextrose in normal saline, 5% Ringer's lactate solution) in hospitalized patients is advocated to prevent the development of hyponatremia.

The higher ratio of surface area to body mass and the decreased subcutaneous fat reserves in infants and young children allow greater heat loss through evaporation and radiation. Maintenance of body temperature is also limited in infants because they do not shiver to generate heat. The compensatory process of metabolizing brown adipose tissue to generate heat is harmful because it results in metabolic acidosis. It is important, therefore, to maintain an appropriate, neutral environment temperature to assure a rectal temperature of 98.6°F (37°C) for the neonate.

2. Glucose

Low glycogen stores and an increased metabolic rate make hypoglycemia more common in infants during stress. A continuous infusion of glucose (5 mg/kg/min) is often necessary. If glucose-containing fluids are withheld, blood glucose should be monitored frequently (at least every 1-2 hours) to avoid hypoglycemia (glucose <65 mg/dL [3.6 mmol/L]). Boluses of 10% glucose 0.5 to 1 g/kg (5-10 mL/kg) in neonates and 25% glucose (2-4 mL/kg) in children will generally correct hypoglycemia.

3. Sodium

Hyponatremia (sodium <135 mmol/L) is the most common metabolic abnormality found in the pediatric hospitalized patient. It occurs when hypotonic oral or intravenous solutions are given to children with increased losses secondary to diarrhea or with diuretic use. Children with cystic fibrosis, adrenal insufficiency, syndrome of inappropriate antidiuretic hormone (SIADH), and obstructive uropathy are also at risk for hyponatremia. Children with severe hyponatremia (sodium <125 mmol/L) will exhibit signs of irritability, poor feeding, nausea and vomiting, lethargy, seizures, and eventually coma and death if left untreated. In children with hyponatremia-induced neurologic symptoms or seizures, 3% hypertonic saline can be titrated until seizures resolve, followed by a slow correction over 24 hours with an isotonic solution. The usual 3% sodium chloride (0.513 mmol/mL) dose range is 3 mL/kg (2.5 mmol/kg). In patients with less severe acute hyponatremia (sodium 125-130 mmol/L), a slow correction over 12 to 24 hours to levels of about 130 mmol/L is recommended. The patient's hydration status must be taken into consideration when treating hyponatremia. Hypovolemic patients must be hydrated with normal saline. In euvolemic or hypervolemic patients with mild hyponatremia, fluid restriction and loop diuretics in addition to the hyponatremia correction might be indicated. Early consultation with a pediatric intensivist and transfer to a pediatric intensive care unit for further monitoring are indicated in symptomatic patients.

Hypernatremia (sodium >145 mmol/L) results from excessive free-water losses in gastroenteritis, inadequate amounts of free-water intake, withholding of water, or nephrogenic or central diabetes insipidus. Infants are more susceptible to hypernatremia. Hypernatremic dehydration can be detected with signs such as irritability, high-pitched cry, mental status changes, hypertonia, and seizures. Isotonic fluids (normal saline) are recommended in these patients during the initial resuscitation phase to correct hypovolemia or shock. In children, the free-water deficit can be calculated as 4 mL/kg for every 1 mmol/L sodium >145 mmol/L. The serum sodium should be lowered no faster than 0.5 mmol/L/h over a period of 48 to 72 hours. Five percent dextrose half-strength normal saline (D5 0.45% sodium chloride) can be used in patients whose serum sodium is <165 mmol/L, allowing for the sodium to drop no faster than 1 mmol/L/h. A more conservative approach should be considered in patients with serum sodium >165 mmol/L. In these situations, the solution of choice may be dextrose 5% normal saline (D5 0.9% sodium chloride), provided an adequate hydration state was achieved. Central diabetes insipidus should be suspected in patients with brisk urine output after severe head injury or recent intracranial surgery. Early consultation with a pediatric neurosurgeon and or pediatric intensivist is advised.

4. Potassium

Hypokalemia (potassium ≤3.5 mmol/L) is usually the consequence of renal losses (diuretic therapy), renal tubular disorder resulting from chemotherapy, gastrointestinal losses (vomiting, fistulas), or decreased intake. In children with life-threatening hypokalemia (arrhythmia, paralysis), potassium chloride can be administered intravenously at a rate of <1 mmol/kg/h (maximum 20 mmol/h) with continuous electrocardiographic monitoring. The usual replacement rate of potassium is 0.2 to 0.3 mmol/kg/h. Serum potassium levels must be monitored at frequent intervals during the replacement phase.

Hyperkalemia (potassium >5.5 mmol/L) is most often the result of decreased losses, increased intake, or kidney dysfunction. Recommended treatment for hyperkalemia in children is listed in **Table 16-11**.

Table 16-11 Treatment of Hyperkalemia

If significant electrocardiographic abnormalities are present (peaked T waves, QRS widening, PR-interval prolongation):

- Administer calcium gluconate (10%) 50 mg/kg intravenously OR
- Administer calcium chloride (10%) 10 mg/kg intravenously via central line

For redistribution of potassium:

- Administer sodium bicarbonate 1 mmol/kg intravenously AND/OR
- Administer 25% dextrose 2-3 mL/kg (0.5-1 g/kg) + regular insulin 0.1 U/kg intravenously (1 U for each 5 g dextrose)
- Administer inhaled β_2-agonists (albuterol 2.5-5 mg per dose has been used successfully)

To remove potassium:

- Administer loop diuretic: furosemide 0.5-1 mg/kg
- Administer sodium polystyrene sulfonate 1 g/kg per dose orally/rectally every 6 h
- Perform dialysis

5. Calcium

Critically ill newborns are susceptible to hypocalcemia (total calcium <8.5 mg/dL [2.2 mmol/L], ionized calcium <1 mmol/L) because they experience a sudden withdrawal from the high rate of calcium intake associated with normal maternal-to-fetal transfer of calcium during gestation. In neonates with congenital heart disease, hypocalcemia may be the presenting sign for DiGeorge syndrome (22q11 microdeletion). Children with hypocalcemia may present with tetany, carpopedal spasm, laryngeal stridor, apnea, convulsions, hypotension, and congestive heart failure.

To correct life-threatening hypocalcemia in children, calcium gluconate 100 mg/kg per dose should be injected through a small needle into a large vein at a rate of approximately 1.5 mL/min if central venous access is not available. Calcium chloride 20 mg/kg per dose may be administered instead of calcium gluconate only if central venous access is available. Maintenance doses of calcium gluconate or calcium chloride may be delivered every 6 hours intravenously or by mouth (calcium gluconate 200-500 mg/kg/day) in cases of persistent hypocalcemia.

Hypercalcemia (total calcium >11 mg/dL [>2.75 mmol/L], ionized calcium >1.3 mmol/L) is rare in the pediatric population but suspicious for an underlying malignancy. Treatment is similar to that for adults: normal saline infusion 10 to 20 mL/kg followed by furosemide 1 to 2 mg/kg every 6 to 12 hours.

6. Magnesium

Hypomagnesemia (magnesium <1.8 mg/dL or 1.5 mEq/dL [0.75 mmol/L]) is commonly associated with malnutrition or malabsorption syndromes in children and with poor gut function in critically ill infants receiving prolonged intravenous fluid administration. It can be seen in patients with a renal tubular disorder resulting from chemotherapy for the treatment of bone tumors. Clinical manifestations of hypomagnesemia overlap those of hypokalemia and hypocalcemia. Life-threatening hypomagnesemia may be treated with magnesium sulfate 25 to 50 mg/kg intravenously over 5 to 15 minutes.

7. Phosphorus

Hypophosphatemia (phosphate <2.5 mg/dL [0.81 mmol/L]) is relatively uncommon in children and is usually associated with malnutrition, malabsorption syndromes, or renal tubular defects. Life-threatening hypophosphatemia, which may be signaled by muscle weakness, respiratory failure, coma, and seizures, can be treated with sodium phosphate or potassium phosphate 0.4 mmol/kg infused over 6 hours (maximum 21 mmol).

D. Immune System

The following factors increase the risk of infection in neonatal patients:

- Decreased polymorphonuclear white cell function and storage reservoir
- Reduced delivery of phagocytes to inflammatory sites
- Decreased antibody synthesis
- Passive maternal immunity that is depleted by 2 to 5 months after birth, and amounts of immunoglobulins comparable to adult levels are not reached until 4 to 7 years of age

Because of their incompletely developed immune systems, children are treated with empiric antibiotic therapy more frequently than are adults. For the same reason, antibiotics are considered an emergency drug, particularly for febrile infants younger than 2 months. Before the age of 3 years, the risk of occult bacteremia is increased if the temperature is >104°F (>40°C) or white blood cell count is <500 cells/mm^3 or >15,000 cells/mm^3. Absolute neutrophil count <1,000 cells/mm^3 or significant bands of 25% to 30% are also markers of severe bacterial infection in children. In such situations, a full workup is recommended that should include blood culture, urine culture, and lumbar puncture, if clinically indicated. The stages of physiologic compromise due to infection in pediatric patients are similar to adult stages of sepsis, with some modifications. The systemic manifestations of sepsis are age adjusted for heart rate, blood pressure, and leukocyte count. Criteria for severe sepsis include cardiovascular dysfunction or acute respiratory distress syndrome or two or more other organ dysfunctions. Septic shock is defined by the presence of cardiovascular dysfunction

In neonates, group B streptococci, *Escherichia coli, Listeria,* and *Enterococcus* often cause life-threatening bacterial infections. The following organisms should be considered in children ages 2 months to 2 years: *Streptococcus pneumoniae, Haemophilus influenzae, Neisseria meningitides,* and *Salmonella.* The organisms associated with serious infections in children and the suggested treatments are summarized in **Table 16-12.**

Table 16-12 Most Common Serious Infections in Infants and Children

Site	Organism	Treatment[a]
Neonates		
Bacterial meningitis	Group B streptococci, *Escherichia coli* (and other enteric gram-negative organisms)	Cefotaxime 50 mg/kg/dose
	Listeria and *Enterococcus*	Ampicillin 50 mg/kg/dose
Viral meningitis	Neonatal HSV and HSV encephalitis	Acyclovir 15 mg/kg/dose
Children		
Bacterial meningitis	*Haemophilus influenzae,* *Streptococcus pneumoniae,* *Neisseria meningitidis,* *Salmonella*	Cefotaxime 50 mg/kg OR ceftriaxone 50 mg/kg; dexamethasone 0.15 mg/kg for *H influenzae* and *S pneumoniae*
Viral meningitis	HSV encephalitis	Acyclovir 15 mg/kg
Epiglottitis	*H influenzae*	Cefotaxime 50 mg/kg OR ceftriaxone 50 mg/kg
Bacterial tracheitis	*Staphylococcus* *Streptococcus* *Moraxella catarrhalis*	Nafcillin 50 mg/kg/dose OR clindamycin 10 mg/kg/dose and cefotaxime 50 mg/kg/dose
Retropharyngeal abscess	*Staphylococcus aureus* Group A streptococci (may be mixed infection) Gram-negative enteric organisms Anaerobes	Nafcillin 50 mg/kg OR Clindamycin 10 mg/kg and gentamicin 2.5 mg/kg OR ampicillin/sulbactam 50-100 mg/kg (based on application) and gentamicin 2.5 mg/kg
Croup	Parainfluenza Influenza	Supportive care
Peritonitis	Gram-negative organisms: *Escherichia coli, Klebsiella* Gram-positive organisms: Pneumococcus, *Staphylococcus,* α-hemolytic *Streptococcus,* *Enterococcus* Anaerobes: *Bacteroides*	Cefotaxime 50 mg/kg, clindamycin 10 mg/kg, and ampicillin 50 mg/kg OR ampicillin 50 mg/kg, gentamicin 2.5 mg/kg, and clindamycin or metronidazole 7.5 mg/kg

Table 16-12 Most Common Serious Infections in Infants and Children (continued)

Children		
Immunocompromised patients	Gram-positive organisms: coagulase-negative *Staphylococcus*, α-hemolytic *Streptococcus, Enterococcus,* coryneform bacteria	Vancomycin 10-15 mg/kg
	Gram-negative organisms: *Klebsiella, Bacillus, Pseudomonas, E coli*	Cefepime 50 mg/kg OR ceftazidime 50 mg/kg
	Fungi: *Candida, Aspergillus*	Fluconazole: Loading dose 10 mg/kg; maximum loading dose 400 mg Amphotericin B: 0.25-1 mg/kg/day OR caspofungin: 50 mg/m²/dose q 24 h; maximum dose 50 mg

Abbreviation: HSV, herpes simplex virus
[a]These recommendations are general guidelines only. Specific antibiotic choices should be individualized, taking into consideration clinical circumstances (renal function, liver function), patient age, immunization status, and local microbial virulence, sensitivities, and patterns of resistance. The antibiotic closing interval and frequency should be discussed with a pediatric intensivist or pediatric infectious disease expert.

E. Nervous System

The Glasgow Coma Scale (GCS) is difficult to apply in children, even when it is adapted for age, as shown in **Table 16-13** (see **Chapter 8** for adult GCS). When assessing the need for further intervention, careful attention should be paid to the pupillary responses, the patient's ability to maintain the airway, the motor score, and the fontanelle fullness in infants. Any young child with a depressed level of consciousness, seizures, and/or coma should be evaluated for the possibility of occult trauma (eg, child abuse, especially shaken baby syndrome), even if there are no outward signs of injury. Infectious, metabolic, or toxic etiologies also should be considered. Boluses of 10% glucose in neonates and 25% glucose in children will generally correct hypoglycemia-induced coma and/or seizures (see earlier section). Hyponatremia, hypoglycemia, and hypocalcemia should be considered in small children with seizures. Diazepam may be administered rectally to children with ongoing seizure activity and no intravenous access (0.5 mg/kg per dose; use injectable or gel preparation). Lorazepam, midazolam, or diazepam can be used in the initial treatment of seizures at a dose of 0.05 to 0.1 mg/kg given intravenously. Subsequently, a full intravenous loading dose of phenytoin or fosphenytoin 15 to 20 mg/kg should be administered if a second dose of benzodiazepine is ineffective. If the patient is already on phenytoin or the loading dose was ineffective, phenobarbital 15 to 20 mg/kg per dose should be

> **!** *Early airway intervention and close neurologic monitoring is recommended in children with seizures.* **!**

considered. The physician caring for these patients should be aware of the cumulative respiratory depression potential of these medications and the resulting need for early airway support. Endotracheal intubation and general anesthesia should be considered in the event that seizures persist despite adequate treatment. Neuromuscular blocking agents are used only to facilitate endotracheal intubation. Early consultation with a pediatric neurologist and pediatric intensivist is recommended.

Table 16-13 Glasgow Coma Scale Modified for Infants and Children

Clinical Parameter	Infants (Ages 0-12 Months)	Children (Ages 1-5 Years)	Points[a]
Eye opening	Spontaneous	Spontaneous	4
	Response to speech	Response to speech	3
	Response to pain	Response to pain	2
	No response	No response	1
Verbal response	Coos/babbles	Appropriate words	5
	Irritable cries	Inappropriate words	4
	Cries	Persistent cry	3
	Moans	Grunts	2
	No response	No response	1
Best motor response	Normal	Spontaneous	6
	Withdraws to touch	Localized pain	5
	Withdraws from pain	Withdraws from pain	4
	Flexor response	Flexor response	3
	Extensor response	Extensor response	2
	No response	No response	1

[a]Total Glasgow Coma Scale score = eye + verbal + motor points; best possible score = 15; worst possible score = 3

The unique features in the care of infants and children highlight the very small margin for error in treating critically ill or injured pediatric patients. Specialty consultation should, therefore, be requested early.

Key Points

Critical Care in Infants and Children: The Basics

- Irritability is an early sign of changes in mental status in the young child.
- In children, early signs of respiratory distress include tachypnea, grunting, and nasal flaring.
- Ensuring a patent airway is the most important first step in treating a child with respiratory compromise.
- Important airway anatomic differences between a child and an adult must be considered when intubating an infant or child.
- Suggested initial ventilator settings for children are tidal volume 8 to 10 mL/kg in normal lungs and 6 mL/kg in acute lung injury or acute respiratory distress syndrome. Respiratory rates in children may need to be higher than those in adults to maintain acceptable $Paco_2$ levels.
- The perfusion status in children is best assessed initially by capillary refill and extremity temperature. Hypotension is a late finding in children with shock. Those with hypovolemic shock may require 40 to 60 mL/kg of isotonic fluids (normal saline, Ringer's lactate solution).
- Vasopressor support with norepinephrine is indicated in patients with fluid-refractory vasodilated shock. Dopamine is indicated in patients with low cardiac output (vasoconstricted shock) after adequate fluid resuscitation is delivered.
- Obstructive shock in infants is commonly caused by congenital lesions that interfere with outflow from the left ventricle, such as coarctation of the aorta or interrupted aortic arch.
- Intracranial hemorrhage in the young infant can cause hemodynamically significant blood loss.
- Hypoglycemia is common in infants during stress and must be corrected promptly.
- Infants do not maintain body temperature well, and care must be taken to avoid hypothermia.
- Young infants are at increased risk of infection due to their immature immune systems.
- Empiric antibiotics are considered an emergency drug for febrile infants younger than 2 months.
- Diazepam may be administered rectally to children with ongoing seizure activity and no intravenous access.

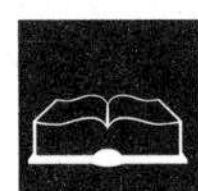

Suggested Readings

1. Brierley J, Carcillo JA, Choong K, et al. Clinical practice parameters for hemodynamic support of pediatric and neonatal septic shock: 2007 update from the American College of Critical Care Medicine. *Crit Care Med.* 2009;37:666–688.

2. Goldstein B, Giroir B, Randolph A, and International Consensus Conference on Pediatric Sepsis. International pediatric sepsis consensus conference: Definitions for sepsis and organ dysfunction in pediatrics. *Pediatr Crit Care Med.* 2005;6:2-8.

3. Mejia R, Greenwald B, Fields A, et al, eds. *Pediatric Fundamental Critical Care Support.* 1st ed. Mount Prospect, IL: Society of Critical Care Medicine; 2008.

4. Smith L, Hernan L. Shock states. In: Fuhrman BP, Zimmerman JJ, eds. *Pediatric Critical Care.* 3rd ed. St. Louis, MO: Mosby; 2006:394.

5. Thompson AE. Pediatric airway management. In: Fuhrman BP, Zimmerman JJ, eds. *Pediatric Critical Care.* 3rd ed. St. Louis, MO: Mosby; 2006:485.

6. Wood EG, Lynch RE. Electrolyte management in pediatric critical illness. In: Fuhrman BP, Zimmerman JJ, eds. *Pediatric Critical Care.* 3rd ed. St. Louis, MO: Mosby; 2006:939.

Appendix 1

Rapid Response System

I. Introduction

Rapid response systems (RRS) have emerged as important resources that focus on the hospitalized patient with unexpected sudden deterioration in condition from any cause. Typically, crisis teams are activated only after a significant event occurs, like cardiac arrest. Previously, there was no organized approach to rescuing the at-risk hospitalized patient in order to prevent an untoward event. Most patients who have a cardiac arrest while in the hospital demonstrate identifiable signs of deterioration during the previous 8 hours. These serious events are neither sudden nor unpredictable in the vast majority of cases. Early recognition of deterioration and timely intervention can reduce the incidence of cardiac arrest or need for intensive care.

Unfortunately, the early indicators of clinical deterioration can be difficult to identify. Assessing a patient's physiologic reserve is challenging. Rapid response systems bring additional experienced providers with advanced monitoring tools to the patient's bedside. If needed, more advanced monitoring and therapy can be initiated immediately, and a decision can be made about the most appropriate care level. The most important action in the process is the call for help.

The RRS model can be divided into four components, each of which plays an integral role in the success of the system (**Figure A1-1**). The administrative arm oversees appropriate staffing and resourcing of the team, drafts protocols and guidelines, and ensures staff education regarding the presence and utility of the service. The afferent arm is composed of methods and personnel to detect impending deterioration, while the efferent arm is focused on rendering therapy and mobilizing additional resources quickly. Lastly, the performance improvement arm seeks to identify recurrent patterns of deterioration and assess improvement in quality measures following system-wide interventions.

Figure A1-1. Rapid Response System Structure[a]

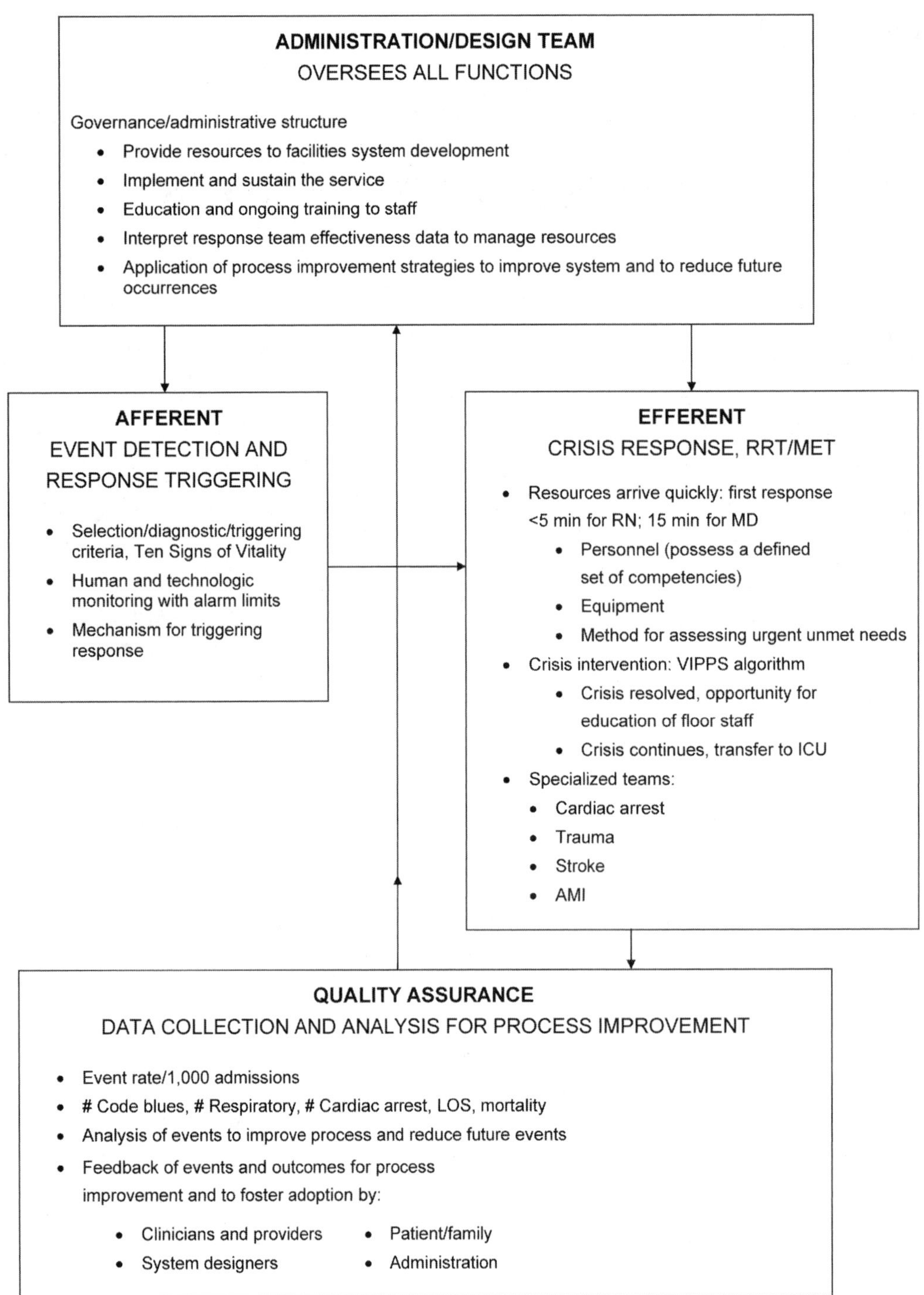

Abbreviations: RRT, rapid response team; MET, medical emergency team; RN, nurse; MD, physician; VIPPS, ventilation, infusion of volume, pressors/pump, pharmacy, and specific interventions; AMI, acute myocardial infarction; LOS, length of stay.

[a]Adapted from Sebat F, ed. *Designing, Implementing, and Enhancing a Rapid Response System.* Mount Prospect, IL: Society of Critical Care Medicine; 2009:41.

II. BUILDING A MEDICAL EMERGENCY OR RAPID RESPONSE TEAM

A rapid response team (RRT) is the intervention limb of the RRS. By consensus, a medical emergency team (MET) is led by a prescribing clinician (physician or mid-level provider) where an RRT is a led by a nurse and/or respiratory therapist (non-prescribing clinician).

A. Composition of a Medical Emergency or Rapid Response Team

Although there is no one perfect team composition, the most successful METs and RRTs have been developed by leveraging existing hospital resources and targeting them at a particular at-risk patient population. Multidisciplinary, physician-led teams (METs) are prevalent in academic centers with training programs. Nurse-led or nurse–respiratory therapist teams (RRTs) with physician backup (or medical control similar to the emergency medical services model) are more often found in community hospitals without training programs. Regardless of the team composition, effective teamwork skills are essential to the success of the program. The implementation of standardized protocols or standing orders will allow the team to use evidence-based best practices to address commonly identified clinical issues, especially in circumstances where there is difficulty contacting the responsible physician. The RRS administrative leadership should develop these protocols and standing orders in accordance with institutional policies and procedures. Possible members of an MET or RRT are identified in **Table A1-1**.

Table A1-1 Possible Members of a Medical Emergency or Rapid Response Team

Physicians	
Attending, fellow, resident	Intensivist, hospitalist, emergency medicine physician, anesthesiologist, pulmonologist, surgeon, internist
Mid-level providers	
Nurse practitioner, physician assistant	
Nurses	
Staff, advanced practice, clinical nurse specialist	Intensive care unit nurse, postanesthesia care unit nurse, emergency department nurse, telemetry unit nurse, certified registered nurse anesthetist, nursing supervisor
Other providers	Respiratory therapist, electrocardiography technician, emergency medical technician-paramedic

At an academic hospital, the composition of the responding team may include the following combinations of caregivers:

- ICU attending and/or fellow, ICU nurse, respiratory therapist, pharmacist
- Medicine resident or mid-level provider, ICU nurse, respiratory therapist
- ICU nurse, respiratory therapist, physician (backup)

At a non-teaching hospital, the team may consist of one of the following combinations:

- Emergency department physician or mid-level provider, ICU nurse, respiratory therapist
- Emergency department nurse, ICU nurse, respiratory therapist
- Postanesthesia care unit nurse, respiratory therapist, physician (backup)

Typically, physician members are trained (or are training) in critical care or emergency medicine. They bring their knowledge of critical illness and skills in the management of life-threatening problems to the patient's bedside. Nurse members usually have many years of bedside experience and most often have extensive critical care training. Team members from other disciplines add value to the MET or RRT with their knowledge of such factors as airway and respiratory management, drug therapies, traumatic injury management, and critical care transport.

Team members usually are expected to maintain current provider status in basic and advanced cardiac life support, pediatric advanced life support (where applicable), and fundamental critical care. Periodic teamwork exercises in mock events or medical simulation centers can hone members' evaluation and management skills. Treatment protocols and standing orders should be reviewed and amended based on feedback from MET or RRT calls and quality improvement data.

B. Response Team Equipment

The use of advanced physiologic monitors and equipment by appropriately trained MET members can provide crucial support to the at-risk patient. This can greatly enhance the team's ability to evaluate and manage signs and symptoms of clinical deterioration. Clearly, the earlier clinical abnormalities are identified and addressed, the greater the potential for a positive outcome and, often, the simpler the needed intervention. The MET or RRT should first evaluate the resources that are readily available in the areas it will support and then create a list of additional needed equipment. The response team must have access to cardiac, respiratory, and simple hemodynamic monitors. Other equipment and medications should be selected based on the patient populations served, the team composition, and local regulations and policies. Since the MET or RRT is expected to respond quickly, any additional needed equipment and supplies should be organized in appropriate bags or carts that can be readily transported to the patient. See **Table A1-2**.

Table A1-2 Medical Emergency Team Equipment List[a]

Physiologic Monitors	Cardiovascular Equipment
Monitor/defibrillator with external pacing capability	Manual blood pressure device
Noninvasive blood pressure device	IV administration kits
Pulse oximetry	IV catheters
Portable capnography (if available)	
Respiratory Equipment	**Miscellaneous**
Portable oxygen tank	Personal protective equipment
Portable suction device	Sterile gloves
High-flow oxygen reservoir face mask	Dressings and bandages
Bag-mask device	Antiseptics
Ventimask®, nasal cannula, and simple face mask	
Nebulizer mask	**Drug Bag (as appropriate for scope of practice)**
Oropharyngeal/nasopharyngeal airways	Vasopressors
Laryngeal mask airways	Inotropes
Laryngoscopes and blades	Vasodilators
Endotracheal tubes with stylets	Sedatives and analgesics
Cricothyrotomy catheter kit	Bronchodilators
Stethoscope	Crystalloid and colloid IV fluid
	Aspirin

[a]Needed equipment and supplies should be available on the patient unit or carried by the team.

III. ACTIVATING THE MEDICAL EMERGENCY OR RAPID RESPONSE TEAM

A. Activation Criteria and Triggers

The most important activation criterion is the concern of the bedside staff or family that something is wrong, even if other indicators are within acceptable limits. This intuition is often quite sensitive and warrants additional assessment. The fact that an intuition or a gut feeling is not very specific should not discourage activation of the MET or RRT.

The distribution of a predefined set of MET or RRT activation criteria may help to focus attention on important early indicators and empower the bedside staff to call for help early. The criteria may be based on the detection of acute changes in physiology, organ system–specific signs and symptoms, and event triggers. Acute changes in physiology may include changes in vital signs that exceed predefined limits, like tachycardia, tachypnea, hypotension, and oliguria. The detection of one or more indicators of organ system dysfunction may trigger activation of the response team. Such pattern recognition may be more effective in detecting clinical deterioration when there is a more gradual change in physiologic variables.

Event triggers help emphasize that some patient incidents or interventions warrant further evaluation. The event may be a sign or a result of a larger issue that could be an ongoing threat to the patient's safety. For example, any administration of naloxone is an indicator that one or more undesirable side effects of opiates may be present. Although naloxone may temporarily reverse these side effects, they can recur as the antagonist effects wane. A more focused evaluation by the MET or RRT may avoid the undesirable consequences of these events. Models of activation criteria and event triggers are presented in **Table A1-3**.

Table A1-3 Models of Activation Criteria

Acute Physiologic Criteria

Acute change in heart rate to <40 or >130 beats/min

Acute change in systolic blood pressure to <90 mm Hg

Acute change in urine output to <50 mL in 4 hours

Acute change in respiratory rate <8 or >30 breaths/min

Acute change in pulse oximetry to <90% despite oxygen administration

Acute change in consciousness

Qualitative deterioration in clinical status

Organ System–Specific Criteria

Airway
- Respiratory distress
- Threatened airway

Breathing
- Respiratory rate >30 breaths/min
- Respiratory rate <6 breaths/min
- Spo_2 <90% on oxygen
- Difficulty speaking

Circulation
- Blood pressure <90 mm Hg despite treatment
- Pulse rate >130 beats/min

Neurology
- Any unexplained decrease in consciousness
- New agitation or delirium
- Repeated or prolonged seizures

Other
- Concern about the patient
- Uncontrolled pain
- Failure to respond to treatment
- Inability to obtain prompt assistance

Event Trigger

Unscheduled naloxone dose administered

Increase in oxygen requirement
- Any change to a 100% reservoir face mask
- Any change in Fio_2 delivery by ≥20%

After 3 unanswered pages to medical/surgical team for any patient in a shift

Table A1-3 Models of Activation Criteria (continued)

Event Trigger
Response time to medical/surgical team page >30 min
Family concern about patient status
Any falls or traumatic injuries
Pain score ≥4 of 10 more than 30 min after highest ordered dose of analgesic
Persistent nausea/vomiting more than 30 min after highest dose of antiemetic
Any newly noted abnormal pulse

B. Response Team Scoring Systems

The use of a scoring system in evaluating the at-risk patient can provide a graded assessment of clinical status and help to determine the level of response needed. An overall score is calculated based on the aggregate of points assigned to various symptoms, vital signs, and laboratory studies. Additional points are assigned to results that vary more greatly from normal. The Modified Early Warning Score (**Table A1-4**), which evaluates vital signs and mental status, has been validated in hospitalized medical patients. A score of 5 or greater has been associated with an increased mortality rate and increased incidence of ICU admission.

Individual MET or RRT programs may choose to define absolute value or trend thresholds that trigger a move to a higher level of care or mobilization of additional clinical resources. Collection and analysis of aggregate scores in patients receiving MET or RRT services can be used for quality improvement efforts, such as evaluation of standing orders, event cluster identification, and resource utilization.

Table A1-4 Modified Early Warning Score[a]

Indicator	3	2	1	0	1	2	3
Systolic blood pressure (mm Hg)	<70	71-80	81-100	101-199		≥200	
Heart rate (beats/min)		<40	41-50	51-100	101-110	111-129	≥130
Respiratory rate (breaths/min)		<9		9-14	15-20	21-29	≥30
Temperature (°C)		<35		35-38.4		≥38.5	
AVPU score				**A**lert	Reacting to **V**oice	Reacting to **P**ain	**U**nresponsive

[a]Reproduced with permission from Oxford University Press.[10]

IV. MEDICAL EMERGENCY OR RAPID RESPONSE TEAM RESPONSE

A. Response Team Interventions

Interventions should be aimed at rapidly stabilizing the patient and preventing further deterioration or full arrest. Studies have shown that the three most common reasons for activating an MET or RRT are hypoxemia, hypotension, and altered mental status. The responding team should identify the primary activating events in their facilities and build protocols to address each rapidly. Respiratory distress is the leading physiologic cause of MET or RRT activation. The reasons for acute changes can be related to fluid status, medications such as narcotics, progression of underlying disease, or patient noncompliance with physician-ordered oxygen therapies. Initial treatment is stabilization of the airway and application of high-flow oxygen to relieve the patient's distress and improve oxygen saturation. Following improvement in patient status, the team can evaluate for potential reversible causes.

Hypotension is a frequent physiologic cause of MET or RRT activation and can be related to volume status (both overall volume and blood volume); medications, including narcotics and antihypertensives; and the potential for sepsis. Initial treatment is administration of fluids to raise systolic pressure and/or immediate reversal of a known cause, such as narcotics. Consideration should be given to empiric antibiotic therapy in cases of suspected severe sepsis or septic shock.

Altered mental status, another common physiologic trigger of MET or RRT activation, is most often associated with hypoxemia, hypotension, or hypoglycemia. These should be evaluated and treated first. Altered mental status unrelated to those issues should be evaluated for either neurologic or medication causes, and treatment, including evaluation with computed tomography scanning, should be guided accordingly.

The responding team should make every effort to involve the patient's primary physician and rounding team in decisions regarding disposition and care. The role of a MET or RRT is not to take the place of the primary team but to act for – and with – them at the bedside in an emergency.

B. Response Team Communications

In the complex hospital environment, the use of a structured communication tool and a common critical language fosters the open communication among caregivers that is essential to the prompt evaluation and management of the at-risk patient. Incorporating the Situation, Background, Assessment, and Recommendation (SBAR) tool into MET or RRT documentation can facilitate effective communication by gathering all pertinent data in one place for any discussions to follow. This tool has proven to be most valuable in the effective communication of critical information (**Table A1-5**).

Table A1-5 SBAR Communication Tool

Situation: *What is happening with the patient?*

Background: *What is the clinical background or context?*

Assessment: *What do I think is the problem?*

Recommendation/interventions: *What would I do to evaluate and correct it?*

C. Response Team Education

One of the primary goals of METs and RRTs is education. The detection limb of the RRS model relies heavily on the early recognition of signs and symptoms of clinical deterioration. Regularly scheduled staff in-services and mock-event drills are effective in maintaining competencies in identifying the at-risk patient. Public posting and discussion of activation criteria can further enhance the use of MET or RRT services and reduce patient clinical crises. Review of aggregate quality improvement data from response team activity also can reinforce education. Post hoc review of a patient event with the entire unit staff after an MET or RRT call serves to raise the entire group's collective knowledge and skill. This may help reduce the likelihood of subsequent problems and increase the likelihood that signs and symptoms of clinical deterioration will be detected at the earliest indication in future patients. Topic-of-the-week presentations, MET or RRT case reviews, and SBAR practice sessions are examples of targeted educational activities.

V. STRATEGIES FOR SUCCESS

Hospitals that use an RRS report various factors that lead to successful team implementation. Some common themes in their success include:

1. Training/Education – The MET or RRT members and the bedside nursing staff have to gain an understanding of when and how to activate the team, and the scope of team capabilities. The response team members will need ongoing training in management of common indicators of "at-risk" patients, and effective intervention and communication strategies. The mentoring of bedside nursing staff in critical assessment skills and effective communication skills is a primary team education objective. High-fidelity simulation in a simulation center is helpful, but not necessary. Low-fidelity simulations with mock medical emergency scenarios or table-top exercises are very effective as well. Scenario-based case presentations using a chalkboard or paper can be offered in any clinical setting.

2. Equipment/Supplies – The equipment and supplies carried by the response team should be tailored to the needs of the patient population served, but then standardized to assure that the appropriate resources reach the bedside with each call. If multiple RRT bags are used, the items should be organized within each bag to facilitate rapid access at the bedside. It is impractical to carry every item available in the ICU. Equipment use should be reviewed as part of the quality improvement program. Seldom-used items should be removed unless they serve an important role in the management of infrequent, but high-risk events. The response team should strive to carry only the necessary equipment and supplies.

3. Culture of Empowerment – Staff nurses should be trained to recognize signs of clinical deterioration before a crisis and to trust their experience and skills. They should be empowered, and supported by leadership to activate the MET or RRT according to established criteria. There should be no penalty for activating the MET or RRT, especially if the findings do not point towards an impending clinical crisis. Such events can identify areas for targeted education in the detection of signs of clinical deterioration or focused review of the risks inherent to that patient population.

4. Evaluation – Data collection should be embedded into the clinical workflow to facilitate monitoring of clinical and service outcomes. Regular reporting of response team activities and outcomes guides rapid cycle improvement of team processes. Patient and family satisfaction data helps prioritize program development and resource allocation. Constant dialogue among the stakeholders to identify improvement opportunities is essential.

VI. SUMMARY

Hospitalized patients can be at risk for clinical deterioration in part due to the complex nature of healthcare delivery systems. The goal of the RRS model is to identify and manage signs and symptoms of clinical deterioration in at-risk patients through detection strategies at the bedside and mobilization of appropriate resources. Important factors in the successful implementation of an RRS include: (1) appropriate team composition; (2) activation criteria based on bedside staff concern, acute changes in physiology, or the use of scoring systems to identify at-risk patients; (3) interventions aimed at rapidly stabilizing the patient; (4) effective communication strategies like SBAR; (5) ongoing education to enhance detection and management of potential clinical crises; (6) availability of appropriate advanced clinical monitors, equipment, and medications to conduct MET or RRT activities; and (7) evaluation and correction of processes and causes that may put patients at risk.

Suggested Readings

1. Bellomo R, Goldsmith D, Uchino S, et al. A prospective before-and-after trial of a medical emergency team. *Med J Aust.* 2003;179:283-287.

2. Buist MD, Moore GE, Bernard SA, et al. Effects of a medical emergency team on reduction of incidence of and mortality from unexpected cardiac arrests in hospital: preliminary study. *BMJ.* 2002;324:387-390.

3. DeVita MA, Bellomo R, Hillman K, et al. Findings of the First Consensus Conference on Medical Emergency Teams. *Crit Care Med.* 2006;9:2463-2478.

4. DeVita MA, Hillman K, Bellomo R, eds. *Medical Emergency Teams: Implementation and Outcome Measurement.* New York, NY: Springer Science + Business Media Inc; 2006.

5. Halvorsen L, Garolis S, Wallace-Scroggs A, et al. Building a rapid response team. *AACN Adv Crit Care.* 2007;18:129-140.

6. Leonard M, Graham S, Bonacum D. The human factor: the critical importance of effective teamwork and communication in providing safe care. *Qual Saf Health Care.* 2004;13 (suppl 1):i85-i90.

7. Murray T, Kleinpell R. Implementing a rapid response team: factors influencing success. *Crit Care Nurse Clin North Am.* 2006;18:493-501.

8. Sebat F, ed. *Designing, Implementing, and Enhancing a Rapid Response System.* Mount Prospect, IL: Society of Critical Care Medicine; 2009.

9. Sebat F, Musthafa AA, Johnson D, et al. Effect of a rapid response system for patients in shock on time to treatment and mortality during 5 years. *Crit Care Med.* 2007;35:2568-2575.

10. Subbe CP, Kruger M, Rutherford P, et al. Validation of a modified Early Warning Score in medical admissions. *QJM.* 2001;94:521-526.

11. Thomas K, VanOyen Force M, Rasmussen D, et al. Rapid response team: challenges, solutions, benefits. *Crit Care Med.* 2007;26:15-20.

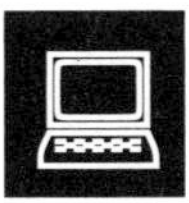

Web Sites

1. International Conference on Medical Emergency Team Response. http://www.metconference.com. *Downloadable files from the conference presentations.*

2. Institute for Healthcare Improvement. http://www.IHI.org/IHI/Programs/Campaign. *Information regarding the Institute for Healthcare Improvement's 5 Million Lives Campaign to improve patient safety, which includes creation of an MET team.*

Appendix 2

Endotracheal Intubation

I. Indications, Patient Evaluation, Manual Mask Ventilation, Patient Preparation

See Chapter 2.

II. Equipment

A. Bag-mask resuscitation unit with oxygen supplementation (with positive end-expiratory pressure valve if indicated)

B. Topical anesthetic spray

C. Medications as selected for analgesia/anesthesia, amnesia, and neuromuscular blockade

D. Towel roll or pad for occipital elevation

E. Pulse oximeter

F. Electrocardiography monitor

G. Automatic blood pressure device or manual blood pressure monitoring device

H. Gloves, mask, eye protection

I. Laryngoscope handle and blade(s): usually sizes #3 and #4 curved, #2 and #3 straight

J. Endotracheal tubes: usually 7.0- or 7.5-mm for adult women and 8.0-mm for adult men

K. Malleable stylet

L. Yankauer and tracheal suction catheters, suction device

M. Magill forceps

N. 10-mL syringe to inflate cuff

O. Water-soluble lubricant

P. Qualitative CO_2 detector, CO_2 monitor, or esophageal detector device

Q. Tape or tracheal tube stabilization device

R. Resuscitation cart

III. ROUTE OF INTUBATION

A. Orotracheal intubation via direct laryngoscopy

- This route is generally favored in most circumstances, including when cervical spine injury is suspected.

B. Blind nasotracheal intubation

- The nasotracheal route using a blind approach can only be attempted in a spontaneously breathing patient and may be favored by experienced operators in select patients and situations. This technique has the advantage of allowing continued spontaneous ventilation and generally requires less sedation than direct laryngoscopy. It is more time-consuming than direct laryngoscopy and therefore is less useful in emergent intubation. Endotracheal tubes used for nasotracheal intubation have smaller diameters than those used for orotracheal intubation. Nasotracheal intubation should be avoided if basilar skull fracture is suspected and in the presence of coagulopathy. Nasotracheal intubation is discouraged in infants and small children due to anatomic differences compared with adults.

IV. OROTRACHEAL INTUBATION

A. Preparation

1. Don gloves, mask, and eye protection for universal precautions.

2. Explain the procedure, if patient is conscious.

3. Assure patent airway and optimal oxygenation and ventilation (**Chapter 2**).

4. Assure intravenous access.

5. Apply pulse oximeter, electrocardiography, and blood pressure devices.

6. Assemble all equipment and ensure proper working order.

7. Prepare the endotracheal tube.

    a. Check cuff integrity by inflating and fully deflating.

    b. Insert stylet into endotracheal tube, bend to predicted configuration to assist glottic entry. Ensure the distal tip of the stylet does not protrude past the end of the endotracheal tube.

    c. Apply water-soluble lubricant to the cuff end of the tube.

8. Connect laryngoscope blade to handle.

    a. Select blade type (operator's choice).

        1. Straight blade — used to elevate the epiglottis anteriorly

        2. Curved blade — inserted into the vallecula

    b. Select blade length — #3 blade is proper unless patient's neck is very long.

    c. Assure that light is sufficiently bright.

9. Place pad or towel under occiput if cervical spine injury is not suspected.

10. Use topical anesthetic on the patient's oropharynx.

11. Preoxygenate with 100% oxygen for 2 to 3 minutes if time permits.

12. As necessary, proceed with sedation and neuromuscular blockade (**Chapter 2**).

B. Technique

1. The operator stands at the head of the bed, and the bed is raised to a position of comfort for the operator. The head of the bed may be flat or raised slightly per operator preference.

2. When no cervical injury is suspected, a small pad is placed under the occiput (the "sniffing" position) and the neck is gently extended (**Figure A2-1**). When cervical spine injury is possible, these steps are omitted, the neck is stabilized by an assistant (as described in **Chapter 2**), and the anterior portion of the cervical collar is removed.

Figure A2-1. Positioning for Orotracheal Intubation

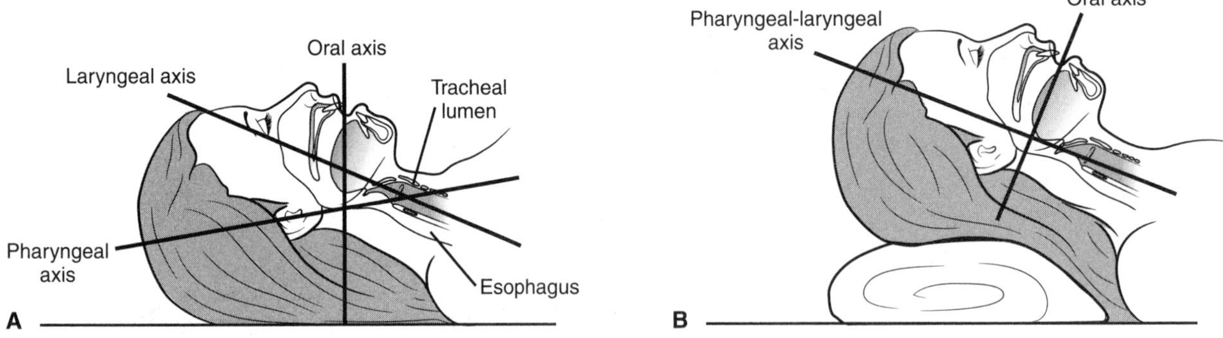

The axial planes of the neck are not lined up with the head in a neutral position (**A**). Slight extension and forward movement of the neck will line up the pharyngeal-laryngeal axis and place the oral axis perpendicular to this line, thereby allowing visualization of the vocal cords (**B**). Note that this positioning is contraindicated in patients with possible cervical spine injury.

3. Regardless of the operator's dominant hand in other contexts, the laryngoscope is always held in the left hand.

4. Cricoid pressure should be gently but firmly applied by an assistant as soon as consciousness is lost and should be sustained until endotracheal tube placement is confirmed and the cuff inflated.

5. Mouth opening in the sedated/relaxed patient may be assisted by a cross-finger technique wherein the thumb of the right hand is placed on the front lower teeth of the mandible and the first finger on the front upper teeth (maxilla). The mouth is gently opened by a "reverse scissor" movement of the fingers, and the laryngoscope is introduced into the mouth.

6. The tip of laryngoscope blade is inserted into the right side of the patient's mouth (**Figure A2-2**); the blade is advanced to the base of the tongue.

7. The tongue should be swept to the left; proper tongue control is key to laryngeal visualization.

8. The blade is gently advanced further to its proper position. A straight blade is placed beneath the epiglottis; a curved blade is placed into the vallecula above the epiglottis.

9. Caution! Traction should be applied only along the long axis of the laryngoscope handle as the laryngoscope lifts the tongue upward away from the larynx, revealing the glottic opening. A rocking or rotating motion of the blade and handle may damage teeth, gingiva, or lips. The base of the laryngoscope blade should never contact the upper teeth!

Figure A2-2. Insertion of Laryngoscope

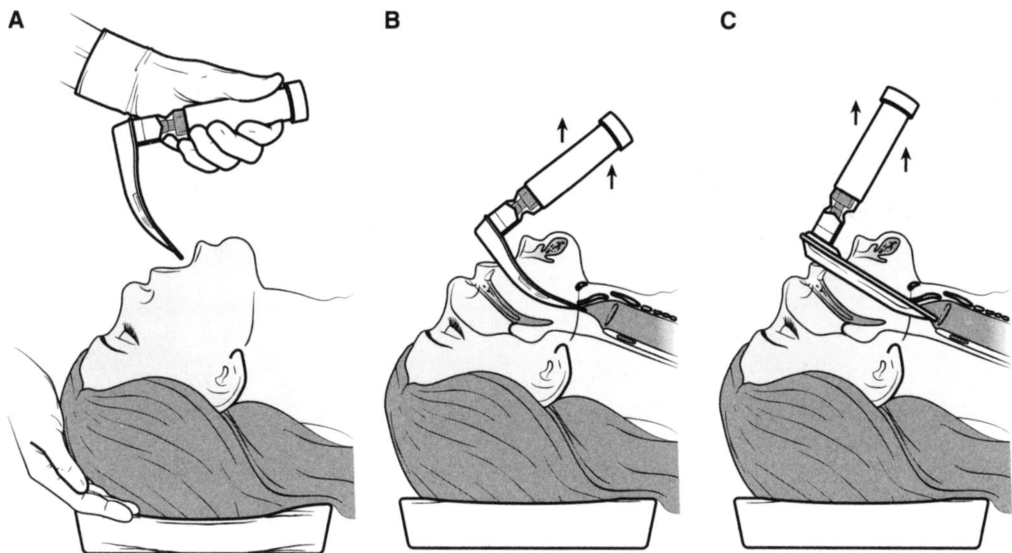

(A) The blade of the laryngoscope is inserted into the patient's mouth and pushes the tongue to the left. **(B)** The curved blade follows the base of the tongue and is inserted into the vallecula and **(C)** the straight blade is inserted beneath the epiglottis.

10. The vocal cords and glottic opening should be visualized.

11. If the vocal cords and glottis cannot be visualized, it may be helpful for an assistant to grasp the thyroid cartilage between the thumb and index finger and exert pressure in the following sequence: Pressure is applied backward against the cervical vertebrae and then in an upward direction to shift the larynx superiorly. Additional pressure is applied to shift the thyroid cartilage no more than 2 cm to the right side of the patient's neck. This procedure can be remembered by the acronym BURP (backward, upward, and rightward pressure on the thyroid cartilage).

12. The endotracheal tube is inserted gently through the vocal cords (**Figure A2-3**), holding the tube/stylet with the right hand. The stylet, if angled, may interfere with passage of the tube into the trachea. If resistance is encountered as the tube is advanced, consider having an assistant remove the stylet while the operator holds the endotracheal tube firmly in the glottic opening.

13. The stylet and laryngoscope should be removed carefully (**Figure A2-3**). The operator must continue to hold the endotracheal tube firmly and position it such that the external centimeter length markers on the tube show 21 cm (female) or 23 cm (male) adjacent to the front teeth.

Figure A2-3. Placement of Endotracheal Tube

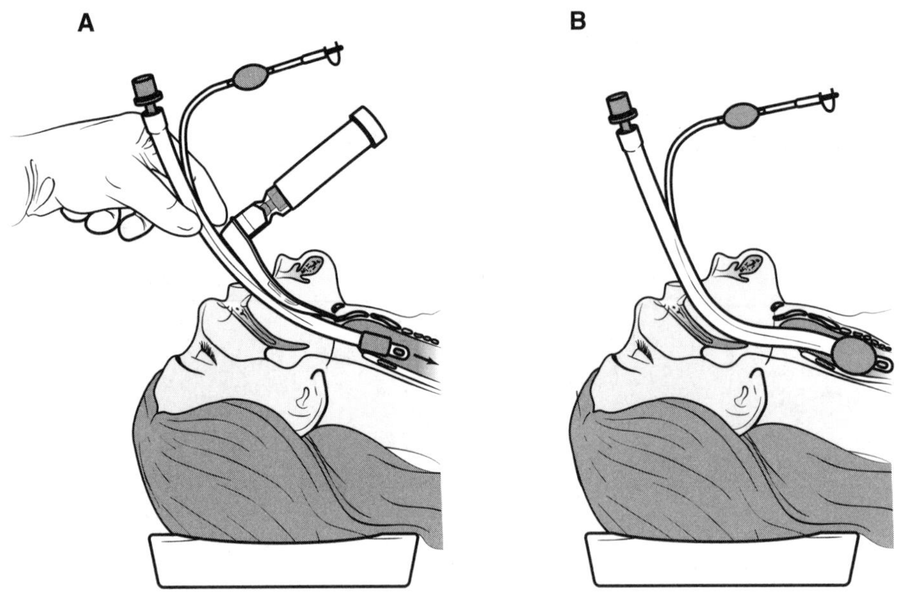

(A) The endotracheal tube is inserted through the vocal cords until the distal end rests approximately 2 to 3 cm above the carina. **(B)** Once the endotracheal tube is in the proper position, the laryngoscope and stylet are removed and the cuff is inflated.

14. The cuff is inflated.

15. To ensure proper position of the tube:

    a. Auscultate the epigastrium; inspect and auscultate chest to assure equal bilateral gas entry.

    b. Use qualitative CO_2 detector or monitor or esophageal detector device. Lack of color change with a qualitative CO_2 detector or low exhaled CO_2 measurement may occur with a correctly placed tracheal tube in the patient with poor pulmonary perfusion, such as during cardiac arrest or profound hypotension.

    c. Observe for condensation in the endotracheal tube during exhalation.

    d. Listen for breath sounds through the endotracheal tube as the patient is breathing spontaneously.

    e. Obtain chest radiograph (tube tip 2 to 3 cm above carina).

16. Secure endotracheal tube with tape or endotracheal tube stabilization device.

V. BLIND NASOTRACHEAL INTUBATION

A. Preparation

1. See Section IV-A, for preparation for orotracheal intubation, steps 1-8.
2. Position the patient's head on a small towel with the neck in a slightly extended position.
3. Preoxygenate with 100% oxygen for 2 to 3 minutes if time permits.
4. Use topical anesthetic on the nasal passages and pharynx and lubricate the nasal passages.

B. Technique

1. The operator stands at the head of the bed, and the bed is raised to a position of comfort for the operator. The head of the bed may be flat or raised slightly per operator preference. The patient should have spontaneous ventilation and an adequate tidal volume.
2. The larger naris should be used if there is significant deviation of the nasal septum.
3. A well-lubricated endotracheal tube without a stylet is inserted gently through the nasal passage into the posterior oropharynx.
4. Oxygen may be administered by face mask/blowby or by intermittently connecting the oxygen source to the endotracheal tube.
5. The oropharynx should be inspected to assure that the endotracheal tube is in the midline.
6. The amount of air movement at the endotracheal tube connector is assessed by either listening to air movement through the tube, using a specially designed "whistle," or using an exhaled CO_2 monitor.
7. The endotracheal tube is advanced slowly while feeling and listening for air movement at the connector end of the endotracheal tube. Advancement continues if air movement increases through the tube. If air movement decreases, the endotracheal tube should be withdrawn until air movement resumes, re-advancing after repositioning the head.
8. Advancing the tube through the glottis is usually easier during inspiration.
9. The operator must continue to hold the endotracheal tube firmly and position it such that the external centimeter length markers on the tube show approximately 24 cm (female) or 26 cm (male) adjacent to the naris.
10. The cuff is inflated.

11. To ensure proper position of the tube:

    a. Auscultate epigastrium; inspect and auscultate chest to assure equal bilateral gas entry.

    b. Use qualitative CO_2 detector or monitor or esophageal detector device. Lack of color change with a qualitative CO_2 detector or low exhaled CO_2 measurement may occur with a correctly placed endotracheal tube in the patient with poor pulmonary perfusion.

    c. Observe for condensation in the endotracheal tube during exhalation.

    d. Listen for breath sounds through the endotracheal tube as the patient is breathing spontaneously.

    e. Obtain chest radiograph (tube tip 2 to 3 cm above carina).

12. The endotracheal tube is secured with tape or endotracheal tube stabilization device.

VI. PEDIATRIC CONSIDERATIONS

A. Anatomic differences between adults and children:

1. The larynx is more cephalad in infants than in adults, making it appear more anterior and resulting in a more difficult visualization during laryngoscopy.

2. Cricoid pressure is valuable during laryngoscopy because of the position of the larynx and assists in preventing aspiration.

3. In young children, the narrowest part of the airway is at the level of the cricoid cartilage, not at the larynx, making an anatomic "cuff" below the vocal cords.

4. In general, the diameter of the small finger approximates the properly sized endotracheal tube. A full-term neonate can accept a tube with a 3.5-mm internal diameter.

5. Cuffed tubes therefore are usually limited to use in children >8 years old (endotracheal tube size >6.0-mm internal diameter); uncuffed tubes are generally used in younger children.

B. Technique differences between adults and children:

1. Head position: a towel roll under the head is often needed in adults to achieve the sniffing position; a shoulder roll is usually needed to achieve this position in infants.

2. Laryngoscope blade selection: operator may choose a straight or curved blade; however, most clinicians do not use curved blades in infants. A common mistake in intubating a child is choosing a blade that is too small. The blade must be long enough to reach the epiglottis.

3. Proper depth of insertion (in centimeters) can be estimated by multiplying the internal diameter of the endotracheal tube by 3 (eg, internal diameter = 4.0; depth of insertion = 4.0 × 3 = 12.0 cm).

4. Appropriately sized equipment (eg, face mask, laryngoscope, endotracheal tube, suction catheter) should be used.

VII. PRECAUTIONS/COMPLICATIONS

A. Hypoxia, hypercapnia during procedure

B. Cardiovascular compromise during and immediately after procedure

C. Damaged teeth, lips, gingiva

D. Malpositioned tube (esophagus, right main-stem bronchus)

E. Pharyngeal, laryngeal, tracheal damage

F. Gastric distension and aspiration of gastric contents

G. Bronchospasm

H. Pneumothorax

Suggested Readings

1. Balk RA. The technique of orotracheal intubation. *J Crit Illness.* 1997;12:316-323.

2. Knill RL. Difficult laryngoscopy made easy with a "BURP." *Can J Anaesth.* 1993;40:279-282.

3. Lavery GG, Jamison CA. Airway management in the critically ill adult. In: Parrillo JE, Dellinger RP, eds. *Critical Care Medicine: Principles of Diagnosis and Management in the Adult.* 3rd ed. Philadelphia, PA: Mosby Elsevier; 2008:17.

4. Wheeler DS, Spaeth JP, Mehta R, et al. Assessment and management of the pediatric airway. In: Wheeler DS, Wong HR, Shanley TP, eds. *Pediatric Critical Care Medicine: Basic Science and Clinical Evidence.* London, England: Springer-Verlag; 2007:223.

Appendix 3

Airway Adjuncts

I. LARYNGEAL MASK AIRWAY

A. Indications

1. Provide an airway and ventilation when bag-mask ventilation is difficult
2. Provide a temporizing airway when endotracheal intubation is unsuccessful

B. Equipment

1. Bag-mask resuscitation unit with high-flow oxygen source
2. Pulse oximeter
3. Electrocardiographic monitor
4. Blood pressure monitoring
5. Gloves, mask, eye protection
6. Laryngeal mask airway (LMA) of appropriate size (**Table A3-1**)
7. Syringe for cuff inflation
8. Water-soluble lubricant
9. Qualitative CO_2 detector or CO_2 monitor
10. Resuscitation cart

Table A3-1 Laryngeal Mask Airway Size and Cuff Inflation

LMA Size	Patient Size	Maximum Cuff Volume	Largest ETT ID (mm)[a]
1	Neonate/infant to 5 kg	Up to 4 mL	3.5
1.5	5-10 kg	Up to 7 mL	4.0
2	10-20 kg	Up to 10 mL	4.5
2.5	20-30 kg	Up to 14 mL	5.0
3	>30 kg/small adult	Up to 20 mL	6.0 cuffed
4	Average adult	Up to 30 mL	6.0 cuffed
5	Large adult	Up to 40 mL	7.0 cuffed

[a]Largest endotracheal tube size (ETT ID) that will fit through laryngeal mask airway (LMA) tube lumen.

C. Preparation for insertion

1. Don gloves, mask, and eye protection.
2. Assure patent airway and optimal oxygenation and ventilation.
3. Assure intravenous access.
4. Apply pulse oximeter, electrocardiographic and blood pressure monitors.
5. Select appropriate size LMA.
6. Check cuff integrity by inflating and fully deflating.
7. Lubricate only the posterior aspect of the deflated mask with a water-based lubricant.
8. Preoxygenate with 100% oxygen for 2 to 3 minutes if time permits.

D. Technique (**Figure A3-1**)

1. The cuff is deflated completely so that it forms a spoon shape and there are no folds in the mask.

2. The operator stands behind the head of the bed, and the bed is raised to a position of comfort for the operator.

3. The patient is placed in the sniffing position (ie, head extended, neck flexed), unless potential or definite cervical spine injury prevents neck extension.

4. Cricoid pressure is not recommended during placement of the LMA because it may interfere with correct placement.

5. The mask is positioned with the bowl facing anteriorly. Hold the device like a pencil, with the index finger of the dominant hand at the junction of the bowl and tube, pressing against the palate and pharyngeal wall with the index finger.

6. The cuff is inserted into the hypopharynx until definite resistance is felt.

7. Without the operator holding the device, the cuff is inflated with enough air to obtain a seal around the laryngeal inlet. This results in an outward movement of the tube.

8. The cuff is inflated with enough air to obtain a seal (intracuff pressure of approximately 60 cm H_2O). Maximum volumes are listed in **Table A3-1**, but lesser volume may provide an adequate seal.

9. A manual ventilation device is attached, and chest movement and breath sounds are verified in both lung fields. Correct position should be confirmed with a qualitative or quantitative end-tidal CO_2 detector.

10. If chest movement is inadequate, or if a large air leak is present, the device should be removed and reinserted.

11. When the LMA is positioned appropriately, the tube is secured with tape.

Figure A3-1. Insertion Technique for Laryngeal Mask Airway[a]

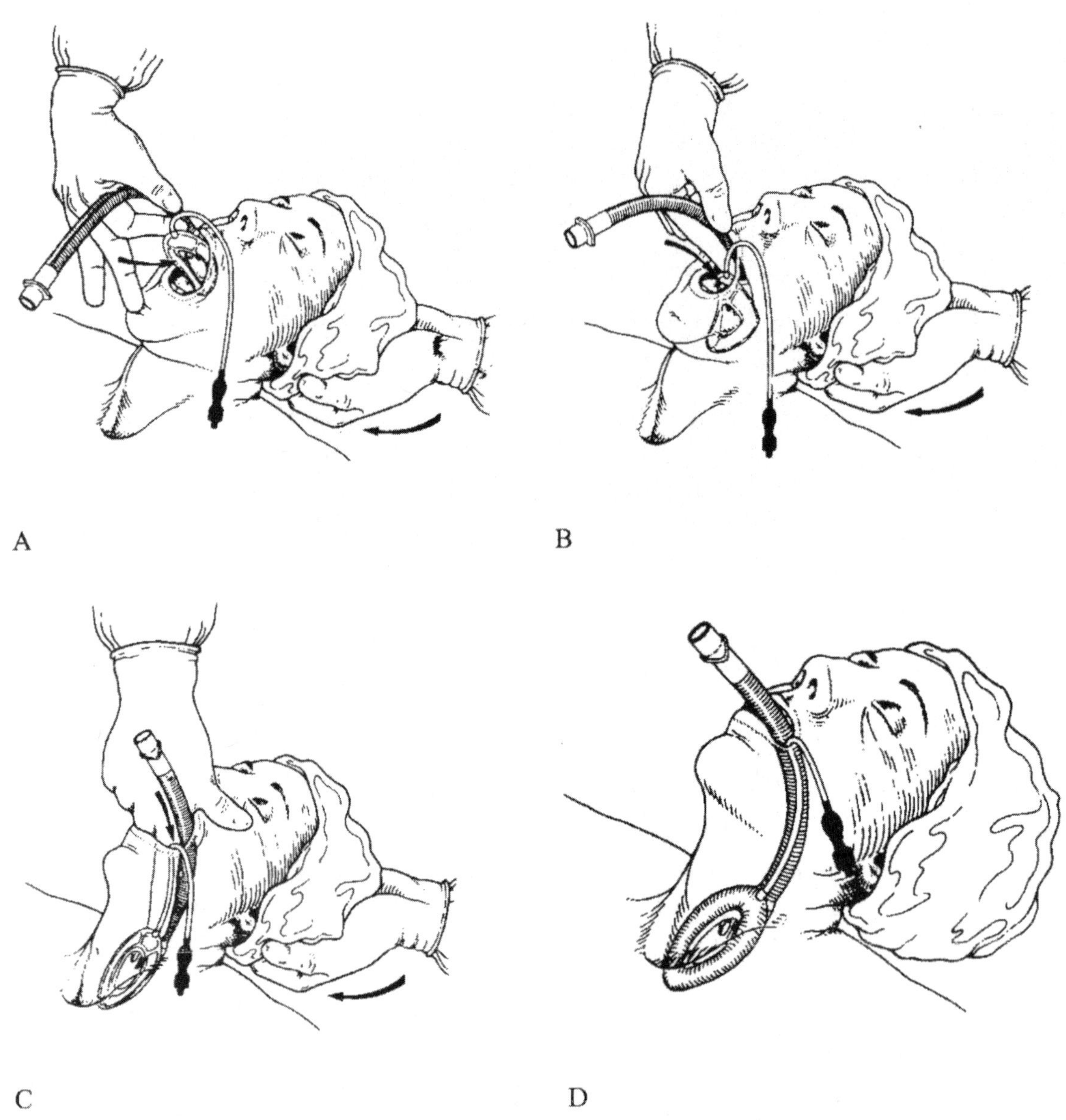

(A) Insert lubricated and deflated mask into the open mouth with the bowl facing anteriorly. **(B)** Hold the device like a pencil, pressing against the palate and pharyngeal wall with the index finger. **(C)** Continue inserting the cuff behind the tongue into the hypopharynx until definite resistance is felt. **(D)** Without holding the device, inflate cuff with enough air to obtain a seal. Attach manual ventilation device and ensure chest movement.
[a]Reproduced with permission from Intravent Direct.[1]

II. ESOPHAGEAL-TRACHEAL DOUBLE-LUMEN AIRWAY DEVICE

A. Indications

1. Cardiorespiratory arrest and inability to provide an airway by other means

B. Equipment

1. Bag-mask resuscitation unit with high-flow oxygen source
2. Pulse oximeter
3. Electrocardiographic monitor
4. Blood pressure monitoring
5. Gloves, mask, eye protection
6. Esophageal-tracheal double-lumen device
7. Syringe for cuff inflation
8. Water-soluble lubricant
9. Qualitative CO_2 detector or CO_2 monitor
10. Resuscitation cart

C. Preparation for insertion

1. Don gloves, mask, and eye protection.
2. Assure patent airway and optimal oxygenation and ventilation.
3. Assure intravenous access.
4. Apply pulse oximeter, electrocardiographic and blood pressure monitors.
5. Select appropriate size device. The available sizes for the device are 41 and 37 French. Use the 41 French for patients taller than 5 feet (152 cm) and the 37 French for patients less than that height.
6. Check integrity of both cuffs by inflating and fully deflating.
7. Preoxygenate with 100% oxygen for 2 to 3 minutes if time permits.

D. Technique (**Figure A3-2**)

1. The cuffs should be deflated completely.

2. The operator stands behind the head of the bed, and the bed is raised to a position of comfort for the operator.

3. The patient is placed in a neutral or sniffing position (ie, head extended, neck flexed), unless potential or definite cervical spine injury prevents neck extension.

4. The patient's tongue and jaw are grasped between the thumb and index finger, and the device is inserted blindly. It is advanced until the placement ring markers on the tube are positioned as indicated by the manufacturer. Do not force the tube if resistance is met. A laryngoscope can be used to assist with placement.

Figure A3-2. Esophageal-Tracheal Double-Lumen Airway Device

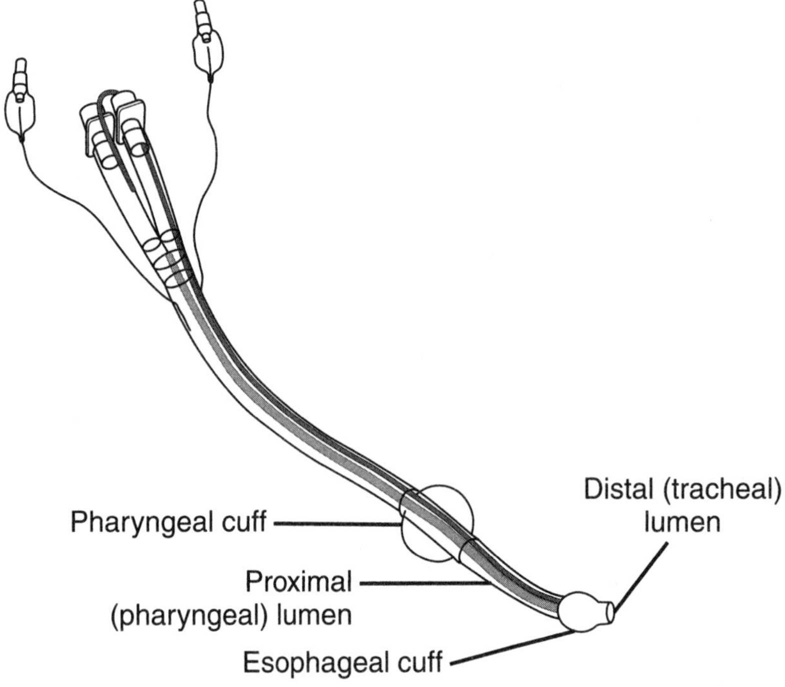

Some tubes have two pilot balloons to allow for independent inflation of the pharyngeal and esophageal cuffs, whereas other tubes have a single pilot port and simultaneously inflate both cuffs. Detection of end-tidal CO_2 in the proximal lumen suggests that the tube is in the esophagus. In the rare instance that the tube enters the trachea, ventilation is only possible via the distal lumen and end-tidal CO_2 will not be detected from the proximal lumen.

5. The pharyngeal cuff is inflated first to seal the posterior pharynx.

6. The distal cuff is then inflated.

7. Ventilation should be attempted first through the pharyngeal lumen, and the chest should be auscultated for breath sounds and observed for movement. The tube enters the esophagus approximately 95% of the time.

8. If breath sounds are absent, ventilation should be attempted through the tracheal lumen while auscultating for breath sounds.

9. Use of the correct lumen for ventilation should be confirmed with a qualitative/quantitative end-tidal CO_2 or esophageal detector device.

10. When the device is positioned appropriately, the tube is secured with tape.

III. VIDEO LARYNGOSCOPE

A. Indications

1. Endotracheal intubation in known or presumed difficult airway

2. Known or suspected cervical spine injury

B. Equipment

1. Bag-mask resuscitation unit with high-flow oxygen source

2. Pulse oximeter

3. Electrocardiographic monitor

4. Blood pressure monitoring

5. Gloves, mask, eye protection

6. Video laryngoscope with appropriate blade

7. Endotracheal tube (ETT) of appropriate size for patient

8. Syringe for cuff inflation

9. Water-soluble lubricant

10. Qualitative CO_2 detector or CO_2 monitor

11. Resuscitation cart

C. Preparation for insertion

1. Don gloves, mask, and eye protection.

2. Assure patent airway and optimal oxygenation and ventilation.

3. Assure intravenous access.

4. Apply pulse oximeter, electrocardiographic and blood pressure monitors.

5. Prepare ETT with stylet and check cuff.

6. Turn on video laryngoscope power and check light/camera.

7. Assure proper cable and blade attachment.

8. Position video screen for optimal viewing during laryngoscopy.

9. Preoxygenate with 100% oxygen for 2 to 3 minutes if time permits.

D. Technique (**Figure A3-3**)

Figure A3-3. Video Laryngoscope[a]

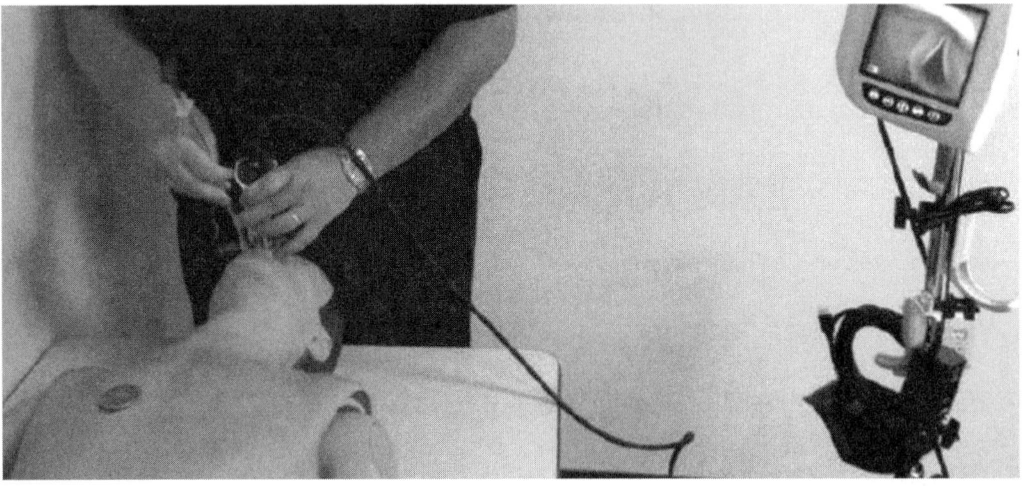

[a]Photo by Jason Emerson, originally published in the Skaneateles Press, August 17, 2011. Used courtesy Eagle Newspapers.

1. The operator stands behind the head of the bed, and the bed is raised to a position of comfort for the operator.

2. The patient is placed in a neutral or sniffing position (ie, head extended, neck flexed), unless potential or definite cervical spine injury prevents neck extension.

3. Consider lubricating the tongue side of the laryngoscope blade prior to insertion. Insert the laryngoscope blade into the oropharynx, and advance into the hypopharynx while watching the video screen for anatomical landmarks.

4. Once positioned in the hypopharynx, lift up and away, then adjust the position until the glottis and vocal cords are seen.

5. Insert and advance the ETT into the hypopharynx until the tip is seen near the end of the laryngoscope blade.

6. Advance the ETT through the glottis opening until the cuff passes the vocal cords. Make small adjustments in laryngoscope and ETT positioning as necessary to intubate the trachea.

7. Gently remove the laryngoscope blade while holding the ETT in place. Be careful not to kink or pinch the camera cable.

8. Inflate the ETT cuff and remove the stylet. Attach the bag-valve device and provide manual ventilation. Confirm bilateral breath sounds and end-tidal carbon dioxide.

9. When the ETT is positioned appropriately, the tube is secured with tape.

IV. OPTICAL LARYNGOSCOPE

A. Indications

1. Endotracheal intubation in known or presumed difficult airway

2. Known or suspected cervical spine injury

B. Equipment

1. Bag-mask resuscitation unit with high-flow oxygen source

2. Pulse oximeter

3. Electrocardiographic monitor

4. Blood pressure monitoring

5. Gloves, mask, eye protection
6. Appropriately sized optical laryngoscope – color coded
7. ETT of appropriate size for patient
8. Syringe for cuff inflation
9. Water-soluble lubricant
10. Qualitative CO_2 detector or CO_2 monitor
11. Resuscitation cart

C. Preparation for insertion

1. Don gloves, mask, eye protection.
2. Assure patent airway and optimal oxygenation and ventilation.
3. Assure intravenous access.
4. Apply pulse oximeter, electrocardiographic and blood pressure monitors.
5. Prepare ETT, check cuff, and lubricate.
6. Choose appropriately sized optical laryngoscope.
7. Turn on laryngoscope light at least 30 seconds prior to use.
8. Load ETT into optical laryngoscope side channel.
9. Assure ETT tip is seen through eyepiece but is not obstructing view.
10. Preoxygenate with 100% oxygen for 2 to 3 minutes if time permits.

D. Technique (**Figure A3-4**)

1. The operator stands behind the head of the bed, and the bed is raised to a position of comfort for the operator.
2. The patient is placed in a neutral or sniffing position (ie, head extended, neck flexed), unless potential or definite cervical spine injury prevents neck extension.
3. Consider lubricating the tongue side of the laryngoscope blade prior to insertion. Insert the laryngoscope blade in the midline over the tongue into the oropharynx and advance into the hypopharynx by rotating the laryngoscope along the tongue until it is perpendicular. Use caution to not displace the tongue posteriorly.

Figure A3-4. Optical Laryngoscope[a]

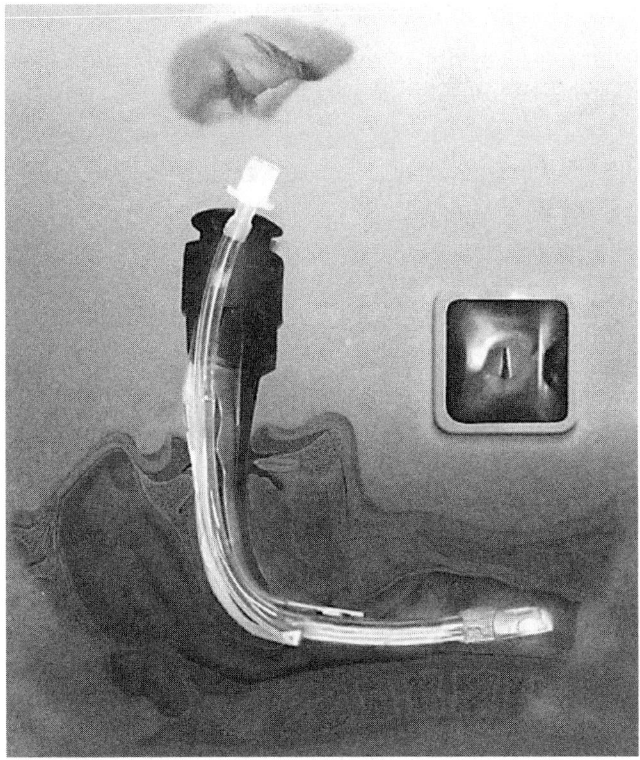

The optical laryngoscope allows the operator to look through the device, whereas the video laryngoscope in **Figure A3-3** is the device with the video camera and screen.
[a]Used with permission from Prodol Meditec SA, Las Arenas Vizcaya, Spain.

4. Once positioned in the hypopharynx, look through the eyepiece and lift up gently. Adjust the position until the glottis and vocal cords are seen. If glottis structures are not seen, gently pull back until seen. DO NOT tilt back or leverage against upper teeth or gums.

5. Advance the ETT through the glottis opening until the cuff passes the vocal cords. Make small adjustments in laryngoscope positioning as necessary to intubate the trachea.

6. Inflate the ETT cuff and separate from the laryngoscope with a gentle spreading or peeling motion. Be careful to not displace the ETT.

7. Gently remove the laryngoscope blade while holding the ETT in place. Rotate in opposite direction from insertion.

8. Attach the bag-valve device and provide manual ventilation. Confirm bilateral breath sounds and end-tidal carbon dioxide.

9. When the ETT is positioned appropriately, the tube is secured with tape.

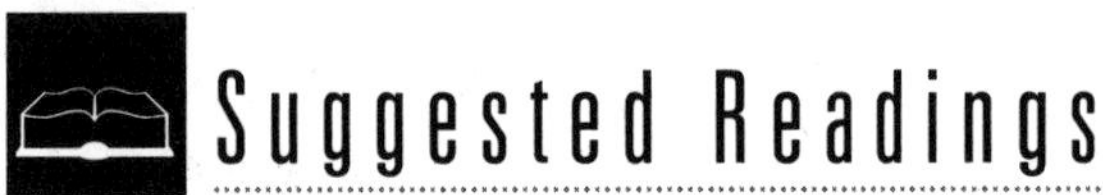

Suggested Readings

1. Brain AIJ. *The Intavent Laryngeal Mask Instruction Manual.* Berkshire, UK: Brain Medical; 1992.

2. Danks RR, Danks B. Laryngeal mask airway: review of indications and use. *J Emerg Nurs.* 2004;30:30-35.

3. Krafft P, Schebesta K. Alternative management techniques for the difficult airway: esophageal-tracheal Combitube. *Curr Opin Anaesthesiol.* 2005;17:499-504.

4. Lu Y, Jiang H, Zhu YS. Airtraq laryngoscope versus conventional Macintosh laryngoscope: a systematic review and meta-analysis. *Anaesthesia.* 2011;66:1160-1167.

5. Mace SE. The laryngeal mask airway: guidelines for appropriate usage. *Resid Staff Physician.* 2001;47:30.

6. Niforopoulou P, Pantazopoulos I, Demestiha T, et al. Video-laryngoscopes in the adult airway management: a topical review of the literature. *Acta Anaesthesiol Scand.* 2010;54:1050-1061.

Advanced Life Support Algorithms

Figure A4-1. Pulseless Arrest Algorithm[a]

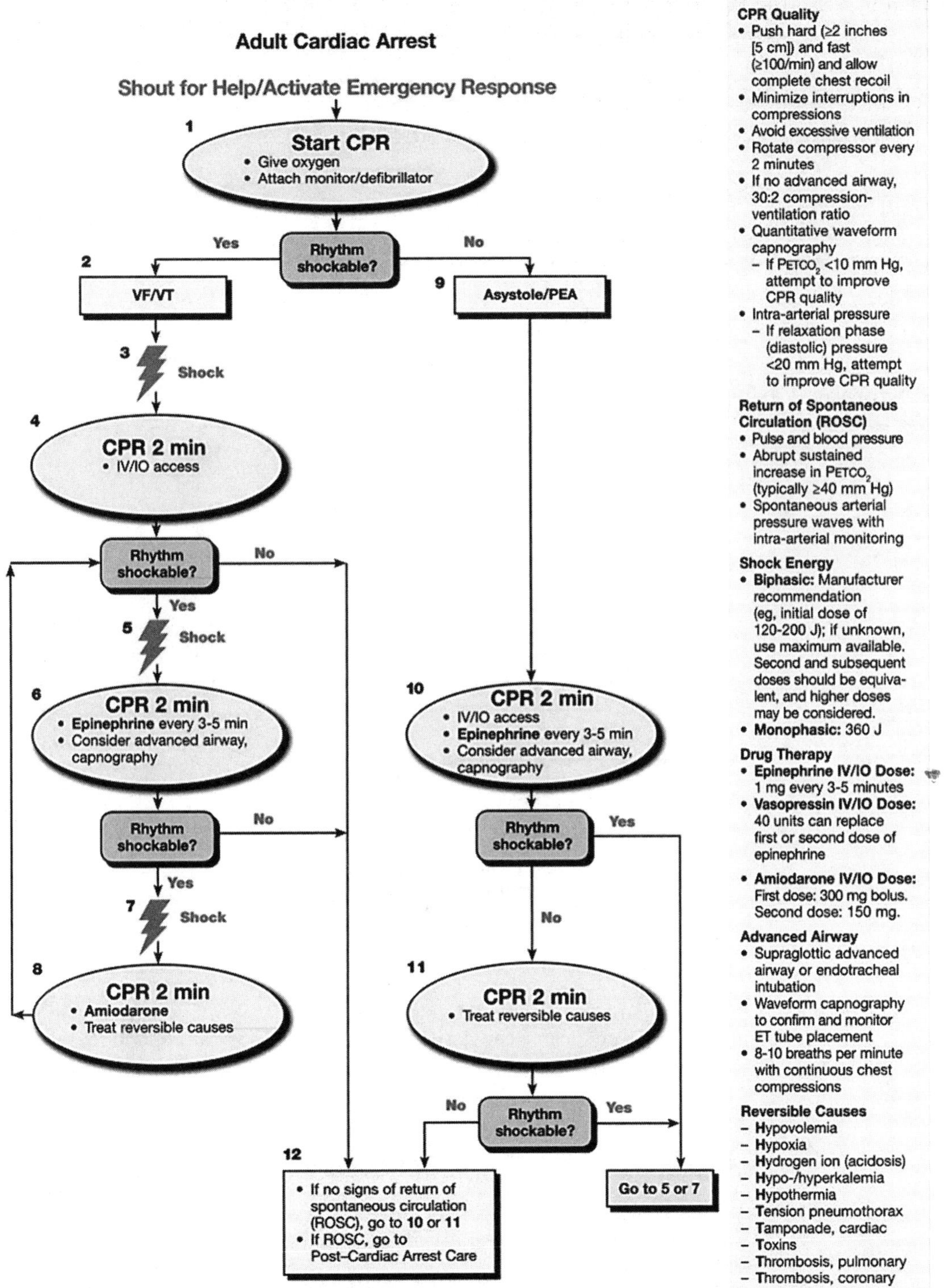

Performance of CPR should be continuous, with interruption only as necessary.

[a]Reproduced with permission from Wolters Kluwer Health. Neumar RW, Otto CW, Link MS, et al. Part 8: Adult advanced Cardiovascular life support: 2010 American Heart Association Guidelines for Cardiopulmonary Resuscitation and Emergency Cardiovascular Care. *Circulation.* 2010;122(18 suppl 3):S729-267.

Figure A4-2. Bradycardia Algorithm[a]

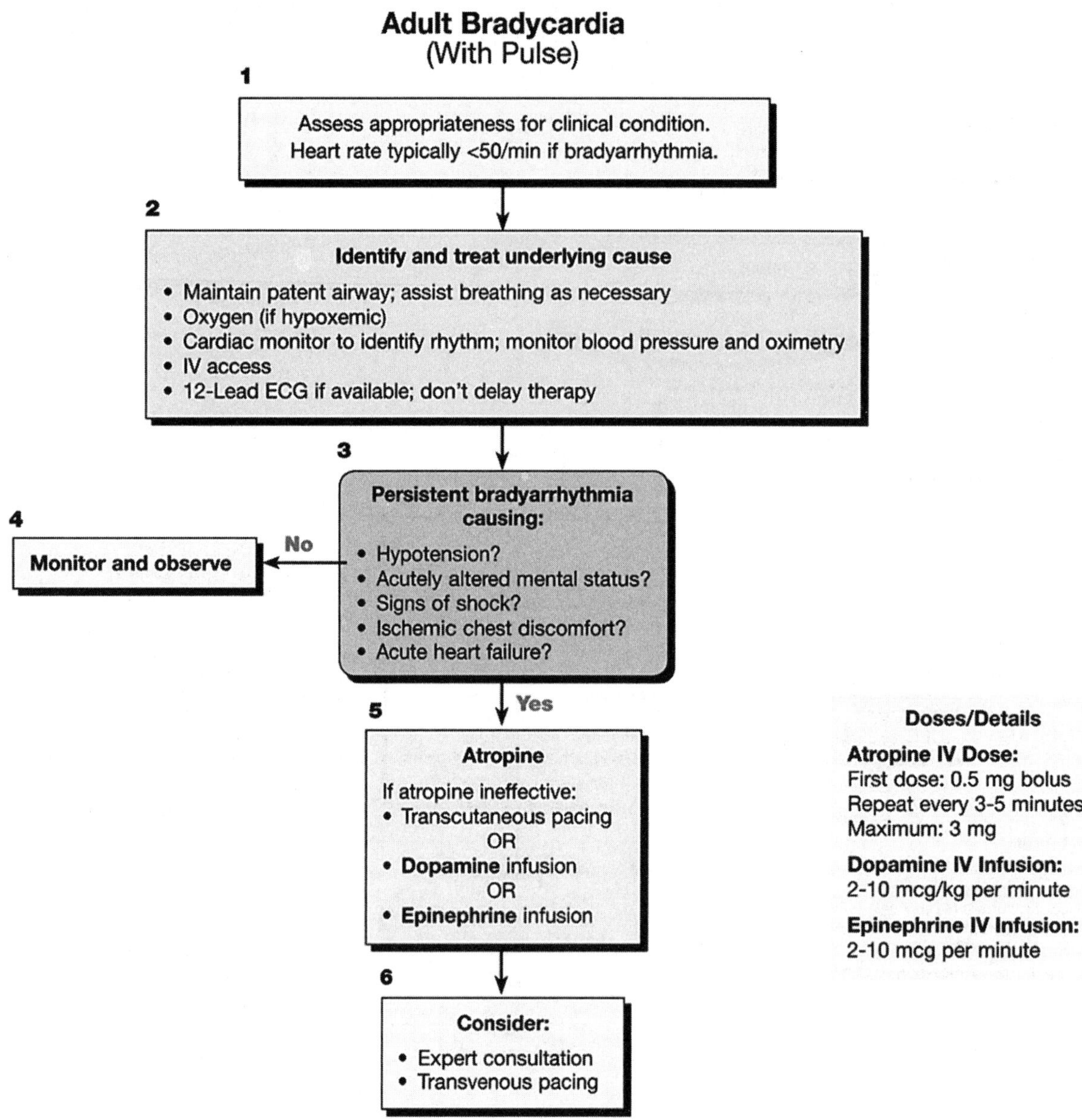

[a]Reproduced with permission from Wolters Kluwer Health. Neumar RW, Otto CW, Link MS, et al. Part 8: Adult advanced Cardiovascular life support: 2010 American Heart Association Guidelines for Cardiopulmonary Resuscitation and Emergency Cardiovascular Care. *Circulation.* 2010;122(18 suppl 3):S729-267.

Figure A4-3. Tachycardia Algorithm[a]

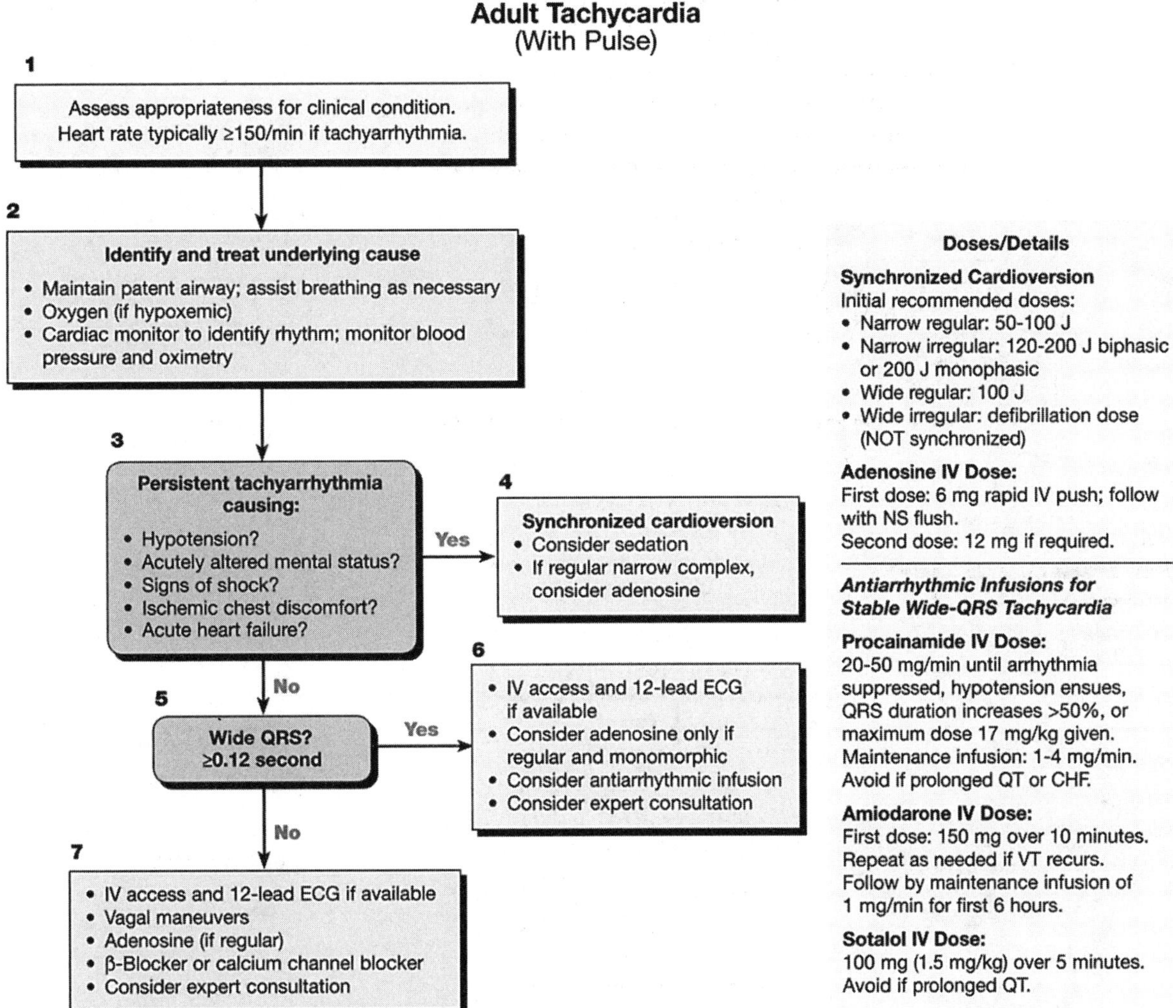

[a]Reproduced with permission from Wolters Kluwer Health. Neumar RW, Otto CW, Link MS, et al. Part 8: Adult advanced Cardiovascular life support: 2010 American Heart Association Guidelines for Cardiopulmonary Resuscitation and Emergency Cardiovascular Care. *Circulation.* 2010;122(18 suppl 3):S729-267.

Figure A4-4. Pediatric Pulseless Arrest Algorithm[a]

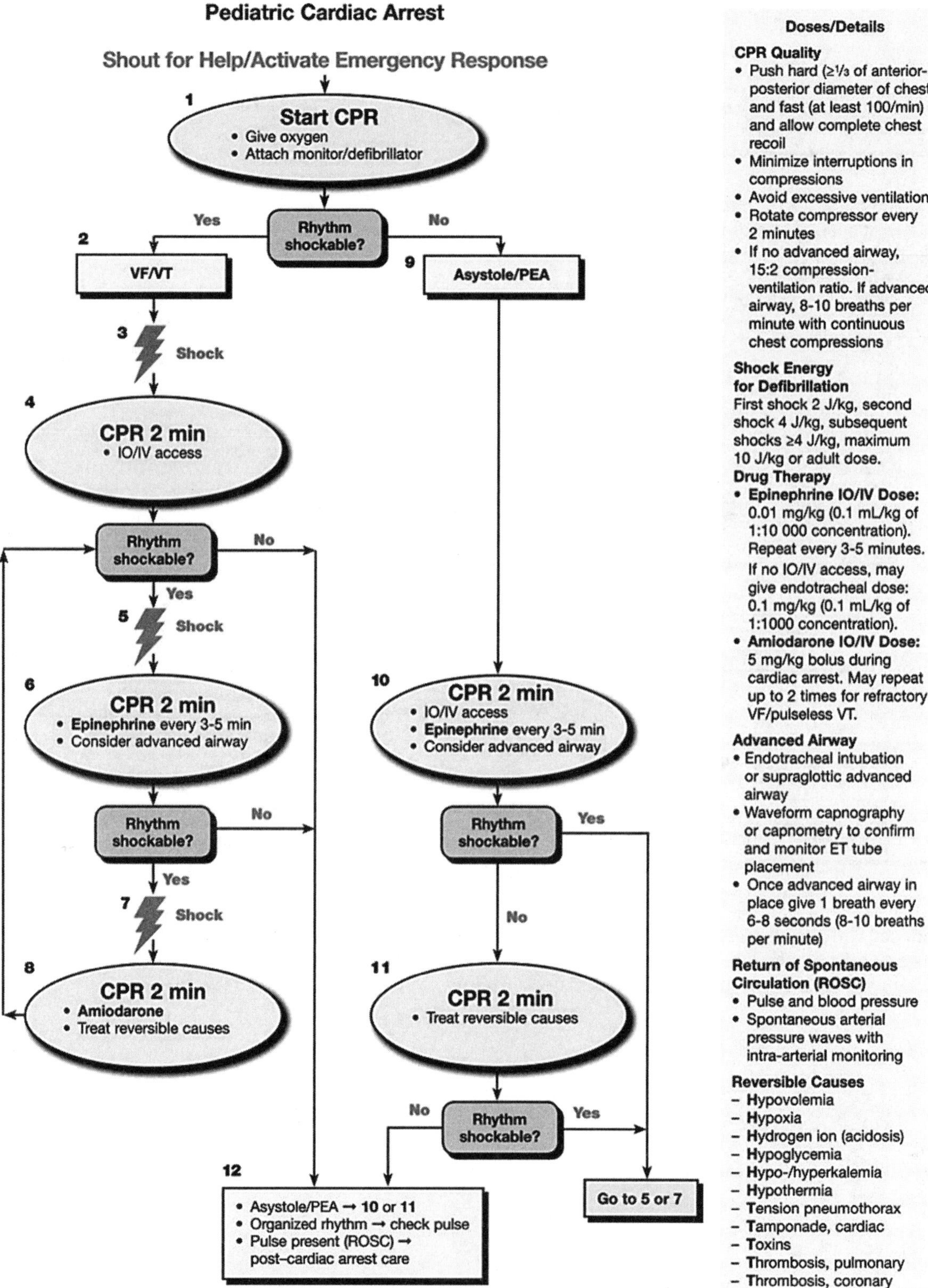

Performance of CPR should be continuous, with interruption only as necessary.

[a]Reproduced with permission from Wolters Kluwer Health. Kleinman ME, Chameides L, Schexnayder SM, et al. Part 14: Pediatric advanced life support: 2010 American Heart Association Guidelines for Cardiopulmonary Resuscitation and Emergency Cardiovascular Care. *Circulation.* 2010;122(18 suppl 3):S876-S908.

Figure A4-5. Pediatric Bradycardia Algorithm[a]

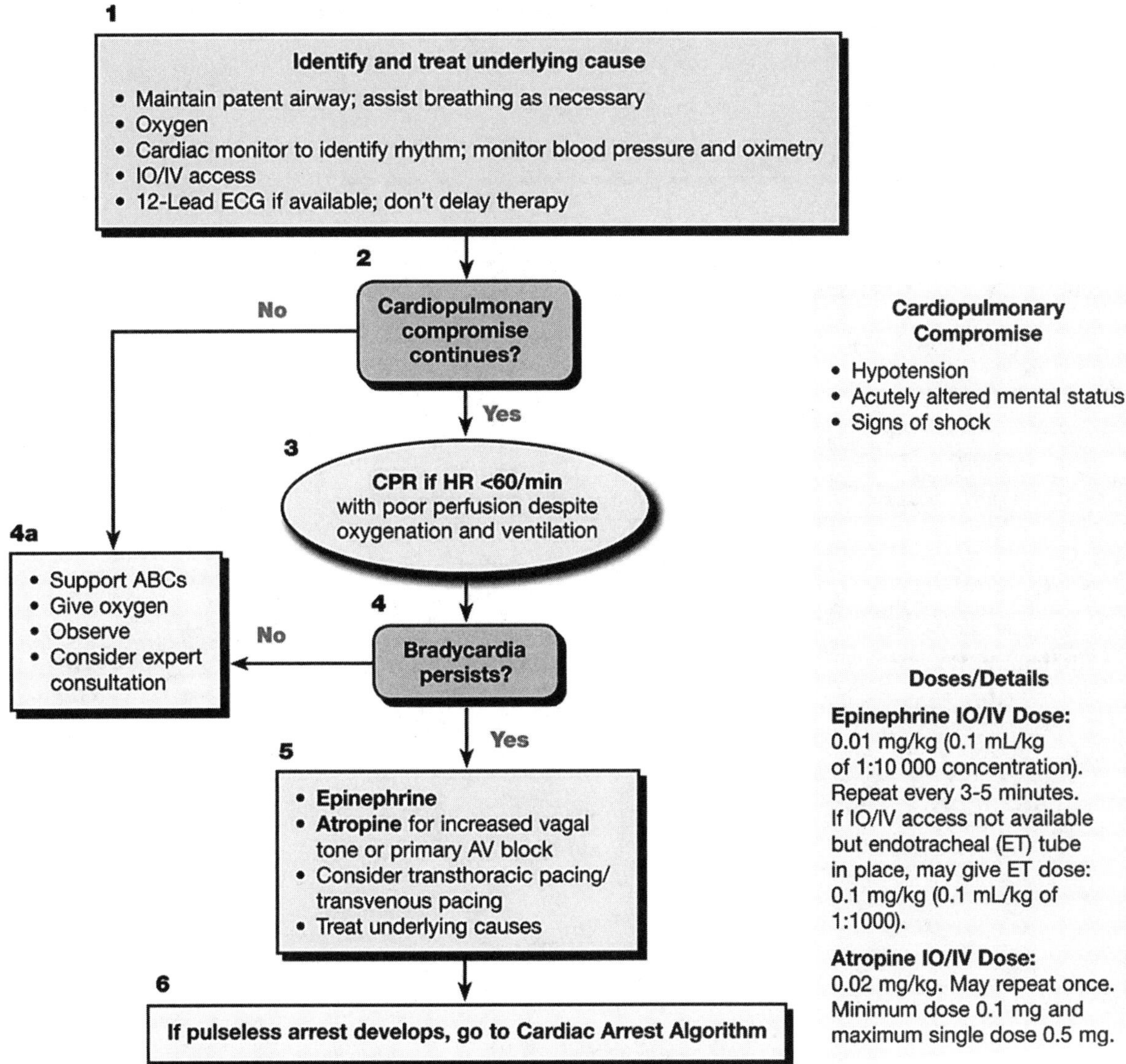

[a]Reproduced with permission from Wolters Kluwer Health. Kleinman ME, Chameides L, Schexnayder SM, et al. Part 14: Pediatric advanced life support: 2010 American Heart Association Guidelines for Cardiopulmonary Resuscitation and Emergency Cardiovascular Care. *Circulation.* 2010;122(18 suppl 3):S876-S908.

Figure A4-6. Pediatric Tachycardia Algorithm[a]

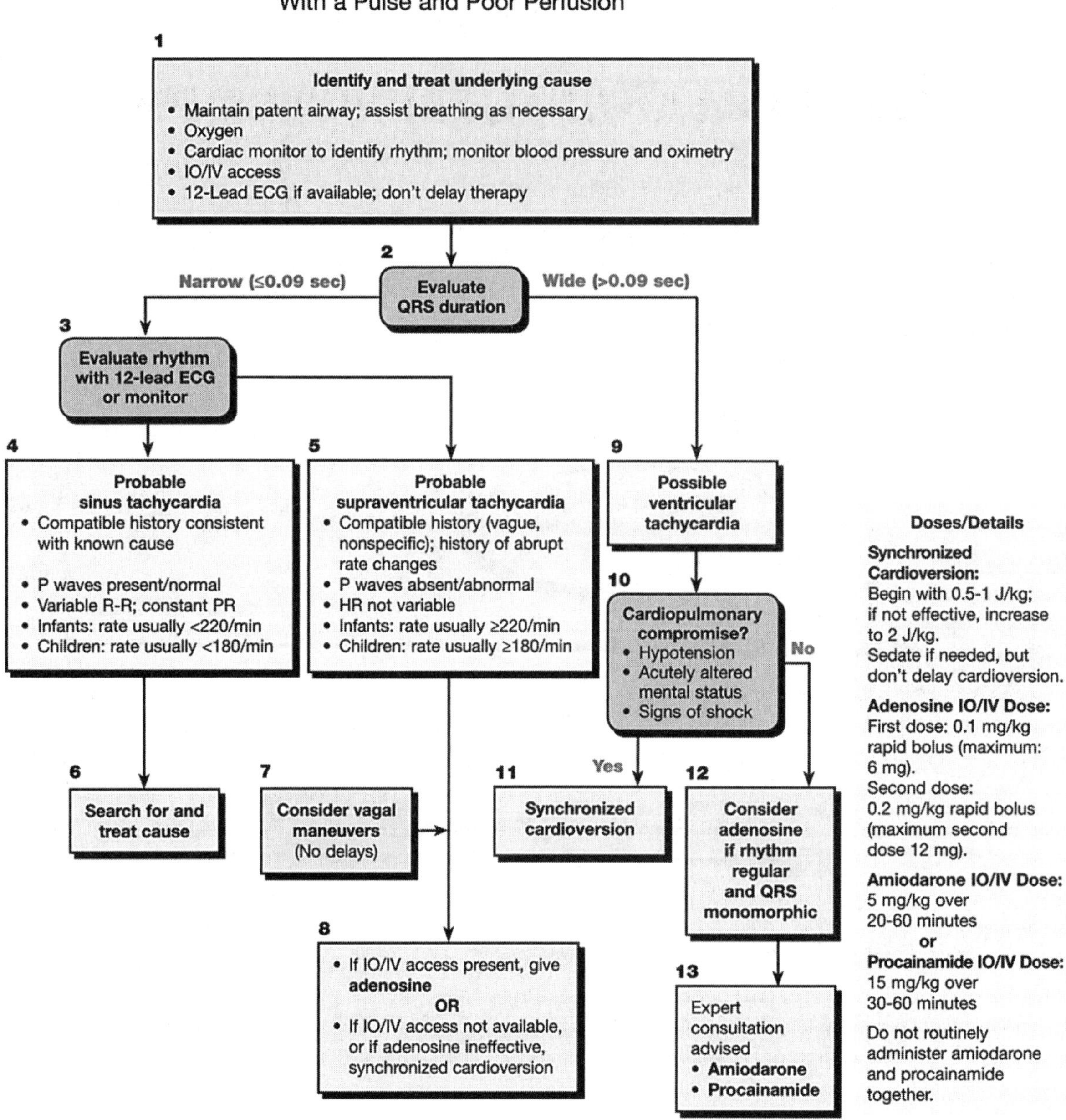

[a]Reproduced with permission from Wolters Kluwer Health. Kleinman ME, Chameides L, Schexnayder SM, et al. Part 14: Pediatric advanced life support: 2010 American Heart Association Guidelines for Cardiopulmonary Resuscitation and Emergency Cardiovascular Care. *Circulation.* 2010;122(18 suppl 3):S876-S908.

Appendix 5

Defibrillation/Cardioversion

I. Indications

A. Defibrillation/unsynchronized cardioversion

1. Ventricular fibrillation
2. Pulseless ventricular tachycardia
3. Polymorphic ventricular tachycardia

B. Synchronized cardioversion

1. Unstable or stable ventricular tachycardia with a pulse
2. Unstable or stable supraventricular tachycardia, atrial fibrillation, or atrial flutter

II. Equipment

A. Conductive gel or self-adhesive defibrillation pads

B. Defibrillator/cardioverter

C. Connecting cable, leads, and electrodes

D. Medication for sedation

E. Supplemental oxygen with bag-mask oxygen delivery device

F. Emergency suction and intubation equipment

G. Pulse oximeter

H. Electrocardiography and blood pressure monitor

I. Intravenous catheter, infusion pump, tubing, fluids

J. Resuscitation cart

III. TECHNIQUE

A. Recognize cardiac rhythm, determine severity of its physiologic effect.

B. In patients with unstable rhythms or adverse physiologic effects on systemic perfusion, begin immediate defibrillation/cardioversion. Initiate cardiopulmonary resuscitation if appropriate.

C. Recognize that time delays under the above circumstances decrease the likelihood of conversion to a stable rhythm.

D. Inform and prepare the patient as clinical situation dictates; sedate if necessary.

E. Assure intravenous access.

F. Provide supplemental oxygen.

G. Monitor pulse oximeter and electrocardiograph.

H. Turn on defibrillator/cardioverter.

I. Attach monitoring electrodes (if needed).

J. Apply conductive gel to paddles or apply conductive pads to chest wall.

1. Male patients with a hirsute chest may require rapid shaving to ensure adequate contact.

K. Paddle/electrode placement

1. Anterolateral (default placement)

   a. One paddle/electrode to right of upper sternum below clavicle

   b. One paddle/electrode *lateral to left nipple* with center in midaxillary line

2. Anteroposterior

   a. One paddle/electrode anteriorly over left precordium, below clavicle

   b. One paddle/electrode posteriorly in left infrascapular location, left of thoracic spine

3. Avoid placement directly over permanent pacer or implantable cardioverter-defibrillator

L. Paddle pressure (if used)

1. Adult — approximately 25 lb of pressure to each paddle

2. Pediatric — ensure good contact with chest wall

M. Activate appropriate switch for synchronized cardioversion or unsynchronized defibrillation.

N. Set energy level of electrical discharge (in accordance with recommendations of the American Heart Association).

1. Adult defibrillation

a. Manual biphasic waveform device: energy level is device-specific (typically between 120 to 200 J). If unknown, use 200 J for initial shock. Subsequent shocks should be same or higher energy level as initial shock.

b. Monophasic waveform device: 360 J, initial and subsequent shocks

2. Adult cardioversion (synchronized)

a. Ventricular tachycardia (stable): with monophasic or biphasic device, 100 J for initial attempt and advance energy level as needed.

b. Polymorphic ventricular tachycardia: treat as ventricular fibrillation (see above).

c. Atrial fibrillation: 200 J with monophasic device; 120 J to 200 J with biphasic device, or consult manufacturer. Escalate energy levels as needed for subsequent shocks.

d. Atrial flutter: 50-100 J; if rhythm persists, advance energy levels as needed.

e. Paroxysmal supraventricular tachycardia: 50 J; if rhythm persists, advance energy levels as needed.

f. If delays in synchronization occur or conditions are critical, use immediate unsynchronized shocks (defibrillation mode).

O. Ensure electrical safety (all personnel clear of contact with the patient, bed, and equipment).

P. Charge capacitors through defibrillator/cardioverter.

Q. Depress discharge button(s) on the device or simultaneously on the defibrillator/paddles (with synchronized cardioversion, the discharge buttons must remain depressed until the energy is released).

R. If defibrillation performed, immediately resume chest compressions; if cardioversion performed, assess patient (respiration, pulse, and rhythm).

S. If unsuccessful, repeat process, following standard Advanced Cardiovascular Life Support protocols.

IV. PEDIATRIC CONSIDERATIONS

A. Manual defibrillator

1. Appropriate paddle size is important; use the largest paddle size possible, assuring good chest contact over its entire area and good separation between the two paddles (about 3 cm).

   a. Infants (<10 kg) — 4.5-cm paddles usually used

   b. Children (>10 kg) — 8.0- to 13-cm paddles usually used

2. Paddle placement is similar to that for adults.

3. Be sure that the defibrillator/cardioverter provides a low-dose range for infants. Some defibrillators do not go below 10 J and therefore should not be used for converting infants/children whose weight <20 kg (5-6 yrs of age).

4. Pediatric defibrillation

   a. 2 J/kg (initial)

   b. Advance to 4 J/kg if rhythm persists

   c. Use adult energy levels in children ≥50 kg

5. Pediatric cardioversion

   a. Stable or unstable ventricular tachycardia: 0.5 to 1.0 J/kg

   b. Stable or unstable supraventricular tachycardia: 0.5 to 1.0 J/kg

   c. Advance to 2 J/kg if unsuccessful

B. AED (automatic external defibrillator)

1. >25 kg (8 years old): Use standard adult AED with adult pad-cable system.

2. <25 kg (>1 year old but <8 years old): Use attenuated dose if a pediatric system is available. Use adult system if pediatric system is not available.

3. <1 year old. There is insufficient evidence to recommend for or against the use of an AED.

V. PRECAUTIONS/COMPLICATIONS

A. During procedure

1. Skin burn may occur if insufficient gel or improper pads are used, poor contact with the chest wall occurs during discharge, or if the pads/paddles are too close to each other.

2. All metal objects should be removed from the patient to avoid skin burns.

3. Patient's environment and chest must be dry to avoid current traveling across water, resulting in a decreased amount of delivered energy.

4. Transdermal patches should be removed as they may impede transmission of current.

5. Medical personnel may sustain electrical shock or burn if safety precautions are not followed.

B. After procedure

1. Arterial embolization

2. Pulmonary edema

3. Postcardioversion arrhythmias; be prepared to institute cardiopulmonary resuscitation

4. Post-shock syndrome (myocardial damage)

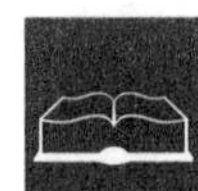

Suggested Readings

1. American Heart Association. *Advanced Cardiovascular Life Support: Provider Manual.* Dallas, TX: American Heart Association; 2010.

2. Part 6. Electrical therapies: Automated external defibrillators, defibrillation, cardioversion, and pacing. 2010 American Heart Association Guidelines for Cardiopulmonary Resuscitation and Emergency Cardiovascular Care. *Circulation.* 2010;122;S706-S719.

3. Wiegand D. *AACN Procedure Manual for Critical Care.* 6th ed. St. Louis, MO: Elsevier Saunders; 2010.

Appendix 6

Intraosseous Needle Insertion

I. INDICATIONS

A. Emergency vascular access in children and adults if intravenous access is delayed

B. Any fluid or medication that can be given intravenously can be given by the intraosseous route in the same dosages with onset and concentrations similar to the venous route

II. EQUIPMENT

A. Sternal or iliac bone marrow aspiration needle (15- to 18-gauge) or disposable intraosseous needle (battery-powered insertion device)

B. Sterile syringes and infiltrating needles

C. Sterile 4 × 4 gauze sponges

D. Medication for local anesthesia

E. Gloves, sterile drapes

F. Skin disinfectant

G. Supplemental oxygen

H. Pulse oximeter

I. Electrocardiography monitor

J. Intravenous tubing, T-connector, and fluid

III. SITE SELECTION

A. Young children

1. In neonates, proximal tibia, just below the growth plate, distal to the tibial tubercle. In infants 6 to 12 months old, insert 1 cm distal to tibial tuberosity. In children >1 year of age, insert 2 cm distal to the tibial tuberosity.

B. Adults

1. Proximal anterior tibia (see below)

2. Distal tibia above the medial malleolus

3. Distal radius and distal ulna

4. Distal femur

5. Anterior-superior iliac spine

6. Sternum

IV. TECHNIQUE (TIBIAL SITE)

A. Apply oxygen, monitor pulse oximeter and electrocardiograph.

B. Restrain leg with a small sandbag or intravenous fluid bag behind the knee for support.

C. Create sterile field.

D. Infiltrate local anesthetic if clinical situation permits.

E. Use proximal anterior tibia, midpoint of the medial flat surface, 1 to 3 cm below the tibial tuberosity (**Figure A6-1**).

F. Insert the needle 60° to 90° to the skin away from the growth plate; advance with a screwing motion.

G. Use the distal tibia only if the proximal tibia is impenetrable (just proximal to the medial malleolus and posterior to the saphenous vein).

H. Confirm entry into the marrow space by noting a lack of resistance after the needle has passed through the cortex.

Figure A6-1. Intraosseous Needle Insertion[a]

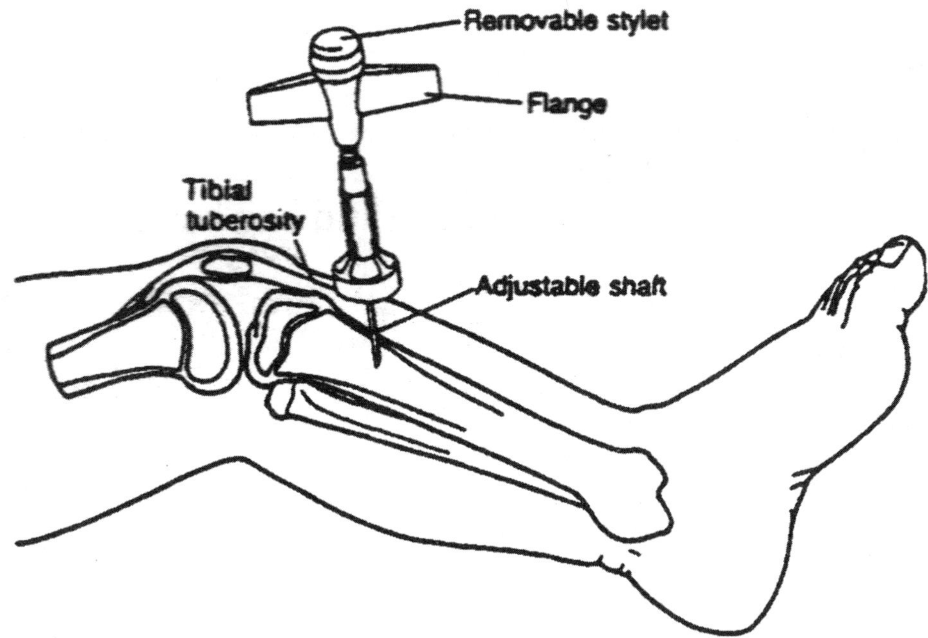

Approach to puncture of the proximal anterior tibia.
[a]Reproduced with permission from the Massachussetts Medical Society.[2] Copyright 1990 Massachussetts Medical Society.

I. Aspirate marrow into the syringe; this should be accomplished easily, but failure to do so does not necessarily indicate improper placement.

J. Infuse fluids; fluids should flow freely.

K. Secure needle by taping flanges to the skin (may require support of external portion of the needle).

L. Consider flushing with heparin-saline solution.

M. Infuse intravenous fluids.

N. Observe for infiltration of fluids.

O. Continue attempts to place intravenous catheter(s).

P. Discontinue intraosseous infusion and withdraw needle after intravenous access is established (preferably within 1-2 hours).

Q. Apply pressure to puncture site for approximately 5 minutes.

R. Apply sterile dressing.

V. PRECAUTIONS/COMPLICATIONS

A. Inability to place needle (approximately 20% of patients)

B. Subcutaneous and/or subperiosteal infiltration of fluid

C. Tibial fracture

D. Compartment syndrome

E. Clotting of marrow within the needle

F. Cellulitis, subcutaneous abscess

G. Osteomyelitis (0.6%)

H. Pain (usually minor)

Suggested Readings

1. Fiorito BA, Mirza F, Doran TM, et al. Intraosseous access in the setting of pediatric critical care transport. *Pediatr Crit Care Med.* 2005;6:50-53.

2. Fiser HD. Intraosseous infusion. *N Engl J Med.* 1990;322:1579-1581.

3. International Liaison Committee on Resuscitation. The International Liaison Committee on Resuscitation (ILCOR) consensus on science with treatment recommendations for pediatric and neonatal patients: Pediatric basic and advanced life support. *Pediatrics.* 2006;117:e955-e977.

4. Part 14. Pediatric Advanced Life Support. 2010 American Heart Association Guidelines for Cardiopulmonary Resuscitation and Emergency Cardiovascular Care. *Circulation.* 2010;122:S876-S908. Available at http://circ.ahajournals.org/content/122/18_suppl_3/S876.full.pdf+html

Appendix 7

Temporary Transcutaneous Cardiac Pacing

I. INDICATIONS/CONTRAINDICATIONS

A. Indications

1. Symptomatic bradycardia (hypotension, chest pain, syncope, altered mental status, heart failure, etc) unresponsive to pharmacologic management

2. Overdrive pacing of tachycardias, refractory to drug therapy or electrical cardioversion

B. Contraindications

1. Severe hypothermia

2. Not recommended for asystole

II. EQUIPMENT

A. Cardiac pacing electrode pads

B. Pulse generator

C. Connecting leads

D. Medication for sedation and/or analgesia, if necessary

E. Supplemental oxygen (cannula, mask, other as necessary)

F. Pulse oximeter

G. Electrocardiography monitor

H. Intravenous catheter, tubing, fluids

I. Resuscitation cart

III. TECHNIQUE

A. Recognize cardiac rhythm, determine severity.

B. Prepare patient.

C. Obtain intravenous access if not done previously.

D. Apply oxygen; monitor pulse oximeter and electrocardiograph.

E. Attempt pharmacologic management, including atropine, epinephrine, and/or dopamine when appropriate (follow Advanced Cardiovascular Life Support guidelines).

F. Assemble equipment.

G. Apply electrode pads.

1. Anteroposterior

    a. One electrode anteriorly over left precordium as close as possible to maximal cardiac impulse, below clavicle

    b. One electrode posteriorly in left infrascapular location directly behind anterior electrode, left of thoracic spine

2. Anterolateral

    a. One electrode to right of upper sternum below clavicle

    b. One electrode *lateral to left nipple* with center in midaxillary line

3. Shaving of excessive body hair may be required to ensure good contact

H. Administer sedation or analgesia as necessary and tolerated by patient

I. Connect leads to pulse generator

J. Turn on pulse generator and monitor

K. Set rate at 60 to 100 beats/min; adjust as needed, based on clinical response

L. Adjust pulse generator output (mA) upward until electrical and mechanical ventricular capture (threshold) occurs (usually 20 to 60 mA). Set output 2 mA above threshold to allow for safety margin. In the setting of severe symptoms, it may be appropriate to start at the maximal output and then decrease if capture is achieved.

M. Criteria for proper electrical capture:

1. Pacer spike followed by a ventricular complex 100% of the time
2. Wide QRS complex
3. T wave in an opposite deflection from baseline as the QRS complex

N. Assess efficacy of mechanical capture — obtain blood pressure and palpate pulse distal to carotid site as electrical muscle stimulation from the pacemaker may mimic a carotid pulse.

O. Arrange for temporary or permanent transvenous pacemaker as necessary.

IV. PEDIATRIC CONSIDERATIONS

A. Bradycardia in children is most often secondary to hypoxemia.

B. Pacing for bradycardic rhythms secondary to hypoxemic insult may be considered after airway management, oxygenation, ventilation, chest compressions, epinephrine bolus (0.01 mg/kg, 1:1,000 concentration) and infusion, and possibly atropine bolus (0.02 mg/kg, may repeat; minimum dose 0.1 mg and maximum total dose for child 1 mg) have been accomplished.

C. The effectiveness of cardiac pacing in this setting is unproven.

D. Even if electrical capture of the heart is accomplished, contractility and myocardial blood flow may not improve without mechanical capture.

E. It is recommended to use the largest available paddles or self-adhering electrode pads that will fit on the chest wall without touching (allow at least 3 cm between paddles or pads).

1. For children >10 kg (>1 year of age), use large adult paddles.
2. For children <10 kg (<1 year of age), use small infant paddles (4.5 cm).

V. PRECAUTIONS/COMPLICATIONS

A. Inability to capture (~20% of patients), usually related to delay in attempting to pace

B. Painful skeletal muscle contraction

C. Skin or tissue damage

D. Temporizing measure only, before transvenous pacing

Suggested Readings

1. American Heart Association. *Advanced Cardiovascular Life Support: Provider Manual.* Dallas, TX: American Heart Association; 2011.

2. Link MS, Atkins DL, Passman RS, et al. Part 6: electrical therapies: automated external defibrillators, defibrillation, cardioversion, and pacing: 2010 American Heart Association Guidelines for Cardiopulmonary Resuscitation and Emergency Cardiovascular Care. *Circulation.* 2010;122(18 suppl 3):S706-719.

3. Wiegand D. *AACN Procedure Manual for Critical Care.* 6th ed. St. Louis, MO: Elsevier Saunders; 2010.

Appendix 8

Thoracostomy

I. Indications/Contraindications

A. Indications

1. Tension pneumothorax
2. Large simple pneumothorax
3. Penetrating thoracic wound with concurrent need for positive pressure ventilation
4. Hemothorax
5. Symptomatic pleural effusion (recurrent, following thoracentesis)
6. Empyema
7. Chylothorax

B. Contraindications

1. Coagulopathy
    a. Correct prior to nonemergent thoracostomy.
    b. Risk of hemorrhage must be accepted with tension pneumothorax.
2. Inability to aspirate fluid or air to confirm a patent pleural space
    a. This dictum holds in all circumstances except a penetrating thoracic wound with need for positive pressure ventilation.
    b. Attempted tube placement in the presence of an obliterated pleural space risks pulmonary injury and potentially fatal hemorrhage.
    c. Aspiration is performed most conveniently through the thoracostomy incisional wound immediately before tube placement.
    d. Aspiration is most important when an apparent effusion presents as "whiteout" on chest radiograph, and its free-flowing nature cannot be confirmed radiographically. Such an apparent effusion in reality may be solid tumor; blunt dissection into such tumor may have devastating hemorrhagic consequences.

II. EQUIPMENT

A. Needle thoracostomy
   1. 14- to 16-gauge catheter over needle
   2. 23-gauge butterfly needle (infants)

B. Tube thoracostomy
   1. Sterile gloves, gown, eye protection, mask, cap, and drapes
   2. Intravenous catheter, tubing, and fluid
   3. Supplemental oxygen
   4. Monitors (echocardiographic, pulse oximeter)
   5. Skin disinfectant
   6. Sterile syringes and infiltrating needles
   7. Local anesthetic
   8. Scalpel with #10 or #15 blade
   9. Forceps
   10. Curved clamp
   11. 24- to 40-French thoracostomy tube
       a. 32- to 40-French thoracostomy tubes are placed in trauma settings to evacuate an acute hemothorax that potentially contains clots. The largest diameter tube accommodated by the intercostal space is used in this circumstance.
       b. For infants and children, see **Table A8-1**.
   12. Water-seal drainage system
   13. Needle holder
   14. 0-silk or 0-polypropylene suture on cutting needle
   15. Suture scissors
   16. 1/4-inch-wide adhesive tape strips or "cable ties" with applicator
   17. Sterile 4 × 4 gauze sponges
   18. Petroleum jelly gauze
   19. Antiseptic ointment
   20. 4-inch-wide impervious tape strips
   21. 1-inch-wide adhesive tape
   22. Resuscitation cart

Table A8-1 Approximate Sizes for Pediatric Thoracostomy Tubes by Age and Weight[a]

Age	Approximate Weight (kg)	Tube Size (French)
Newborn to 9 months	3.5-8	12-18
10 to 17 months	10	14-20
18 months to 3 years	12-15	14-24
4 to 7 years	17-22	20-32
8 years	28	28-32
≥9 years	≥35	28-38

[a]Needle thoracostomy can usually be accomplished on infants with a 23-gauge butterfly needle.

III. TECHNIQUE: SURGICAL CHEST TUBE PLACEMENT

A. Analgesia/Sedation

1. Tube thoracostomy is a painful procedure. In nonemergent and semiurgent circumstances, intravenous narcotic analgesia and a benzodiazepine should be titrated to effect as hemodynamic and respiratory status allow. Local anesthetic should be infiltrated generously throughout the tube thoracostomy tract.

B. Preliminary needle thoracostomy (**Figure A8-1**)

1. Indication: before tube thoracostomy for rapid temporizing treatment of tension pneumothorax.
2. Site
   a. Midclavicular line at the second intercostal space; necessitates that the pectoralis major muscle and possibly breast tissue be penetrated before the intercostal space.
   b. Midaxillary line at the fifth intercostal space; placed in the auscultatory triangle posterior to the pectoralis and anterior to latissimus dorsi muscles where only the thin serratus anterior muscle need be penetrated prior to the intercostal space.
3. Don cap, mask, eye protection, and sterile gloves.
4. Quickly prepare the access site with povidone-iodine solution.
5. Advance 14-gauge catheter over needle with attached syringe immediately over the superior aspect of the rib while aspirating.
6. When air is aspirated, advance catheter completely, and withdraw needle and syringe. Withdraw catheter following completion of tube thoracostomy.
7. Note: 1 mL of saline in the aspirating syringe allows access of intrapleural air to be recognized as bubbles.

Figure A8-1. Sites for Needle Thoracostomy

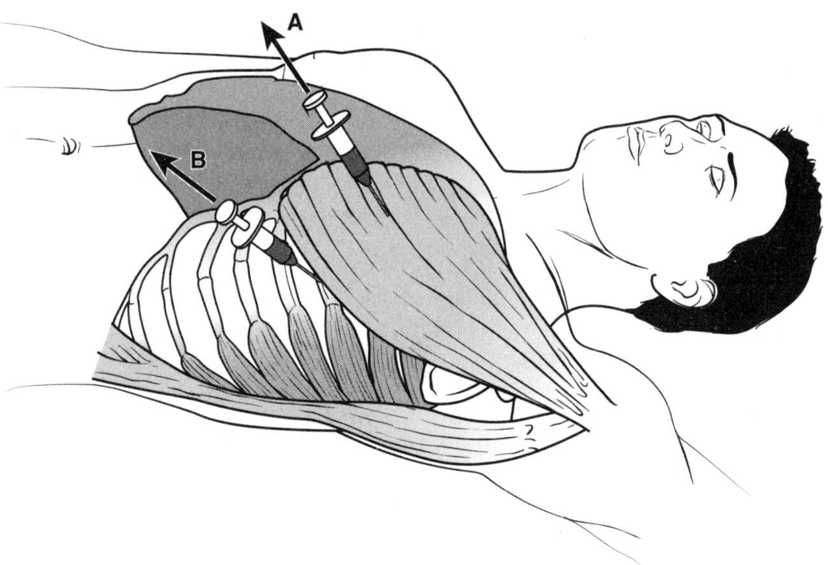

(A) Second intercostal space, midclavicular line. **(B)** Fifth intercostal space, midaxillary line. The latter is also the incision site for placement of a thoracostomy tube and necessitates transgression of much less chest wall musculature and no breast tissue.

C. Preparation for tube thoracostomy
   1. Provide supplemental oxygen.
   2. In nonemergent circumstances, establish intravenous access, electrocardiographic monitoring, and pulse oximetry.
   3. Assemble the following nonsterile materials: water-seal drainage system, 1/4-inch-wide strips of adhesive tape or cable ties to secure thoracostomy tube to drainage system, 4-inch-wide impervious tape strips to secure dressing.
   4. Ensure adequate lighting.
   5. Place patient in supine position with ipsilateral arm extended.
   6. Don cap, mask, eye protection, and sterile gloves.
   7. Paint patient's anterior and lateral chest wall with antiseptic solution. Remove gloves.
   8. Don sterile gown and gloves.
   9. On a sterile work space, lay out, from left to right, the following sterile instruments and materials in sequence: syringe with infiltrating needle loaded with local anesthetic, scalpel with blade, forceps, curved clamp, thoracostomy tube, needle holder loaded with suture, suture scissor, dressing composed of gauze 4 × 4 sponges, petroleum jelly gauze, and antiseptic ointment. These instruments and materials will be used in this sequence.

D. Insertion

Instrument	Maneuver
1. Syringe and needle with local anesthetic	a. Raise cutaneous wheal at incision site. b. Deeply infiltrate underlying subcutaneous tissue.
2. Scalpel	a. 3-cm incision at position *B* in **Figure A8-1** through the skin and subcutaneous tissue of the fifth intercostal space. b. Deepen incision to level of chest wall musculature. Note: The skin incision parallels the intercostal space. It should be placed one interspace below the intended level of pleural entry so that a tract deep to subcutaneous tissue can be created for the tube. This tract closes spontaneously upon tube removal.
3. Syringe and needle with local anesthetic	a. Through wound, infiltrate subcutaneous tissue cephalad to incision.
4. Forceps	a. Using left hand, retract subcutaneous tissue cephalad away from chest wall to create tension at junction of subcutaneous tissue and chest wall musculature **(Figure A8-2)**.
5. Curved clamp	a. Continue to apply above traction with forceps. b. With curved clamp in right hand, spread at junction of subcutaneous tissue and chest wall musculature to open this plane **(Figure A8-2)**.
6. Syringe and needle with local anesthetic	a. Through incisional wound, infiltrate musculature and pleura of fourth intercostal space. b. Advance needle into pleural space while aspirating syringe. c. Confirm presence of air or fluid in the pleural space.

7. Curved clamp	a. With curved clamp in right hand, hold tips against superior aspect of fifth rib with concavity of clamp facing pleural space. b. Perform intercostal dissection immediately superior to a rib to avoid injury to the neurovascular bundle that lies inferior to each rib. c. Advance curved clamp through musculature (serratus anterior and intercostal muscles) and pleura into the pleural space (**Figure A8-3**). Note: This maneuver may need to be forceful but must always be restrained. A dramatic loss of resistance will signal entry into the pleural space and will be followed by egress of fluid and/or air. d. Ensuring that the tips of the clamp remain on the superior aspect of the fifth rib, widely separate the jaws of the clamp to create a generous opening through the serratus anterior muscle, intercostal muscles, and pleura. e. Insert the left index finger into the pleural space as the clamp is withdrawn. Palpation of the smooth pleura confirms the intrapleural location. Sweep the finger through 360° to ensure the absence of adhesions between parietal and visceral pleura. Such adhesions and obliteration of the pleural space would predispose to pulmonary injury during tube insertion.
8. Thoracostomy tube	a. Keep the left index finger in the pleural space. b. With the right hand, advance the thoracostomy tube over the tip of the left index finger into the pleural space (**Figure A8-4**). Passage of the tube over the tip of the intrapleural index finger ensures intrapleural placement of the tube. c. Advance the tube until resistance is encountered (approximately 15 to 25 cm). The last side hole of the tube should reside 2 cm within the pleural cavity. Ideally, the tip of the tube lies at the pleural apex. d. ***Alternative Method - After confirming appropriate access site to the pleural space, the chest tube can be directed superiorly and posteriorly by using initial guidance with the curved clamp. With the tube safely in the pleural space and directed appropriately, the clamp is released and the tube advanced toward the apex of the hemithorax.*** **(See Figure A8-5.)**
9. Water-seal drainage system	a. Connect the thoracostomy tube to the drainage system.

10. Needle holder and suture	a. Place a suture of 0-nonabsorbable material through the wound on either side of the thoracostomy tube. b. Tie each suture to close the wound. c. Tie each suture about the thoracostomy tube to secure it. d. Place additional sutures as necessary to close the wound.
11. 1/4-inch adhesive tape or cable ties	a. Secure connection between chest tube and drainage system tubing **(Figure A8-6)**. b. Tape should never be placed in such a manner as to obscure the connection from view. One must be able to see that the connections are intact at all times.
12. Dressing of gauze, 4 x 4 sponges, petroleum jelly gauze, antiseptic ointment, and impervious tape	a. Place dressing over thoracostomy site. b. Secure dressing with impervious tape.
13. 1-inch adhesive tape	a. Secure chest tube and drainage system tubing to patient's trunk.

Figure A8-2. Blunt Dissection for Thoracostomy

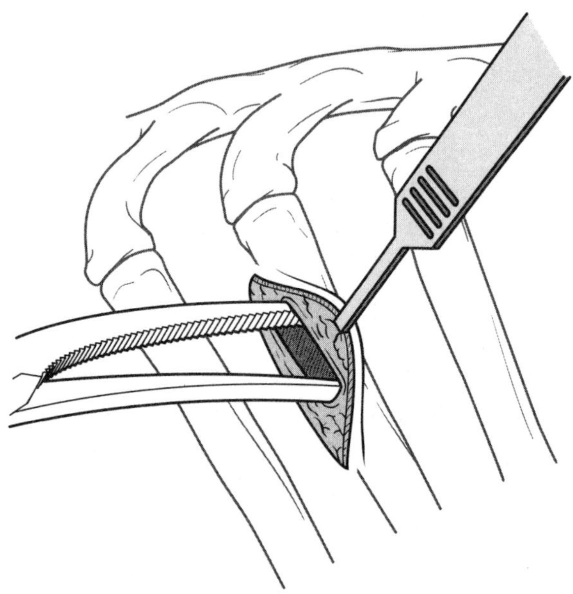

Retraction of skin and subcutaneous tissue with blunt dissection of subcutaneous tissue from chest wall musculature superior to incision.

Figure A8-3. Creation of Pleural Opening

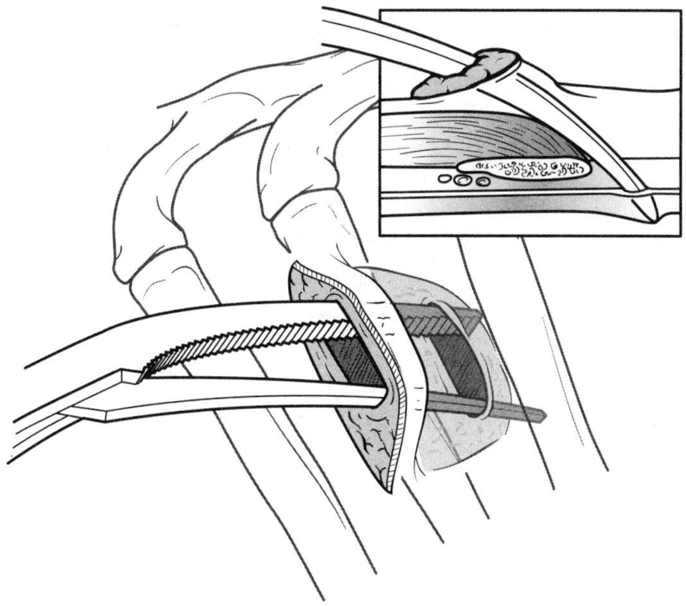

The curved clamp has been advanced into the superior aspect of the incision and advanced through the intercostal musculature and pleura at the superior margin of the fifth rib. The jaws of the clamp are then spread to create a pleural opening. The opening should be generous enough to simultaneously admit a finger and the thoracostomy tube. Insert shows the path of the curved clamp in cross section.

Figure A8-4. Placement of Thoracostomy Tube

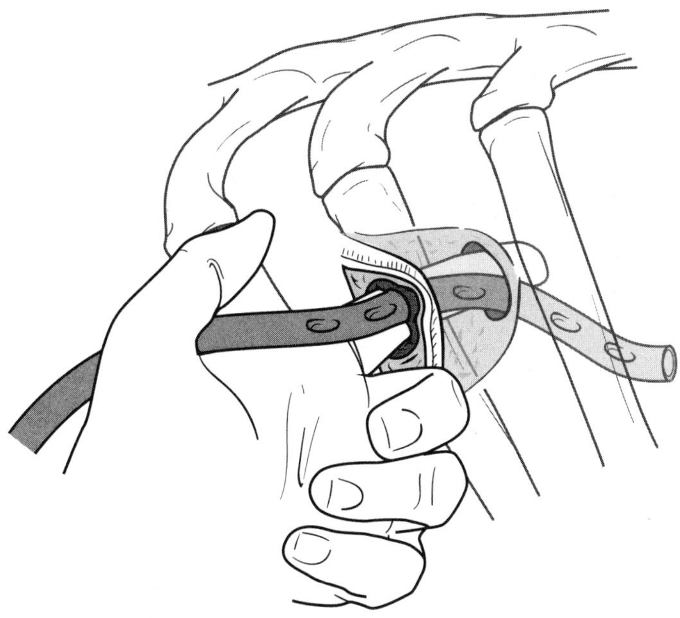

The left index finger replaces the curved clamp and remains within the pleural space as the thoracostomy tube is advanced over the tip of the finger, ensuring intrapleural location.

Figure A8-5. Alternative Thoracostomy Insertion Technique

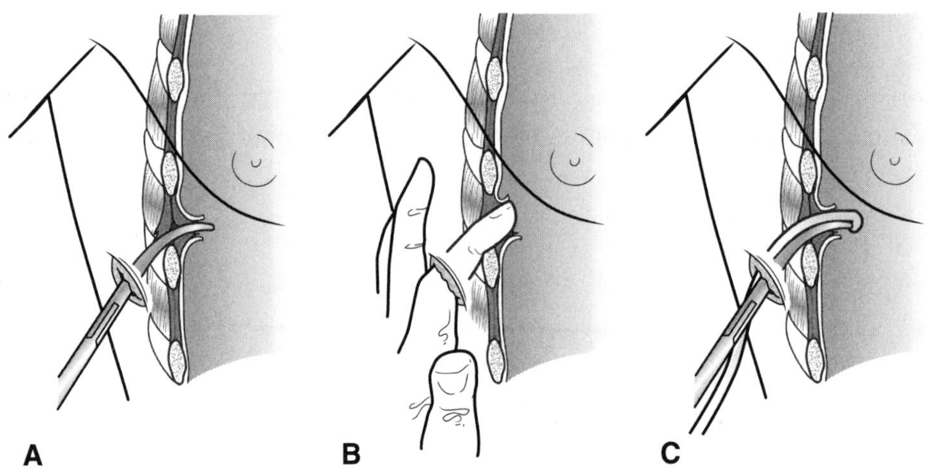

Figure A8-6. Connection of Thoracostomy Tube

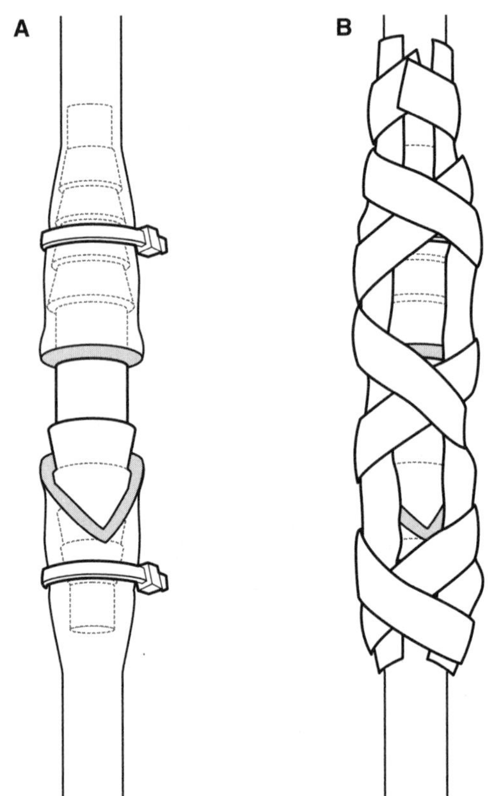

The thoracostomy tube and tubing from the draining system are secured about a conical connecting adaptor with cable ties (**A**) or strips of adhesive tape placed longitudinally and in a spiral fashion (**B**).

E. Pleural decompression

1. Adjust suction to 20 cm H_2O.
2. Consider prophylactic antibiotic coverage.

F. Thoracostomy tube monitoring

1. A thoracostomy tube should be monitored frequently with portable chest radiography to ensure appropriate tube placement and the absence of iatrogenic pneumothorax. The last side hole of the thoracostomy tube lies on a radiopaque line and thus is visible on the radiograph as a gap in this line; the gap should always appear well within the pleural space.
2. Patency of the chest tube is assured by the presence of a to-and-fro movement of fluid with respiration (respiratory variation). This may be detected within the thoracostomy tube, the tubing of the collection device, or the water-seal chamber. As the pleural space is definitively decompressed, the thoracostomy tube will become loculated from the general pleural space by adhesion of visceral and parietal pleura around it; respiratory variation will then be lost.
3. The character and volume of pleural drainage must be assessed frequently. The significance of diminished drainage volume can only be determined in light of concurrent chest radiographic findings. For example, diminishing sanguineous drainage may mean cessation of bleeding or occlusion of the thoracostomy tube by clot; the chest radiograph will reveal increasing effusion/hemothorax in the latter circumstance, but not the former.
4. Air leaks are apparent as air bubbling through the water seal (not the suction regulator). Small air leaks will demonstrate bubbling only during spontaneous expiration or mechanical inspiration. Large air leaks will demonstrate bubbling through both phases of the respiratory cycle. These continuous air leaks may indicate a bronchopleural fistula or tracheobronchial laceration.

G. Thoracostomy tube removal

1. General criteria for thoracostomy tube removal
    a Complete radiographic expansion of the lung
    b. Absence of air leak for 24 hours
    c. Drainage volume <100 mL over 24 hours
2. Prepare a dressing of impervious tape, gauze 4 × 4 sponges, petroleum jelly gauze, and antiseptic ointment.
3. With a sterile scissors, divide the sutures securing the thoracostomy tube.
4. Instruct the patient to take a full inspiration, hold the breath, and perform a Valsalva maneuver. Practice this sequence several times.
5. Repeat the above sequence, briskly withdraw the thoracostomy tube with the patient performing a Valsalva maneuver at full inspiration, and immediately apply the occlusive dressing to the thoracostomy wound.
6. Do not close the thoracostomy site with suture or other material.
7. Obtain an immediate portable chest radiograph to ensure the absence of pneumothorax.

IV. PEDIATRIC CONSIDERATIONS

A. Approximate sizes for pediatric thoracostomy tubes by age and weight are shown in **Table A8-1**.

V. PRECAUTIONS/COMPLICATIONS

A. Possible injury to intercostal artery, vein, or nerve
B. Extrapleural tube position
C. Subcutaneous emphysema
D. Break in water seal, resulting in pneumothorax
E. Chest wall hematoma/ecchymosis
F. Chest wall or intrapleural hemorrhage
G. Infection
    1. Insertion-site cellulitis
    2. Tract infection
    3. Empyema
H. Laceration of diaphragm or intrathoracic/intra-abdominal viscera
I. Recurrence of pneumothorax (upon removal, secondary to entrained room air or rupture of pulmonary bulla/bleb).
J. Clamping a chest tube in the presence of an air leak may result in life-threatening tension pneumothorax.

Suggested Readings

1. Etoch SW, Bar-Natan MF, Miller FB, et al. Tube thoracostomy. Factors related to complications. *Arch Surg.* 1995;130:521-525.

2. Lotano VE. Chest tube thoracostomy. In: Parrillo JE, Dellinger RP, eds. *Critical Care Medicine: Principles of Diagnosis and Management in the Adult.* 3rd ed. Philadelphia, PA: Mosby Elsevier; 2008:271.

3. Martino K, Merrit S, Boyakye K, et al. Prospective randomized trial of thoracostomy removal algorithms. *J Trauma* 1999;46:369-371.

4. Richardson JD, Spain DA. Injury to the lung and pleura: In: Mattox KL, Feliciano DV, Moore EE, eds. *Trauma.* 4th ed. New York, NY: McGraw-Hill, 2000; 523-543.

Appendix 9

Brain Death and Organ Donation

I. Brain Death (Death by Neurologic Criteria)

Brain death is usually a clinical diagnosis based on total and irreversible cessation of all brain function, including that of the brainstem. To diagnose brain death, physicians must verify the presence of unresponsive coma, the absence of brainstem reflexes, and the absence of respiratory drive after a CO_2 challenge. To assure that cessation of brain function is irreversible, physicians must determine the cause of the coma, exclude medical conditions that could mimic coma, and observe the patient for a period of time to exclude the possibility of recovery. Diagnostic criteria and methods in brain death may be established by national, state, or hospital policies and vary among institutions and political jurisdictions. Common requirements are summarized in **Table A9-1**. A physician experienced in brain death certification, hospital policy, and relevant laws should always participate in this process.

Local, regional, and national regulations play a significant role in the organ donation process. Clinicians determining the propriety of organ donation must do this with consideration of applicable standards.

Most hospitals have the capability to perform and interpret an electroencephalogram, nuclear medicine scan, or cerebral angiogram. These may be considered the preferred tests in confirming physical findings consistent with brain death. In some jurisdictions, ancillary tests are utilized when uncertainty exists about the reliability of components of the neurologic examination or when the apnea test cannot be performed.

Special interpretation is required for each of these ancillary tests. In adults, ancillary tests are not needed for the clinical diagnosis of brain death and cannot replace a neurologic examination.

Table A9-1 Clinical Criteria for Brain-Death Certification

1. Identifiable cause of coma
2. Exclusion of reversible central nervous system depression
   - Absence of hypothermia (core temperature >96.8°F [36°C])
   - Systolic blood pressure >100 mm Hg
   - Absence of drugs (eg, ethanol, barbiturates, sedative hypnotics, neuromuscular blocking agents)
   - Absence of metabolic abnormalities that could potentiate central nervous system depression (eg, abnormalities in electrolytes, osmolality, serum ammonia, hypercapnia, hypoxemia)
3. Absent cortical function
   - Unresponsive to painful stimuli administered via cranial nerves (spinal cord reflexes may persist in brain death)
   - No spontaneous muscular movements
   - No posturing, shivering, or seizure activity
4. Absent brainstem function
   - Pupils nonreactive
   - No corneal reflexes
   - No gag or cough reflexes
   - No oculocephalic reflexes
   - No oculovestibular reflexes
5. Documentation of apnea
   - Absence of spontaneous breathing after a $Paco_2$ >60 mm Hg (>8.0 kPa) or 20 mm Hg (2.7 kPa) above normal baseline values has been reached during apnea testing
6. Additional confirmatory studies (optional in adults but may be required in some situations)
   - Cerebral blood flow study (four-vessel angiogram preferred/required in some countries or radionuclide imaging) – absent cerebral blood flow
   - Nuclear cerebral perfusion scan
   - Electroencephalogram – no activity recorded at full gain (consult with a neurophysiologist)

II. ORGAN DONATION

A. Brain Death

Organs and tissues obtained from donors who fulfill brain-death criteria can be used in transplantation. This is facilitated by a local organ procurement organization representative, the procurement transplant coordinator, who can provide information about eligibility criteria for specific organs or tissues. The coordinator can assist in or conduct the process of requesting donation from the family.

Immediate goals for stabilizing the brain-dead organ donor include establishing baseline organ function and stabilizing physiology. In general, a central venous catheter and arterial catheter are required. Cultures are obtained with baseline chemistries to rule out immediate infectious and metabolic complications. Chest radiography, echocardiography, bronchoscopy, and coronary angiography may be indicated. Blood type and cross-match are performed.

Initial fluid management includes crystalloid administration guided by central venous pressure. Vasoactive drugs are often required to maintain perfusion pressure. **Table A9-2** lists standard physiologic goals for initial resuscitation. Other aspects of donor management are more controversial. Donors frequently suffer from panhypopituitarism secondary to ischemia. Vasopressin levels may be extremely low. Dysfunction of the anterior pituitary also may be seen with hormone administration to counteract the loss of corticotropin and thyroid-stimulating hormone. Thyroid hormone and insulin are sometimes given. Insulin therapy is titrated to a blood glucose level of 120-180 mg/dL.

Table A9-2 Suggested Parameters for Optimal Donor Organ Function Before Procurement
Systolic blood pressure >90 mm Hg
Mean arterial pressure >60 to 65 mm Hg
Central venous pressure 4 to 10 mm Hg
Urine output 100 to 200 mL/h, or 1 to 4 mL/kg/h
Arterial oxygen saturation ($Sa{O_2}$) >95% or $Pa{O_2}$ >100 mm Hg (13.3 kPa)
Hematocrit >30%
Temperature 97.7° to 99.5°F (36.5° to 37.5°C)
Normal electrolyte levels
Serum glucose 120 to 180 mg/dL (6.6 to 9.9 mmol/L)
Eyelids taped shut/eye drops

B. Cardiac Death

Organs may be procured from donors after cardiac death. Upon determination of futility and the decision to withdraw care, families and appropriate patients may be approached regarding the possibility of organ donation after cardiac death. This process is also facilitated by the local organ procurement organization.

Organ harvesting takes place in the operating room, where support is withdrawn and a period of asystole typically ensues. The duration of asystole required is directed by local policy; typically, a 2- to 10-minute asystolic interval (pulselessness, apnea, unresponsiveness) is observed. Up to 10% of potential donors maintain cardiac activity for 60 minutes after discontinuation of life support. Normally, these individuals are not organ donors and receive ongoing end-of-life care.

Two common contingencies may be encountered in donation after cardiac death: unexpected cardiac arrest while awaiting withdrawal of care, and failure to progress to cardiac arrest after withdrawal of support. Management of these episodes is based on patient and family wishes regarding resuscitation and end-of-life care.

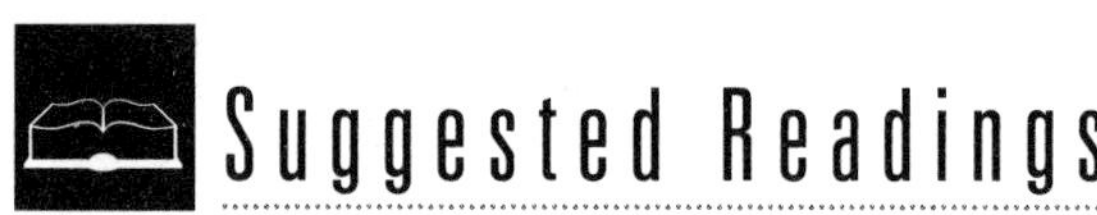

Suggested Readings

1. Shemie SD, Doig C, Dickens B, et al. Severe brain injury to neurological determination of death: Canada forum recommendations. *CMAJ.* 2006;174:S1-13.

2. Shemie SD, Ross H, Pagliarello J, et al. Organ donor management in Canada: recommendations of the Forum on Medical Management to Optimize Donor Organ Potential. *CMAJ.* 2006;174:S13-32.

3. Wijdicks EF. Brain death worldwide: accepted fact but no global consensus in diagnostic criteria. *Neurology.* 2002;58:20-25.

4. Wijdicks EF. The diagnosis of brain death. *N Engl J Med.* 2001;344:1215-1221.

5. Wijdicks EF, Varelas PN, Gronseth GS, et al. Evidence-based guideline update: determining brain death in adults. Report of the Quality Standards Subcommittee of the American Academy of Neurology. *Neurology.* 2010;74:1911-1918.

6. Wood KE, Becker BN, McCartney JG, et al. Care of the potential organ donor. *N Engl J Med.* 2004;351:2730-2739.

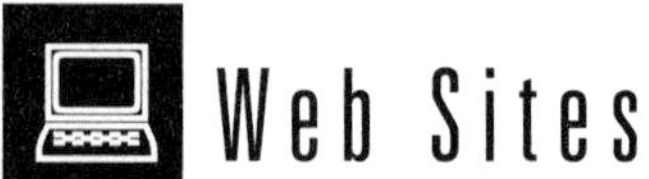

Web Sites

1. United Network for Organ Sharing. http://www.unos.org. *General resource for organ donation.*

2. UK Transplant. http://www.uktransplant.org.uk/ukt/about_transplants/donor_care/donor_care.jsp. *Contains chapter on organ donor management from the Intensive Care Society guidelines for adult organ and tissue donation.*

Appendix 10

Infection Control Measures

*See **Table A10-7** for tetanus prophylaxis.*

Healthcare-associated infections (HAI) are caused by a wide variety of common and unusual organisms. Medical advances have brought lifesaving care to patients in need, yet many of those advances come with a risk of infection that can be devastating and even deadly.

Wherever patient care is provided, adherence to infection prevention guidelines is needed to ensure that all care is safe care, whether delivered in traditional hospital settings, outpatient surgery centers, long-term care facilities, rehabilitation centers, or community clinics. Guidelines cannot always account for individual variation among patients and are not intended to supplant physician judgment with respect to individual patients or clinical situations.

The following is a summary of the strategies to prevent HAI, compiled from leading resources in infection control, including the Centers for Disease Control and Prevention (CDC), the Infectious Diseases Society of America (IDSA), and the Society of Critical Care Medicine (SCCM). Application of these guidelines can help decrease the risks associated with HAI.

Table A10-1 Prevention of Central Line-Associated Bloodstream Infections

Prevention and Monitoring for All Acute Care Hospitals	
Basic Practice	
Before insertion	Educate healthcare personnel involved in the insertion, care, and maintenance of central venous catheters
At insertion	Use a catheter checklist to ensure adherence to infection prevention practices and hygiene Avoid using the femoral vein for central venous access Use an all-inclusive catheter cart or kit Use maximal sterile barrier precautions during insertion Use a chlorhexidine-based antiseptic for skin preparation Use antimicrobial/antiseptic-impregnated catheters and cuffs to help decrease rate of infection
After insertion	Disinfect catheter hubs and injection ports before accessing the catheter Remove nonessential catheters Change the dressings and perform site care with a chlorhexidine-based antiseptic every 5-7 days; change gauze dressings every 2 days Replace administration sets not used for blood, blood products, or lipids at intervals no longer than 96 hours Perform surveillance for central line-associated infection Use antimicrobial ointments for hemodialysis catheter insertion sites Consider possible role of anticoagulants in the prevention of infection
Special Approaches for High-Risk Patients Despite Precautions	
	Bathe patients with a chlorhexidine preparation on a daily basis Use antiseptic- or antimicrobial-impregnated central venous catheters Use chlorhexidine-containing sponge dressings for central venous catheters Use antimicrobial locks for central venous catheters
Approaches That Should NOT Be Considered a Routine Part of CLABSI Prevention	
	Antimicrobial prophylaxis for short-term or tunneled catheter insertion or while catheters are in situ Routine replacement of central venous catheters or arterial catheters Routine use of positive pressure needleless connectors with mechanical valves before a thorough assessment of risks, benefits, and education in proper use

Abbreviation: CLABSI, central line-associated bloodstream infections
More information and a full review can be found in guidelines from the Infectious Diseases Society of America (IDSA) and the Centers for Disease Control and Prevention (CDC):
http://www.idsociety.org/content.aspx?id=4434 - prevention_of_catheter;
http://www.guidelinecentral.com/viewers/HAI.html;
http://www.cdc.gov/mmwr/preview/mmwrhtml/rr5110a1.htm

Table A10-2 Prevention of Ventilator-Associated Pneumonia

Basic Practice	
Education	Educate healthcare personnel and clinicians who care for patients undergoing ventilation
Surveillance	Observe for compliance with VAP bundles
	Conduct active surveillance for VAP
Practice	Implement policies and practices for disinfection, sterilization, maintenance of respiratory equipment, hand hygiene and gloving
	Use orotracheal rather than nasotracheal intubation
	Place patient in a semirecumbent position (30°) unless contraindicated
	Provide regular antiseptic oral care
	Promote the use of noninvasive ventilation and limit amount of time on invasive ventilation
	Use sterile water for rinsing reusable semicritical respiratory equipment
	Change the ventilator circuit when it is visibly soiled or mechanically malfunctioning, and periodically drain and discard any condensate that collects in the tubing system
	Avoid gastric overdistention
Special Approaches for High-Risk Patients Despite Precautions	
	Use an endotracheal tube with in-line and subglottic suctioning for eligible patients
	Monitor beds for angle of incline
Approaches That Should NOT Be Considered a Routine Part of VAP Prevention	
	Administration of intravenous immunoglobulin, white cell–stimulating factors, enteral glutamine, or chest physiotherapy
	Kinetic or continuous lateral rotational therapy beds
	Prophylactic aerosolized or systemic antimicrobials
	Routine change of breathing circuits with humidifiers on the basis of duration of use

Abbreviation: VAP, ventilator-associated pneumonia
More information and a full review can be found in guidelines from the Infectious Diseases Society of America (IDSA) and the Centers for Disease Control and Prevention (CDC):
http://www.cdc.gov/mmwr/preview/mmwrhtml/rr5303a1.htm;
http://www.idsociety.org/content.aspx?id=4430 - HAP;
http://www.guidelinecentral.com/viewers/HAI.html

Table A10-3 Example of Ventilator Bundle

Intervention			
Deep vein thrombosis prophylaxis	Yes	No	Subcutaneous heparin/SCD
Peptic ulcer prophylaxis	Yes	No	Recommended for patients with risk of stress ulcer development
Head of bed elevation	Yes	No	Semirecumbent position (30°-45° elevation of the head of the bed)
Sedation vacation	Yes	No	Daily documentation of consideration of sedation interruption and assessment of readiness to wean or contraindication
Spontaneous breathing trial	Yes	No	Daily assessments of readiness to wean and use of weaning protocols
Hand hygiene	Yes	No	
Antiseptic oral care	Yes	No	Daily documentation of regular oral care according to product instructions

More information and a full review can be found in guidelines from the Infectious Diseases Society of America (IDSA) and the Centers for Disease Control and Prevention (CDC):
http://www.jstor.org/stable/10.1086/591062

Table A10-4 Prevention of Surgical Site Infections

Basic Practice	
Surveillance	Observe for any signs of infection Provide feedback on surveillance and process measures to surgical and perioperative personnel and leadership Adopt the use of automated data
Practice	Administer antimicrobial prophylaxis in accordance with evidence-based standards and guidelines Do not remove hair at the operative site unless its presence will interfere with the operation; do not use razors Control blood glucose level during the immediate postoperative period for patients undergoing cardiac surgery
Education	Educate surgeons and perioperative personnel about prevention techniques Educate patients and families about infection prevention strategies
Special Approaches for High-Risk Patients Despite Precautions	
	Expand surveillance to determine the source and extent of the problem
Approaches That Should NOT Be Considered a Routine Part of SSI Prevention	
	Routine use of vancomycin for antimicrobial prophylaxis Delayed surgery to provide parenteral nutrition

Abbreviation: SSI, surgical site infection
More information and a full review can be found in guidelines from the Infectious Diseases Society of America (IDSA) and the Centers for Disease Control and Prevention (CDC):
http://www.idsociety.org/Content.aspx?id=4434#HAIS;
http://www.guidelinecentral.com/viewers/HAI.html;
http://www.cdc.gov/ncidod/dhqp/pdf/guidelines/SSI.pdf

Table A10-5 Prevention of Methicillin-Resistant *Staphylococcus aureus* Transmission

Basic Practice	
	Execute risk assessment and monitoring program
	Employ contact precautions for MRSA-colonized or infected patients
	Clean and disinfect equipment and the environment
	Educate healthcare personnel
	Educate patients and their families
	Initiate a laboratory-based alert system
	Comply with Centers for Disease Control and Prevention guidelines
Special Approaches for High-Risk Patients Despite Precautions	
	Employ active surveillance testing for patients
	Use active surveillance testing for healthcare personnel
	Perform routine bathing with chlorhexidine
	Initiate decolonization therapy for MRSA-colonized persons
	Administer vancomycin for patients with sternotomy

Abbreviation: MRSA, methicillin-resistant *S aureus*
More information and a full review can be found in guidelines from the Infectious Diseases Society of America (IDSA) and the Centers for Disease Control and Prevention (CDC):
http://www.guidelinecentral.com/viewers/MRSA.html;
http://www.idsociety.org/content.aspx?id=4432 - mrsa;
http://www.cdc.gov/ncidod/dhqp/pdf/ar/mdroGuideline2006.pdf

Table A10-6 Prevention of *Clostridium difficile* Infection

Basic Practice	
	Use contact precautions for infected patients, with a single-patient room preferred
	Use hand hygiene, gloves, and gowns
	Clean and disinfect equipment and the environment
	Initiate laboratory-based alert system and surveillance
	Educate healthcare personnel
	Educate patients and their families about infection prevention strategies
	Comply with Centers for Disease Control and Prevention guidelines
Special Approaches for High-Risk Patients Despite Precautions	
	Perform hand hygiene with soap and water as the preferred method before exiting the room of a patient with CDI
	Place patients with diarrhea under contact precautions while *C difficile* test results are pending
	After the patient becomes asymptomatic, prolong the duration of contact precautions until hospital discharge
	Use sodium hypochlorite (bleach)–containing cleaning agents for environmental cleaning
	Initiate an antimicrobial stewardship program
Approaches That Should NOT Be Considered a Routine Part of CDI Prevention	
	Testing patients with no signs or symptoms of CDI
	Repeating *C difficile* testing after successful therapy in a patient recently treated for CDI

Abbreviation: CDI, *C difficile* infection
More information and a full review can be found in guidelines from the Infectious Diseases Society of America (IDSA) and the Centers for Disease Control and Prevention (CDC):
http://www.guidelinecentral.com/viewers/cdif.html;
http://www.idsociety.org/content.aspx?id=4430 - cd;
http://www.shea-online.org/assets/files/position_papers/Cldiff95.PDF

Table A10-7 Guide to Tetanus Prophylaxis in Routine Wound Management[a]

History of Absorbed Tetanus Toxoid	Clean Minor Wounds (Not Prone to Tetanus[b])		All Other Wounds[b] (Tetanus-Prone[c])	
	Tdap or Td[b]	**TIG[d]**	**Tdap or Td[b]**	**TIG[d]**
Unknown or <3 doses	Yes	No	Yes	Yes
≥3 doses[e]	No[f]	No	No[g]	No

Abbreviations: Tdap, tetanus toxoid, reduced diphtheria toxoid, acellular pertussis vaccine; Td, tetanus toxoid and reduced diphtheria toxoid — for adult use (dose = 0.5 mL); TIG, tetanus immune globulin — human (dose = 250 IU).

[a]Patients who have completed a three-dose primary tetanus vaccination series and have received a tetanus toxoid-containing vaccine <5 years before the injury do not require a tetanus toxoid-containing vaccine for wound management.

[b]Children <7 years = Tdap is recommended; if pertussis vaccine is contraindicated, Td is given. Children 7-9 years or adults >65 years = Td is recommended. Children 10-64 years = Tdap is preferred to Td if the patient has never received Tdap and has no contraindication to pertussis vaccine. For patients >7 years of age, if Tdap is not available or not indicated because of age, Td is preferred to tetanus toxoid.

[c]Such as (but not limited to) wounds contaminated with dirt, feces, soil, and saliva; puncture wounds; avulsions; and wounds resulting from missiles, crushing, burns, and frostbite.

[d]Equine tetanus antitoxin should be used when TIG is not available.

[e]If only three doses of fluid toxoid have been received, a fourth dose – preferably an adsorbed toxoid – should be given. Although licensed, fluid tetanus toxoid is rarely used.

[f]Yes, if ≥10 years since the last tetanus toxoid-containing dose.

[g]Yes, if ≥5 years since the last tetanus toxoid-containing dose; more frequent boosters are not needed and can accentuate side effects.

Suggested Readings

1. Broder KR, Cortese MM, Iskander JK, et al. Preventing tetanus, diphtheria, and pertussis among adolescents: use of tetanus toxoid, reduced diphtheria toxoid and acellular pertussis vaccines recommendations of the Advisory Committee on Immunization Practices (ACIP). *MMWR Recomm Rep.* 2006;55(RR-3):1-34.

2. Gerding DN, Johnson S, Peterson LR, et al. *Clostridium difficile*-associated diarrhea and colitis. *Infect Control Hosp Epidemiol.* 1995;16:459-477.

3. Kretsinger K, Broder KR, Cortese MM, et al. Preventing tetanus, diphtheria, and pertussis among adults: use of tetanus toxoid, reduced diphtheria toxoid and acellular pertussis vaccine recommendations of the Advisory Committee on Immunization Practices (ACIP) and recommendation of ACIP, supported by the Healthcare Infection Control Practices Advisory Committee (HICPAC), for use of Tdap among healthcare personnel. *MMWR Recomm Rep.* 2006;55(RR-17):1-37.

4. O'Grady NP, Barie PS, Bartlett JG, et al. Guidelines for evaluation of new fever in critically ill adult patients: 2008 update from the American College of Critical Care Medicine and the Infectious Diseases Society of America. *Crit Care Med.* 2008;36:1330-1349.

5. Yokoe DS, Mermel LA, Anderson DJ, et al. A compendium of strategies to prevent healthcare-associated infections in acute care hospitals. *Infect Control Hosp Epidemiol.* 2008;29(Suppl 1):S12-21.

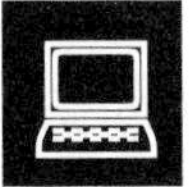

Web Sites

1. Centers for Disease Control and Prevention (CDC)
   http://www.cdc.gov
   http://www.cdc.gov/vaccines/pubs/surv-manual/chpt16-tetanus.pdf
   http://www.cdc.gov/mmwr/preview/mmwrhtml/rr5110a1.htm
   http://www.cdc.gov/mmwr/preview/mmwrhtml/rr5303a1.htm
   http://www.cdc.gov/ncidod/dhqp/pdf/guidelines/SSI.pdf
   http://www.cdc.gov/ncidod/dhqp/pdf/ar/mdroGuideline2006.pdf
   http://www.shea-online.org/assets/files/position_papers/Cldiff95.PDF

2. Infectious Diseases Society of America (IDSA)
   http://www.idsociety.org
   http://www.idsociety.org/content.aspx?id=4434HAIS
   http://www.guidelinecentral.com/viewers/HAI.html

Appendix 11

Unfractionated Heparin Anticoagulation

I. Venous Thromboembolism

1. Make calculations using total body weight in kilograms.

2. Administer heparin, 80 U/kg, as an intravenous bolus.

3. Start intravenous heparin infusion, 18 U/kg/h (20,000 U heparin in 500 mL of 5% dextrose in water = 40 U/mL).

4. Obtain STAT activated partial thromboplastin time (APTT) 6 hours after heparin bolus.

5. Adjust heparin infusion based on sliding scale below.

APTT (s)	Dose Change
<35 (1.2 x control)	80 U/kg bolus, increase drip by 4 U/kg/h
35-45 (1.2 to 1.5 x control)	40 U/kg bolus, increase drip by 2 U/kg/h
46-70 (1.5 to 2.3 x control)	No change
71-90 (2.3 to 3 x control)	Reduce drip by 2 U/kg/h
>90 (>3 x control)	Hold heparin for 1 hour, reduce drip by 3 U/kg/h

Abbreviation: APTT, activated partial thromboplastin time

6. Order APTT 6 hours after dosage change, adjusting heparin infusion based on the sliding scale until APTT is therapeutic. Problems with standardizing APTT monitoring suggest that the therapeutic range should be determined by calibrating reagent lots to APTT values that correlate with therapeutic heparin levels. When two consecutive APTT levels are therapeutic, order APTT (and readjust heparin drip as needed) every 24 hours.

7. Make changes as promptly as possible and round off doses to the nearest mL/h (nearest 40 U/h).

II. CORONARY ARTERY DISEASE

1. Unstable angina and non-ST-segment myocardial infarction

    a. Administer heparin as an initial bolus dose of 60 to 70 U/kg (maximum dose 5,000 U) is recommended.

    b. Start an intravenous heparin infusion of 12 to 15 U/kg/h (maximum 1,000 U/h).

    c. Adjust heparin infusion to maintain a therapeutic APTT value.

2. ST-segment myocardial infarction with use of alteplase, reteplase, or tenecteplase

    a. Administer heparin as an initial bolus dose of 60 U/kg (maximum dose 4,000 U).

    b. Start an intravenous heparin infusion of 12 U/kg/h (maximum 1,000 U/h).

    c. Adjust heparin infusion to maintain a therapeutic APTT value.

3. Percutaneous coronary interventions with use of glycoprotein IIb/IIIa inhibitors

    a. Administer heparin as an initial bolus dose of 70 U/kg.

    b. Provide additional boluses to keep the activated clotting time at >200 s.

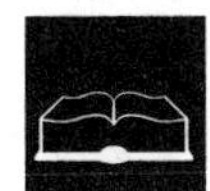

Suggested Readings

1. Anderson JL, Adams CD, Antman EM, et al. ACC/AHA 2007 guidelines for the management of patients with unstable angina/non-ST-elevation myocardial infarction. A report of the American College of Cardiology/American Heart Association Task Force on Practice Guidelines. *J Am Coll Cardiol.* 2007;50:e1-e157.

2. Garcia DA, Baglin TP, Weitz JI, et al. Parenteral anticoagulants: Antithrombotic therapy and prevention of thrombosis, 9th ed: American College of Chest Physicians evidence-based clinical practice guidelines. *Chest.* 2012;141:e24S-e43S.

3. Kushner FG, Hand M, Smith SC, et al. 2009 focused update: ACC/AHA guidelines for the management of patients with ST-elevation myocardial infarction (updating the 2004 guideline and 2007 focused update) and ACC/AHA/SCAI guidelines on percutaneous coronary intervention (updating the 2005 guideline and 2007 focused update). *Circulation.* 2009;120:2271-2306.

4. Raschke RA, Reilly BM, Guidry JR, et al. The weight-based heparin dosing nomogram compared with a "standard care" nomogram. A randomized controlled trial. *Ann Intern Med.* 1993;119:874-881.

Appendix 12

THROMBOPROPHYLAXIS FOR VENOUS THROMBOEMBOLISM

Table A12-1 Pharmacologic and Mechanical Interventions for Venous Thromboembolism Prophylaxis

Clinical Situation	Intervention
General, vascular, and urologic surgery	
Low risk: minor surgery in patients <40 years with no additional risk factors, transurethral procedures, or low-risk urologic or vascular surgery without risk factors	Early, persistent mobilization
Moderate risk: minor surgery in patients with risk factors, major surgery in patients <40 years with no risk factors	Low-dose UFH, LMWH or fondaparinux
High risk: surgery in patients >60 years or >40 years with additional risk factors; major vascular surgery with risk factors; major, open urologic surgery	Low-dose UFH three times daily, LMWH or fondaparinux
General surgery patients with high risk of bleeding	Optimal thromboprophylaxis with CS or IPC
Gynecologic surgery	
Brief procedures (<30 min) for benign disease	Early, persistent mobilization
Laparoscopic procedures with risk factors	Low-dose UFH, LMWH, CS, or IPC
Major gynecologic surgery for benign disease without risk factors	Low-dose UFH, LMWH, or IPC started before surgery and used continuously while patient is nonambulatory
Extensive surgery for malignancy and additional VTE risk factors	Low-dose UFH three times daily, LMWH or IPC started before surgery and used continuously while nonambulatory; or low-dose UFH or LMWH and CS or IPC
Laparoscopic surgery	
Laparoscopic surgery without risk factors	Early, persistent mobilization
Laparoscopic surgery with risk factors	Low-dose UFH, LMWH, IPC, CS, or fondaparinux

Table A12-1 Pharmacologic and Mechanical Interventions for Venous Thromboembolism Prophylaxis (continued)

Clinical Situation	Intervention
Orthopedic surgery	
Elective hip replacement	LMWH at high-risk dose, fondaparinux, or adjusted-dose VKA
Elective knee replacement	LMWH at high-risk dose, fondaparinux, adjusted-dose VKA, or IPC (if pharmacologic prophylaxis is contraindicated)
Knee arthroscopy, elective spine surgery with no risk factors	Early, persistent mobilization
Arthroscopic knee surgery with risk factors	LMWH
Hip fracture surgery	Fondaparinux, LMWH at high-risk dose, adjusted-dose VKA, or low-dose UFH
Elective spine surgery with risk factors	Low-dose UFH, LMWH postoperatively, or perioperative IPC and/or CS
Elective spine surgery with multiple risk factors	Low-dose UFH or LMWH with CS and/or IPC
Neurosurgery	
Intracranial neurosurgery	Optimal use of IPC or low-dose UFH or postoperative LMWH. For high-risk, combination of CS +/- IPC with either LMWH or low-dose UFH
Trauma, burns	LMWH or LMWH and mechanical method of thromboprophylaxis (if no contraindication), or IPC or CS alone (if LMWH is contraindicated); low-dose UFH may be used as an alternative to LMWH in burns
Spinal cord injury	LMWH, low-dose UFH or LMWH with IPC, or IPC ± CS when anticoagulant prophylaxis is contraindicated
Critical care	
ICU patients or medical conditions with moderate risk and/or confined to bed	Low-dose UFH, LMWH, or CS and/or IPC if high risk of bleeding
ICU patients with higher risk	LMWH

Abbreviations: UFH, unfractionated heparin; LMWH, low-molecular-weight heparin; CS, graduated compression stockings; IPC, intermittent pneumatic compression; VTE, venous thromboembolism; VKA, vitamin K antagonist

Suggested Reading

1. Geerts WH, Bergqvist D, Pineo GF, et al. Prevention of venous thromboembolism: American College of Chest Physicians Evidence-Based Clinical Practice Guidelines. *Chest.* 2008;133:381S-453S.

Appendix 12-4

INDEX

Note: Page numbers followed by *f* and *t* indicate figures and tables, respectively.

I

J

K

L

M

Q

R

T

U

V

W

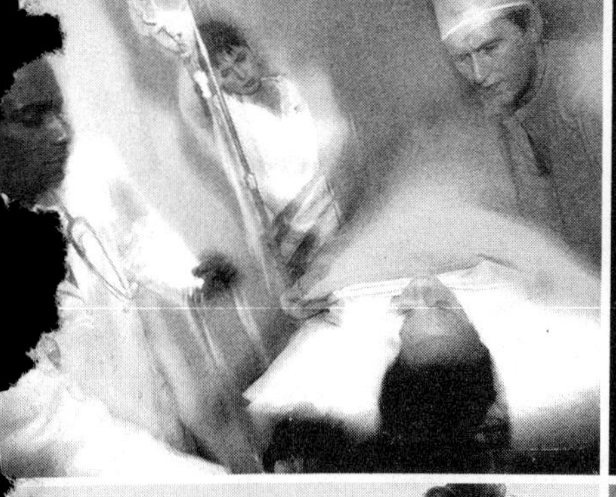

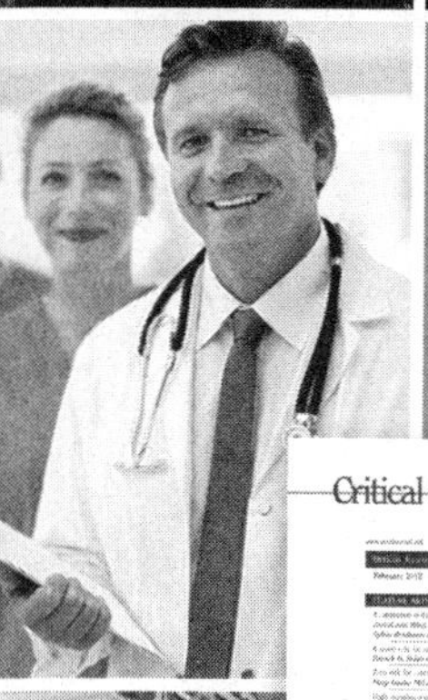

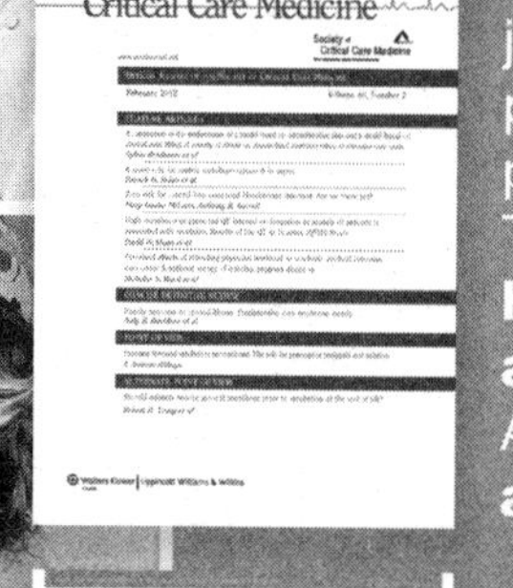

Critical Care Medicine

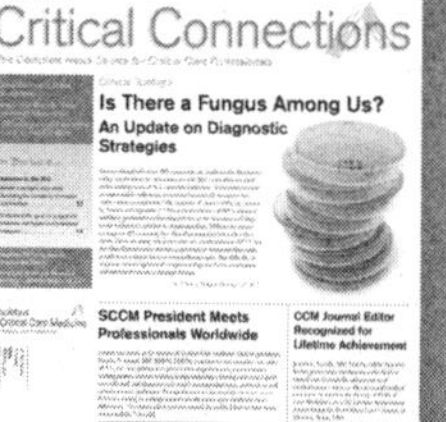

Critical Connections
Is There a Fungus Among Us?
An Update on Diagnostic Strategies
SCCM President Meets Professionals Worldwide
CCM Journal Editor Recognized for Lifetime Achievement

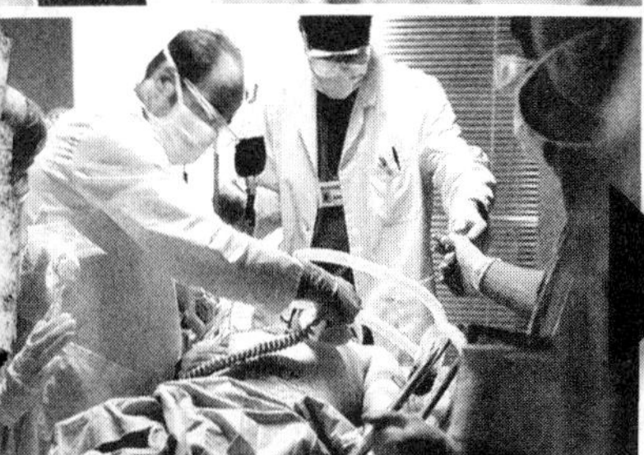

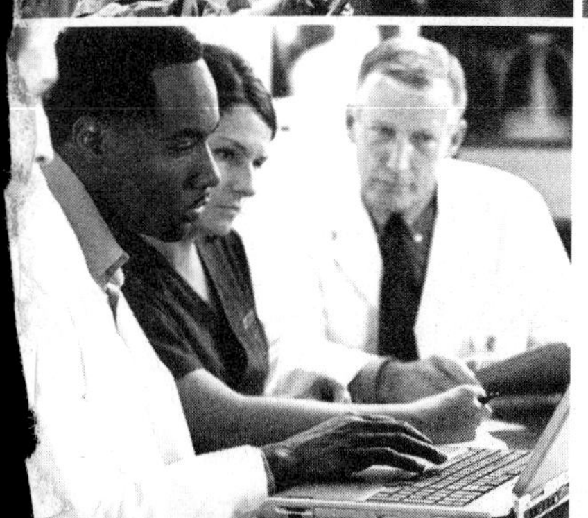